see page 29
medical detective

More Praise for *Why Can't I Get Better?*

"Our world is changing; our parasites are changing, too: small intracellular bacteria, such as the Lyme agent, have learned how to persist in our bodies and to trigger more and more crippling pathologies. This timely book, written by an experienced physician, brings an updated and effective medical solution to a new epidemic."

—Luc Montagnier, winner of the Nobel Prize in Physiology or Medicine for the discovery of HIV

"Modern medicine has lagged behind in confronting a number of chronic illnesses that cause immense suffering and disability for thousands. Dr. Richard Horowitz's insights are a corrective for this glaring gap. *Why Can't I Get Better?* will benefit not only patients, but physicians as well, who are willing to step outside the strictures of ingrained beliefs."

—Larry Dossey, MD, *New York Times* bestselling author of *One Mind: How Our Individual Mind Is Part of a Greater Consciousness and Why It Matters*

"Dr. Horowitz has been, and continues to be, 'in the trenches' in the battle to understand, diagnose, and treat people who, like myself, have suffered or are suffering the effects of Lyme. . . . I can think of no one more qualified to write about this subject."   —Daryl Hall, musician (Hall & Oates)

"This very readable book is the new gold standard on the subject for country doctors, infectious disease specialists, patients, and anyone whose children play outside."

—Jordan Fisher Smith, author of *Nature Noir,* and star of the Lyme disease documentary *Under Our Skin*

WHY CAN'T I GET BETTER?

Solving the Mystery of Lyme
and Chronic Disease

PAIN • FATIGUE • MEMORY AND CONCENTRATION
PROBLEMS • AND MUCH MORE

Richard I. Horowitz, MD

ST. MARTIN'S PRESS ☙ NEW YORK

The names and identifying characteristics of the patients have been changed to protect their privacy.

The information in this book is not intended to replace the advice of the reader's own physician or other medical professional. It is intended for informational purposes only and not for self-treatment and/or diagnosis. You should consult a medical professional in matters relating to health, especially if you have existing medical conditions and before starting, stopping, or changing the dose of any medication you are taking. Individual readers are solely responsible for their own health-care decisions. The author and the publisher do not accept responsibility for any adverse effects individuals may claim to experience, whether directly or indirectly, from the information contained in this book. The information published in this book is not intended to replace or prevent medical treatment and diagnosis. The fact that an organization or Web site is mentioned in the book as a potential source of information does not mean that the author or the publisher endorses all of the information they may provide or recommendations they may make.

Library of Congress Cataloging-in-Publication Data

Horowitz, Richard.
    Why can't I get better? : solving the mystery of lyme and chronic disease / Richard Horowitz, M.D.—First U.S. edition.
        p. cm.
    ISBN 978-1-250-01940-0 (hardcover)
    ISBN 978-1-250-03848-7 (e-book)
    1. Lyme disease—Popular works.   2. Symptoms—Popular works.
    3. Diagnosis—Popular works.   I. Title.
    RC155.5.H67 2013
    616.9'246—dc23   2013013336

To my mother,

EVELYN LOMBARDI,

and my grandparents,

HELEN and SID GORDON,

for their unconditional love and support.

Contents

Acknowledgments

This book represents my life's work, but it couldn't have been written without the help of many people. Jennifer Weis at St. Martin's Press has been an invaluable supporter for many years, and I'm thrilled that I was able to work with her. My good friend, science writer Pam Weintraub, has given me skillful guidance, and Pam Liflander has been helpful in getting my thoughts onto these pages clearly and coherently. I am especially thankful for the expert assistance of Professor Phyllis R. Freeman, PhD, of the State University of New York, New Paltz, who served not only as the preliminary editor but also as the subject matter expert on the biobehavioral aspects of chronic infectious disease diagnosis and management. Dr. Freeman has been a longtime friend, and she encouraged me years ago to write this book. Without her constant support and assistance, this book would not have been possible.

A huge thanks goes out to my wife, Lee, for her understanding and support, as long hours (including on vacation) were needed to get this book into its present form. Her love has graced my life.

My office staff also deserves a special thank you for their dedication, hard work, skill, knowledge, and compassion that has allowed me to help so many stricken with chronic illness. These people include: Gina Edwards; John Fallon, NP; Lisa Haynes; Irene Kaminskaya; Casie Luther; Andrea Mahoney, RN; Jennifer Mastroeni, RN; Kalah Matthews, RN; Christina Novak; Monica Pemberton, MA; Sonja Sideras, LPN; Etheldria Walker,

MA; William Winters, MA; and Lauren Yunker, PA. I would also like to acknowledge Dr. Leo Galland and Dr. Chris Melitis, from the Integrative Health Symposium conference in New York City, who contributed material, as well as Dr. Eva Sapi, from the University of New Haven, who shared her original research on biofilms. A debt of gratitude also goes out to Dr. Alan McDonald for his groundbreaking work on *Borrelia* and permission to reprint his slides on its cystic forms, as well as Dr. Judith Miklossy, who provided photos of the atypical and cystic forms of *Borrelia* in neurological Lyme disease. I also wish to thank Dr. Garth Nicolson for reviewing the initial manuscript and for his assistance in providing extensive scientific literature on mycoplasmal infections and mitochondrial dysfunction. And I would like to recognize the heroes of Lyme disease, who have consistently put their patients before themselves, sometimes at the risk of their own careers. This includes Dr. Joseph Burrascano (who also provided a short history of Lyme disease for this book, and information on Advanced Labs and the new Lyme culture); Dr. Sam Donta; Dr. Charles Ray Jones; Dr. Kenneth Leigner; and many others. Dr. Claire Riendeau provided her insight on biotoxin illness.

I am also grateful for the assistance of several colleagues who lent their expertise and reviewed individual chapters: Allan Warshowsky, MD, for his work on the endocrinology chapter; David H. Haase, MD, for reviewing the GI autonomic nervous system dysfunction, and allergy chapters; Andrea Gaito, MD, for her help with the immunity and inflammation chapters; Sunil Khurana, MD, for helping with the GI and liver function chapters; Fred Harvey, MD, for his assistance in reviewing the chapter on environmental medicine; and David Perlmutter, MD, FACN, who reviewed the brain and pain chapters. Dr. Elizabeth Maloney and Dr. Bea Szantyr also provided their feedback on the manuscript, and I am grateful for their help.

A huge debt of gratitude goes to my spiritual teachers, especially Lama Norlha Rinpoche, who has guided and supported me perfectly through this life.

Finally, thanks to all of the Lyme-MSIDS sufferers, who have been some of the greatest teachers to me in this lifetime. Your courage and perseverance to regain health has inspired me to constantly look for answers, and has been the inspiration for this book.

Foreword

. . . and when the physician's hand on the patient's shoulder or
arm is a shelter against the darkness.

—NORMAN COUSINS, *The Healing Heart: Antidotes to*
Panic and Helplessness

More than twenty-two years ago I struggled with debilitating pain and unending insomnia, symptoms that left me barely able to work or to deal competently with daily life. I saw specialists in internal medicine, orthopedics, ophthalmology, psychiatry, and neurology but still had no definitive diagnosis for my frightening symptoms. My neurologist said that he had heard of a new internist who was gaining attention as a brilliant diagnostician. I made an appointment for a consultation. What did I have to lose?

I vividly remember my first visit with this physician. Dr. Richard Horowitz sat next to me in the exam room. He read the copious laboratory test results I had brought with me, but then he gently asked me to tell him the story of my illness. He listened intently, taking detailed notes, and urged me to slow down, so that I wouldn't feel rushed to get everything out all at once. When I finished he placed his hand on my shoulder and said, "Everything will be OK." That simple act of compassion in response to my narrative was so powerful! For the first time in more than a year I felt that I might regain my former joy and energy; I felt hopeful that I might find a way through the pain and recover my health.

This is a book about diagnosing and treating Lyme and other tickborne infections. But it is also a book about hope. Hope is a central human emotion, misunderstood and often mistaken for optimism, as Jerome Groopman reminds us in *The Anatomy of Hope*. Having true hope, he contends, is not about holding a rosy and unrealistic prospect for the future. It is not: "Just think positive." Rather, hope is clear-eyed. True hope is seeing a viable route out of the darkness while acknowledging the obstacles that might impede your journey.

This book can provide you with a path through the complicated maze of multiple systemic disease diagnosis and management. If you are a health-care provider, this book can remind you of the vital importance of evoking hope in your patients as you face the relentlessly demanding and endlessly challenging practice of twenty-first-century medicine. If you are a multiple systemic disease patient, this book can be the hand on your shoulder that helps you recover true hope and points you toward a passageway out of your suffering.

—Phyllis R. Freeman, PhD
New Paltz, New York
December 2012

Introduction

Exchange yourself with the person you are with. Always think of what would make them happy and what would relieve their suffering. Show loving-kindness and compassion. If you do this, everything will go well.

—LAMA GENDUN RINPOCHE

This book is my story as a medical detective who set out to understand the hidden truth behind chronic illness and its relation to Lyme disease. In my quest I have combined the facts of medical science with thousands of clues I've come across, mostly from listening hard to my patients' stories, reading closely in the chronic disease literature, and trusting deeply in my medical intuition. This led me to uncover surprising clues to solve this challenging medical puzzle.

Like many other physicians, my initial understanding was that Lyme disease is caused by a tick-borne spirochetal bacteria, *Borrelia burgdorferi*, which can progress from a characteristic expanding skin rash, erythema migrans (EM), to a wide variety of nonspecific systemic symptoms that can affect any part of the body. Appropriate and early antibiotic treatment can successfully treat many with the infection. However, in some people a tick bite can lead to disseminated infection and to disabling physical, cognitive, and psychological manifestations. And some people manifest with puzzling multiple systemic symptoms that can occur throughout the body, which lead to complex lab results. Because of this, Lyme disease has been ignored or trivialized by the medical profession for more than a quarter of a century. Many of my patients have seen fifteen to twenty physicians before they walk through the doors of my office, searching for answers for their treatment-resistant symptoms. Their suffering is made worse as they repeatedly face difficulty in obtaining appropriate care from often skeptical medical and insurance communities, as they unknowingly enter one of the most virulent wars between two medical camps that we have seen in our country's history. One camp, the Infectious Diseases Society of America (IDSA), believes that Lyme disease is an easily diagnosable and treatable condition. The other camp, the International Lyme and Associated Diseases Society (ILADS), believes that the blood tests to diagnose Lyme disease are highly unreliable and that thirty days of antibiotics is often insufficient. Chronically ill patients therefore often go from doctor to doctor searching for answers.

A patient's journey typically begins with a primary care physician or a family doctor. A maximum of thirty days of antibiotics is the accepted standard of care for Lyme disease. If patients report back that they are not getting better, they are likely diagnosed as having "post-Lyme syndrome," chronic fatigue syndrome (CFS, which is now often referred to as myalgic encephalomyelitis), or fibromyalgia. They are then given an antidepressant and/or the number of a local psychiatrist, or told to live with their symptoms. When a child contracts Lyme disease and can't concentrate in school and/or shows a decline in their grades and attention span, then the child must have Attention Deficit Disorder (ADD), or perhaps there are problems at home. They are typically given Ritalin, or Strattera, and sent for behavioral therapy. This may help some of the symptoms yet fail to address the root problem.

Desperate patients go from their family doctors to specialists complaining of chronic fatigue, fevers, sweats and chills, stiff neck and headaches, light and sound sensitivities, dizziness, memory and concentration problems, joint aches and muscle aches that migrate around the body, tingling, numbness and burning sensations, chest pain, palpitations and shortness of breath, gastrointestinal problems, resistant urological problems, sleep disorders, and/or a whole host of psychiatric symptoms, including depression, anxiety, and irritability. Or they get saddled with diagnoses of untreatable conditions. Yet the answer might be that they are experiencing multiple systemic problems from Lyme disease and its associated infections. Lyme and other tick-borne disorders have been identified across the globe and are causing untold suffering and disability in millions of people every day. It is no wonder that Lyme and associated tick-borne diseases (TBDs) are called "the great imitators."

Modern medicine is excellent at providing care for acute diseases, such as strep throat, acute bronchitis or pneumonia, urinary tract infections, and acute surgical emergencies. The medical system, however, lacks an understanding of and treatments for a myriad of chronic diseases. I have successfully treated more than twelve thousand people over the past twenty-six years, many of whom had been misdiagnosed and given simplified medical labels. I believe that those I treat are best described as having multiple systemic infectious disease syndrome, or MSIDS. Louis Pasteur's postulate, "one germ, one disease," which has been one of the hallmarks of medical diagnosis for the last century, is no longer applicable, at least in patients with multiple chronic diseases. I've come to believe that we need a new paradigm to diagnose and treat chronic illness. This book provides such a paradigm shift.

Chronically ill, complex patients, no matter which diagnosis we may give them, often have simultaneous multiple bacterial, parasitic, viral, and fungal causes for their illnesses. They also often have associated immune dysfunction with autoimmune markers, large environmental toxin loads, hormonal dysfunctions, mitochondrial dysfunction, allergies with functional metabolic abnormalities, sleep disorders, and underlying psychological dysfunction. I believe my sixteen-point differential diagnostic map, presented in this book, can best be applied to solve the mystery for those individuals with a number of complex chronic medical illnesses and provide treatment options and relief previously not available.

I have spent more than twenty-five years of medical practice treating challenging patients, often with great success. I have shared my clinical and research results with colleagues here in the United States, in Europe, and in Asia at scientific conferences, invited addresses, via video and print forums, and, more recently, as a consultant for medical and patient communities around the world. In addition, a number of physicians have spent a week or more with me in my Hyde Park practice, where I have modeled my perspective on patient care and learned from my colleagues' own insights into patient issues. The public is well aware of the health epidemics of obesity, diabetes, cardiovascular disease, strokes, heart attack, and cancer. But unless you or a family member has faced Lyme disease, you might not know that we are also witnessing epidemics of bacterial, viral, and parasitic illnesses. Today Lyme disease is the number one vector-borne infectious disease in North America, northern Europe, and temperate Asia. This refers to an infection transferred from an arthropod, or tick, to an individual person or animal.

THE BEGINNINGS OF A LYME PRACTICE

I remember the first time that I ever heard about Lyme disease. It was a beautiful spring day in Elmhurst, Queens, in 1987. I was in my third year of an internal medicine residency, and we were called away from our afternoon duties to attend a special grand rounds. I remember thinking what a needed break it would be. I had just finished one of those zombie thirty-six-hour shifts, after which nothing around me seemed real. I sat down next to my buddy, Howie. "What do you think?" I asked. "Another rare disease that we'll never come across in our lifetimes?" Howie had just come off his own thirty-six-hour shift, but his exhaustion was combined with a devilish smile that told of the great pleasures he must have just had in tormenting one of the first- or second-year residents. "Yeah, I'm sure living in Rego Park, Queens, I'm going to come across a lot of this."

So we both listened, intermittently covering our mouths to hide our yawns. It was some strange disease that gave you a bull's-eye rash. Easy to diagnose and treat. Twenty-six years later, unfortunately, that is still the belief of many medical professionals.

Despite my previous seven years of excellent medical school training in Belgium, I didn't remember ever hearing about this disease. However, Lyme disease is known to have been around in Europe since the late 1800s, and was diagnosed as "acrodermatitis chronica atrophicans" (a violaceous skin rash on the hands) or Bannwarth syndrome accompanied by a painful radiculitis (inflammation of the nerves). The neuropsychiatric manifestations of Lyme disease were not discussed at that time.

When I was finishing my residency at Elmhurst Hospital, and just before completing the internal medicine national boards, I received an offer from Vassar Hospital in Poughkeepsie, N.Y., to open an internal medicine practice. I sipped my coffee and dreamed about being a country doc, away from all of the hustle and bustle of the city hospitals. No more running the ER as a third-year resident, pushing IV Lasix on a patient in acute congestive heart failure while the patient in the next bed has an appendix about to burst, while a man with an acute gunshot wound has just been wheeled in on the gurney. No, I would be a country doc. Not a surgeon like my stepfather but an internist.

I also longed for an intellectual challenge in medicine. I loved the notion of being a detective and discovering why people became ill. I would sleuth out their illness. I would be a medical detective! So when I received that call from Vassar Brothers Medical Center in the winter of 1987 to open an internal medicine practice in Dutchess County, New York, I thought to myself, "Ah, this will be paradise." Of course, I now know that if Adam and Eve had lived in this paradise, they both would have had Bell's palsy and forgotten each other's names.

I always had a fondness for "the country." While I was growing up in Rego Park, Queens, my father and mother would take me up to my uncle Morty's hotel in Ellenville, New York, for the summers. My ninety-four-year-old grandfather, Max Horowitz, would get up at 3:00 A.M. to bake bread for the three hundred guests at the hotel. Fresh baked challah, rolls, and babka would await the lucky guests in the morning. It was a nosher's paradise. I used to go up to the hotel during my summers home from Northwestern, and would wait tables from July to Labor Day weekend. I spent many summers at the Melbourne Hotel, and the country held many special memories for me. I can especially remember seeing hunters driving on the roads with deer attached to the top of their cars toward the end of the season. I thought to myself, "Poor deer." My reactions to deer have certainly changed since my teenage years. Many of us in the country battle to keep them away from our plants and the front bumpers of our cars. And, of course, they are a major carrier for the deer tick associated with the disease that has become my life's work. Of course, when I decided to move to the country I didn't know that Dutchess County had the highest incidence of Lyme disease in New York State.

When I first opened my private medical office, I did what every young physician does: advertise. I had been working in the Vassar Brothers' emergency department for several months. Although my practice was slowly growing, from referrals and on-call admissions, I thought it would also help to advertise in the local Hyde Park newspaper. The advertisement I wrote read: "Hyde Park welcomes Dr. Richard Horowitz. Board Certified in Internal Medicine. Accepting All Insurance." My first response to that ad was a local urologist, who cornered me in the medical lounge at the hospital. "Who welcomed you to Hyde Park?' he asked. "I certainly didn't." Many thoughts crossed through my mind: "Was this a sign from the universe?" "Would it be helpful if I obtained a roster of people who actually liked me and had them contact him?" "Was this some type of strange country doc initiation, where if I can make it here, I can make it anywhere?" Although the urologist from Hyde Park did eventually warm up to me, we never got to the point that I would allow him to do a prostate exam on me. We never got that close.

Luckily, the head nurse in the Vassar ER was my best advertisement. Roseanne helped me build a medical practice quickly. About three thousand internal medicine patients joined my practice within my first three years. I became so busy that I closed my practice to new patients—except to Lyme patients.

During my first few years of medical practice, I worked out of a small seventeen-hundred-square-foot office on Route 9, several miles from Poughkeepsie and less than ten minutes from the local hospitals. Hyde Park is well-known for its historical ties with the Roosevelts and the Vanderbilts. FDR would broadcast fireside chats during World War II from his Hyde Park residence. The Roosevelt library holds wonderful memorabilia of a difficult time in American history and how we had the courage to overcome great obstacles. I would often drive by the sign leading into the Roosevelt estate and read its message while hurrying to the hospital for an emergency: THE ONLY THING TO FEAR IS FEAR ITSELF. Really? Roosevelt probably never dealt with insurance companies or health maintenance organization (HMO) medical directors, or walked in the woods in Hyde Park. After treating so many very ill patients, I was even afraid to walk on my own lawn.

In the early days of my practice I was seeing a fairly classic mix of internal medicine patients. I was treating people with diabetes who were overweight, uncontrolled hypertension, stroke, and congestive heart failure. I treated and counseled patients still eating pizza and other fast food despite elevated cholesterol, those with asthma and chronic obstructive pulmonary disease (COPD) who continued to smoke, and the usual upper-respiratory and lower-urinary-tract infections that are the bread and butter of most internists, about thirty to thirty-five patients each day. Some patients just came for preventive care, but many didn't care about prevention. It was an exhausting schedule, since I was practicing without a nurse and even called patients in the evening with their test results. The practice kept growing and growing and I found myself needing more help.

As my medical practice, the Hudson Valley Healing Arts Center, was becoming much larger, I now needed to expand my support staff. The first physician's assistant (PA) I hired was clearly very bright, but I couldn't understand anything he said. It was English, and medical terms were inserted intermittently in sentences, but somehow it made no sense to me. His speech was like a flowing Zen koan. My mind went blank every time I listened to him. So I let him go, due to his unintelligible speech.

The next PA I hired had completely unintelligible handwriting. He was extremely bright and an excellent PA, but his handwriting looked like diagonal lines on a piece of paper that would've given a hieroglyphics expert gray hair and a migraine. If he wasn't around, no one could read his charts.

And so it was that over the first few years, I had PAs come and go in my practice.

Fortunately, two years into the process of looking for a PA, Dylan responded to my ad in *The New York Times*. He was about to graduate from a PA school in Pennsylvania. Dylan had a bright, self-assured energy and was eager to learn. I told him that I would teach him everything I knew about internal medicine and make him a great PA. He was excited. "I just have one question for you Dylan," I said, "before I can hire you. I treat a lot of Lyme disease here. Do you want to save the world?"

Without even a moment's hesitation, Dylan turned to me. "Absolutely, Dr. Horowitz," he said. "If you're Batman, I'm your Robin." I hired him on the spot.

Early on, Lauren also entered the picture. She was bright and tough as nails. Army tough. She was in the reserves and could drop down and give me twenty anytime I asked. Of course, I never asked, but I figured anyone who jogged five miles a day and was used to army discipline should have no difficulty surviving Horowitz boot camp. Many had not survived before her, but she looked like a promising candidate. I have never been disappointed. She has been a blessing to our practice.

After Lauren and Dylan were well established, Dylan called me into his office one day quite upset. "Doc," he said, "I have some bad news." I prepared myself. I had never seen Dylan so sad. "Angie just got accepted to the Yale postdoctorate program in psychology. We are going to have to move." I felt my heart sink to the bottom of my stomach. I had grown very attached to Dylan, and he was an integral part of our practice. "When are you going to have to leave?" I asked. "In two months," he said. "I'm so sorry. I love it here." I let Dylan know that I understood and wished him well, and walked out of the office with my head spinning. I couldn't adequately take care of all of my patients and Dylan's at the same time; the load would be impossible to carry, due to the time and effort required in treating these complex patients. I called up my spiritual teacher, Lama Norlha Rinpoche, of the Tibetan Buddhist lineage, and asked him what I should do. He told me to come down and visit him at the monastery and have some soup. Lama regularly made soup for dinner, and some of our greatest conversations have taken place over his surprisingly delicious mix of leftovers. I drove to the monastery and walked up the stairs to my teacher's room.

I told him of my predicament, and Lama responded: "I think John Fallon would be excellent for your medical center." John was an old student of Lama's. He was very bright and very devoted to Lama, but I had asked him about joining our practice several times in the past, and he had declined my offer. I told Rinpoche that John had not wanted to in the past. "Oh, things different now," he said. "I think very good he join." I could tell that John was about to receive a Tibetan offer that he couldn't refuse. "Thank you, Lama," I said. "I really appreciate all of your help."

John joined our practice one month later, after giving notice to Beth Israel Medical Center in New York City, where he was working on the urology ward. He moved into the PA's room and started training with Dylan and me. After he was there for several days I asked for his impression of our office. "Less prostate exams," he said. "Well," I said, "there will be an occasional one here in the office. There is, however, a protocol that I need you to follow." I then proceeded to tell him the most important thing to ask the men before performing the prostate exam. "Make sure you tell them that if they like it, you won't tell anybody." John looked perplexed. I could tell that passing on my sense of humor was going to be a painful process. However, after six years John has gotten used to my jokes, and has even developed a sense of humor all his own. We have grown close, often stay late discussing cases, and he has been a great blessing. You can often see his car in the parking lot at 10:00 P.M. John is still at his desk, calling patients and caring deeply for them. I am extremely fortunate to have John and Lauren on my medical team.

My professional life became busier and more complicated when, as my internal medicine practice grew, I accepted the position of assistant director of medicine at Vassar Brother's hospital. I had already joined the medical staff at St. Francis Hospital, where I was head of their quality assurance committee for several years, and I also served on their alternative medicine committee. Medical rounds for patients were, therefore, punctuated with occasional committee meetings and rendezvouses with colleagues in the local medical lounge, where we would discuss cases and problems. It was at that time that I was convinced by my local colleagues and medical society to join the new HMO forming in our area. I was told that it was going to be doctor- and patient-friendly. What they meant, of course, was friendly to the doctors who worked on their administrative staff and hostile to everyone else. So after accumulating a patient load of about three thousand internal medicine patients, I decided that it was time to slow down and join this local HMO. My colleagues, who were older, wiser, and more experienced than I was, surely would know what was best for me! It now turns out that these older, wiser doctors weren't so wise after all. Of course, none of us could see the changing face of medicine in the early nineties, when decisions for our patients would start being made by administrators who followed strict medical and financial guidelines.

As I watched many of my colleagues' burn out, slowing down my practice seemed to be the wisest course to take. This was also just as I was starting to see several patients each week appear with a bull's-eye rash, the classic sign of Lyme disease. I had not realized that my practice was located in one of the most Lyme-endemic areas in the United States, one known for hosting a large tick population. No one mentions this in the travel brochures, but residents now know to pay close attention to the possibility of tick attachment while hiking in the woods and walking in tall grasses during the spring, summer, and autumn months.

So in the course of a routine day in the early 1990s, a patient would come in with a tick bite, and some of them had the characteristic rash. I always had my pair of medical tweezers nearby, and I often had to teach patients that applying a match, Vaseline, gasoline, or a variety of other noxious petroleum-based chemicals to the tick was not the correct method for removal. The medical wisdom at the time was to not treat tick bites but to use a wait and see approach. I learned ultimately that that meant wait and see how sick a patient got, and then hope that your treatment worked!

I decided early on that prophylactic treatment made more sense than wait and see. What I observed was that some patients did not adequately respond to antibiotic treatment if we waited and saw. In addition, early on I found that while a ten- or twenty-one-day course of doxycycline would work for the large majority of patients who presented with an EM rash, it was still unclear why it did not work for some patients. And how should I treat patients demonstrating multiple Lyme-like symptoms but who never presented with an EM rash? I was intrigued and challenged: I wanted all of my patients to get better. Why did roughly 75 percent of the patients treated early on get better but 25 percent appeared to develop chronic symptoms? These patients presented with a strange litany of symptoms, such as fatigue, aches and pains that migrated around their bodies, tingling and numbness, memory and concentration problems, and a host of other unexplained symptoms. I asked my colleagues for input, but no one seemed to know the answers. I searched the medical literature but could only find an occasional article demonstrating the failure of classical antibiotic treatment, and even fewer proposing the persistence of the Lyme spirochete, a spiral-shaped bacteria resembling syphilis.

I began to find that re-treating these patients with antibiotics helped them regain their predisease functioning. While on medication their problems all improved, but many quickly relapsed once the antibiotics were stopped.

Then, one patient changed the course of my practice. Eve first came to see me in 1992, complaining of multiple physical and neurological symptoms. She was a bright professional woman who was strongly motivated to get better from a bout of Bell's palsy (facial paralysis), which can be a neurological manifestation of central nervous system Lyme disease. Local neurologists couldn't find the cause for her symptoms. They had screened her with an ELISA (enzyme-linked immunosorbent assay) antibody test for Lyme disease. Her results were negative: no Lyme disease. Through my reading, however, I had learned that another blood test, the Western blot, will often show *Borrelia*-specific bands (the outer surface proteins of an organism, in this case *Borrelia burgdorferi*, the causative agent of Lyme disease), even if the ELISA is negative, thus making it a more sensitive and specific test than the ELISA for Lyme disease. I sent off a Western blot that came back positive; she had been exposed to Lyme disease. I treated her with antibiotics, and her symptoms improved, although there still was a residual Bell's palsy. Classic medical wisdom teaches that 95 percent of Bell's palsy sufferers improve with time. Was she one of the 5 percent whose symptoms linger? Or could her symptoms be manifestations of an ongoing infection that was not helped by her initial round of antibiotics?

Eve told me about a Lyme conference sponsored by the Lyme Disease Foundation in Boston, and she strongly encouraged me to attend. This conference changed my professional life. It wasn't until the very last session on the second day that I got answers for my clinical dilemmas. I felt like a starving man finally being given a morsel to eat at a feast. I was introduced to the methodologies of: Dr. Sam Donta, an infectious disease specialist at Boston University; Dr. Kenneth Leigner, an internist in Armonk, New York; and Dr. Joseph Burrascano, an internist from South Hampton, Long Island, who each discussed the clinical manifestations of Lyme and the utility of using longer-term antibiotic regimens. I drove home from the conference armed with some answers to my medical questions and some new weapons in the fight against Lyme disease.

When I returned to my medical practice and implemented these new ideas, I found that, in fact, increasing the dose of the antibiotics, and/or extending the length of treatment, clearly did help a certain percentage of my patients. Their fatigue, headaches, joint and muscle pain, and cognitive symptoms improved. However, each time we stopped the antibiotics many patients experienced reoccurrences of their symptoms. My teachers taught me to always get to the source of the problem and treat patients the way I wanted to be treated myself. Certainly I would not want to have the symptoms they complained of, and my Hippocratic oath was to serve to the best of my ability.

Dutchess County, New York, is also IBM country. When an IBMer, for example, complains that he/she can't remember keystrokes and forgets basic programming, but once on antibiotics they are able to return to work and function, others take notice. So as I began to help these patients, word spread that Dr. Horowitz was discovering new treatments to help the sick patients in Dutchess County. And it was at this point that I closed my medical office to regular internal medicine patients and only kept it open to those with Lyme symptoms that classical medical treatment was unable to help.

I was excited about the results I was seeing and wanted to share this information with colleagues who had to be facing the same dilemmas. So I did what every extremely naïve, well-meaning physician would do: I shared the information with my local HMO and accepted invitations to lecture at medical conferences. Yet to my amazement, the HMO didn't seem to share the same enthusiasm that I had. Instead, they told me that chronic Lyme disease didn't exist! I was reminded about their HMO Lyme treatment guidelines, which were reviewed and approved by a local infectious disease specialist.

Despite showing them that the continuing medical education credits I received from attending these conferences were sanctioned by the state of New York, they continued to insist that their treatment protocols were the only correct way to diagnose and treat this disease. The more patients who came to see me with unresolved Lyme disease symptoms, and the more I circled Lyme disease on my insurance submission forms, the more intense our conversations became. The Lyme war had begun.

Luckily, many patients have not been passive during this battle. The Lyme Disease Association (LDA), the Lyme Disease Foundation (LDF), the Lyme Research Alliance (formerly known as Time for Lyme), the Tick-Borne Disease Alliance (TBDA), as well as numerous local Lyme support groups have joined the fight. One clear thing I have learned from watching these groups form: Don't get parents angry. They will fight back with a vengeance when the health-care system tells them it has nothing to offer and that their children must suffer endlessly without answers.

These advocacy groups have told their stories to sympathetic politicians. Joel Miller, then a Republican Assembly member from Dutchess County, New York, and Nettie Mayersohn, then a Democratic Assembly member from Queens, fought for patients' rights in New York State. Several years ago, then New York State governor George Pataki also entered the battle, and he sent a memo to the New York State Department of Health and Office of Professional Medical Conduct (OPMC) to stop pursuing physicians who chose to use longer-term antibiotics in the fight against Lyme disease. The attorney general of Connecticut, the Honorable Richard Blumenthal (now a U.S. senator from Connecticut) held insurance hearings and announced that his antitrust investigation had "uncovered serious flaws in the Infectious Diseases Society of America's (IDSA) process for writing its 2006 Lyme Disease guidelines." The IDSA agreed to reassess their guidelines. Blumenthal had found "undisclosed financial interests" and that the IDSA guidelines panel "improperly ignored or minimized consideration of alternative medical opinion and evidence regarding chronic Lyme disease, potentially raising serious questions about whether the recommendations reflected all relevant science." This was a landmark political event. No politician in the history of the United States had ever challenged guidelines set by an infectious disease medical society. It took great courage, strong ethics, and the ability to listen carefully with an open mind and open heart to the people he serves to take such action. Senator Blumenthal is an example of courageous, caring politics at its best. Other politicians, such as Congressman Chris Gibson, have also been paying attention to the suffering of their constituents and have organized congressional public hearings in New York to try and find solutions to this growing epidemic. Congress is hearing the call of the people.

Doctors have also been forced to enter the battle. Many have already been forced out of medicine, lost their licenses, or been forced to undergo medical monitoring, because they have not followed IDSA guidelines sanctioned by medical licensing boards. They have spent hundreds of thousands of dollars in legal fees to uphold their licenses. Dr. Joseph Burrascano went to Congress to testify about the effects of unresolved Lyme disease symptoms on his own patients. Dr. Steven Phillips testified at the insurance hearings in Connecticut years ago. I went to Rhode Island with Dr. Kenneth Leigner and others several years ago to testify at a congressional hearing, and also just traveled to Vermont to testify before their Senate and House on the effects of these infections on the patients in our practice. In our testimony we described how patients were forced to travel great distances to see us, because they could not obtain proper medical care in their own states. Consequently, many states, including Rhode Island and California, have formally recognized that it is not professional medical misconduct to use longer-term antibiotics to treat Lyme disease.

I listen closely to my patients' stories every day. I also listen to the doctors who are fearful of treating Lyme patients, because they face losing their medical licenses. The ineffectual testing and ineffective paradigms that modern medicine offers provide no satisfactory answers. Without a paradigm shift, the present poly-ticks of this epidemic ensure that the suffering will continue.

I believe that the identification of MSIDS, multiple systemic infectious disease syndrome, may prove to be the missing link to end this war once and for all. It incorporates a broad-based solution for Lyme and co-infections that provides a bridge for the two competing groups (IDSA and ILADS), so that they can come together and deliver patients the help they desperately need. My model presumes that everybody who is involved in this controversy is partially correct. Instead of positing another divisive and confrontational position, I am trying to open a door, to move forward. My model suggests that on some fronts the IDSA is accurate. On other fronts, ILADS is accurate.

My ideas about MSIDS began in 1998, when I started presenting my clinical results at national and international conferences. The pieces of the puzzle were slowly coming together. One year it was the clue that led to the identification of a strain of babesiosis, *Babesia microti*, a malaria-like illness that could explain the fevers, chills, and day and night sweats and that account for some of their resistant symptoms. Once treated, some patients using wheelchairs could stand and walk. Next was the discovery of cat scratch disease symptoms, or *Bartonella*, which could explain their resistant neurological symptoms, such as treatment-resistant neuropathy or encephalopathy. Next was the uncovering of *Mycoplasma fermentans*, the organism suspected in Gulf War syndrome and possibly a contributor to some of my patients' ALS-type symptoms. And more recently we have been able to link the presence of heavy-metals, such as mercury, lead, arsenic, cadmium, and aluminum, with patients' overlapping symptomatology. This led me to begin using medications that help remove chemicals, toxins, and heavy metals from the body, such as IV glutathione and oral chelation regimens to detoxify treatment-resistant patients. The results have been no less than astounding, which is why I'm writing this book. You need to know that your symptoms are not only real and identifiable, but they are treatable.

HOW THIS BOOK WORKS

This book is a compilation of everything I've discovered about Lyme disease and, subsequently, about chronic disease in general. By reading this and learning from the many patient anecdotes, my hope is that you will be able to identify your own symptoms and work with your doctor for the best possible treatment outcome. My treatment protocol is based on my sixteen-point differential diagnostic map, which is what I use to solve the mystery of Lyme disease for my patients who present with any number of complex chronic medical illnesses, and provides me with a path toward treatment and relief previously not available.

I believe that those I treat are typically suffering from Lyme disease as well as other illnesses, which is why I describe their condition as multiple systemic infectious disease syndrome, or MSIDS. Through this diagnostic model I have been able to determine that patients with complex, chronic illnesses, no matter which diagnosis we may give them, often have simultaneous bacterial, parasitic, viral, and fungal causes for their illness. Many times they also have associated immune dysfunction, large environmental toxin loads, hormonal dysfunctions, mitochondrial dysfunction, allergies, sleep disorders, or underlying psychological dysfunction.

My overall goals for this book are fourfold. First, my hope is that it will demonstrate how I have reached my understanding of Lyme disease as a medical detective focused on patient outcomes. Second, I hope that the reader will understand the strengths but also the dangerous weaknesses of the present medical system, and that the MSIDS model presents a substantial plan to address the rapidly expanding Lyme crisis and to reduce the burden of chronic disease in this country. This should appeal to the insurance industry in particular. Third, I present a model that if adopted could serve as a bridge between the two opposing diagnostic and treatment perspectives. And last, it is my hope that the MSIDS model will help in the global effort to combat tick-borne diseases and serve as a guide to those seeking answers for any chronic persistent illness. Let us move medicine into the twenty-first century.

PART I

The Mystery of Lyme Disease

ONE

Identifying Lyme Disease

The History of Medicine:

2000 BCE: *Here, eat this root. It will make you strong.*

1080 BCE: *Throw out that root and drink this potion; it is better for you.*

250 AD: *Get rid of that potion; it is bad for you. Take this herb instead.*

1910: *Get rid of this herb and take this potion; it is more effective.*

1950: *That potion is bad for you; here, take this drug.*

2000: *That drug is no longer effective; here, eat this root.*

How is it possible that an epidemic of tick-borne diseases could be spreading without getting the proper attention? How could patients throughout the United States continue to be desperate for help? To understand the answer to this dilemma, you need to understand the intricacies of Lyme disease and the constructs of the medical paradigm that doctors and health authorities work under.

First of all, we must look at the history of medicine. Medicine is a continuously changing and expanding field, and it is said that almost half of everything that we learn in medical school will usually be proven to be wrong every five to ten years. There are numerous examples of the undeniable blessings of modern medicine: antibiotics and other pharmaceuticals; new high-tech diagnostic machines and tests; groundbreaking surgeries; and public health initiatives have extended human life (most especially in infancy) and increased well-being in the general population. But along the way to modern medicine, some medical pioneers have been dismissed or even attacked for what others believed were their heretical ideas.

For example, consider Dr. Ignaz Philipp Semmelweis, a nineteenth-century Hungarian physician, who is now known as an early pioneer of antiseptic procedures described as the "savior of mothers." Semmelweis made an important scientific observation: When he washed his hands before delivering babies, the women in his clinic did not die as often from puerperal sepsis (a bacterial infection that kills women shortly after giving birth) as those in another clinic in the same hospital, which had a death rate of 10 percent. When he shared this important observation with his colleagues, he was ridiculed. As patients abandoned his colleagues and begged to deliver in his clinic, he was ostracized by his medical society and driven out of medicine. He was committed to an asylum, where ironically, he died of septicemia only fourteen days later, possibly the result of being severely beaten by his guards.

Dr. Louis Pasteur was another example of a scientist who was ridiculed. It was years before his theory of the germ origins of illness was proven to be correct.

Helicobacter pylori were first discovered in the stomachs of patients with gastritis and stomach ulcers in 1982 by Australian doctors Barry Marshall and Robin Warren. The conventional thinking at the time of their research was that no bacterium could live in the strong acid environment of the human stomach. They also proposed that treatment with antibiotics rather than the practices then in use, which included stomach removal, were best for ulcer patients. Their discovery was ignored for almost twenty years, while patients had their stomachs removed because of bleeding ulcers, or were told to drink large quantities of milk, or were cautioned that their ulcers were due to stress alone.

There is a long list of other examples available for anyone who wants to explore the history of medicine. Many of these pioneers pushed the boundaries until the paradigm of that specific disease process was transformed. Are things different today? Have we learned to listen to those challenging the medical establishment? Certainly not with respect to Lyme disease and associated tick-borne disorders.

To understand Lyme disease, we need to go back to the mid 1970s, when portrait painter Polly Murray first noticed an outbreak of what had been called "juvenile rheumatoid arthritis" in the town of Lyme, Connecticut, that had affected her and her children from decades earlier. Dr. Alan Steere, a rheumatologist at Yale University, was called in to investigate the epidemic, as were researchers from the National Institutes of

Health (NIH) and Rocky Mountain Labs. Dr. Willy Burgdorfer, a researcher at Rocky Mountain Labs, identified a microscopic spirochete, a spiral-shaped bacteria that resembles the one that causes syphilis. This was eventually identified as the causative agent of the newly identified disease, and the spirochete was named *Borrelia burgdorferi* (Bb) after Dr. Burgdofer's discovery, and the related disease was called Lyme, after its initial outbreak in the town of Lyme, Connecticut.

Although patients may have had other manifestations of the disease, Dr. Allan Steere primarily investigated patients with rashes and rheumatologic manifestations, including hot, swollen joints, for the Connecticut Department of Public Health. He was instrumental in determining that many became ill in summer or early fall and lived in geographic clusters in mostly rural areas. He did recognize that patients were very ill and not just psychologically disturbed. But what caused this mysterious illness?

This mysterious illness was actually not a new discovery at all. Lyme disease had already been reported in Europe in the late 1800s, as a rash of the hands: Dr. Alfred Buchwald described a skin lesion; others in Europe and the United States reported the same lesion as part of a condition called Bannwarth syndrome, a triad of radiculitis (a pain radiating along a nerve), with Bell's palsy (the sudden onset of facial paralysis), and meningitis (an inflammation occurring in the membranes covering the brain and spinal cord). In 1909, Dr. Arvid Afzelius described an expanding ring-like skin rash, later named erythema chronicum migrans, or ECM (in 1990, dermatologist Dr. Bernard Berger recognized that the rash was not chronic in all cases and renamed it *Erythema Migrans* or, simply, EM). Ten years later, Afzelius connected the disease with joint problems and speculated that they are somehow related to the bite of a tick. In 1922 the disease was found to be associated with neurological problems, and in 1930 the diagnosis further included psychiatric disturbances. A few years later, arthritic problems were added. In 1965 Dr. Sidney Robbin, a semiretired internist living in Montauk, New York, described expanding circular rashes that responded to penicillin treatment that appeared in conjunction with a peculiar type of arthritis that he named Montauk knee. Five years later, Dr. Rudolph Scrimenti, a Wisconsin dermatologist, published the first report of an ECM rash in the United States. As Dr. Robbin had observed, he too reported that the rash responded to penicillin.

No one, however, had put all the pieces together. And no one yet connected these symptoms to the patients who were so ill in rural Connecticut. Was this a new illness, and, if so, where did it come from and how should we treat it? By 1977, Dr. Steere was reporting a whole host of specific and often bizarre signs of this new disease, including fever, fatigue, headache, migratory joint pains, as well as multiple cardiovascular and neurological abnormalities. As the result of treating patients with antibiotics for (only) seven to ten days, many patients went on to develop other symptoms. It appeared that antibiotics just wouldn't help Lyme patients. Perhaps Lyme was caused by a virus, or was an autoimmune disorder.

When you have been trained in a particular medical specialty, you see the world through certain lenses and diagnostic paradigms. A gastroenterologist, for example, sees the world through the lens of the gastrointestinal (GI) tract and tries to link up a patient's symptoms to diseases known in their specialty. This is the same for neurology or infectious disease or, in the case of Dr. Steere, a rheumatologist, for diseases of the joints, which include autoimmune diseases. It is not that the thinking of these doctors and subspecialists is necessarily wrong, but it may be that their worldview only includes part of the whole picture. There is relative truth, and then there is absolute truth. When the three blind men are feeling the elephant, they each describe a different part. One describes the elephant as having a long, movable nose, another tough skin with thick legs and big nails, and the third might just describe a thin, coarse tail. Each has described a certain relative truth, and none is incorrect, but none of them have seen the big picture: It's an elephant!

So it is with Lyme disease. The initial paradigm created for diagnosis and treatment of these patients was through a rheumatologist's narrowly focused eyes. Soon the infectious disease doctors claimed Lyme disease as part of their turf.

I was trained as an internist to be a medical detective, with a wide diagnostic perspective: We have to know something about all of the medical subspecialties. The vision of an internist must be broad and inclusive of all possibilities, since his or her job is to diagnose patients to effectively determine who needs to be referred to subspecialists. An internist, therefore, will not necessarily have some of the inherent biases or diagnostic schema associated with subspecialists. As Lyme diagnosis and treatment fell into the domains of the rheumatologists and infectious disease doctors early on, a paradigm was forming based on the way these subspecialists viewed the world. In addition, traditional medical education has always taught doctors to find one cause for all of the patient's symptoms. This is deeply ingrained in every physician's education. We generally are not taught to look for multifactorial causes of an illness. Therefore, if a Lyme disease patient presents with thirty-five different symptoms, the established paradigm would be to try and explain these complaints according to the accepted medical model: one primary diagnosis. If the doctor could not find a single etiology, or cause, for your symptoms, it must be because it is psychological in nature, and you are crazy. Or the answer might be elusive because the symptoms can't be understood in the HMO-dictated fifteen-minute time frame. Or perhaps the physician hasn't looked hard enough, or just sees the world through one narrow diagnostic lens.

Let's embark on a journey together as medical detectives to see how we might diagnose and treat one of the most pressing epidemics facing us in the twenty-first century.

GETTING TO THE SOURCE OF CHRONIC ILLNESS

Although solving such an enormous problem like multiple systemic infectious disease syndrome (MSIDS) might seem a very daunting, or even an unreachable, goal, as a physician I have found that communicating well with my patients is a key ingredient. Searching for clues by listening intently to their symptoms allows even the most seriously ill multisystem-affected patient to achieve greater health and wellness. After accumulating all of the necessary information from the patient, and reviewing the laboratory results, we need to blend medical knowledge with deeper intuitive wisdom.

Tell me again: What do you feel? When did it begin? What makes it better or worse? As I probe each time, their stories prompt me to search for new clues: The mystery unfolds through our dialogue. Of course, this technique doesn't ensure that we can discover the answers for all the problems of all our patients all the time. Nor does it mean that this strategy will cure illnesses that have plagued patients for years (although this might be possible). But it does allow the medical detective to register some clue that hadn't seemed important before.

The second piece of the strategy of being an insightful medical detective is attitude. And by this I mean developing a strong desire to benefit the patient who is suffering. We can achieve this by imagining exchanging ourselves with another and doing for them exactly what we would want done for ourselves. Rather than take an all-knowing physician stance, I believe the best medical strategy is developing a strong and unwavering compassion for others. Any success I have had in my practice rests on this guiding principle. Although this might sound like a new credo for modern medicine, it is, in fact, implied in the Hippocratic Oath that all physicians take. It has doctors pledge respect for human life, and to treat patients as fellow human beings, not medical conditions.

Adopting compassion as the foundation of our health-care system challenges the time-efficient models and financial incentive–driven perspectives of modern health care. Yet many patients, physicians, and insurance directors are unhappy with our current health-care system. Even patients with health insurance coverage suffer with chronic undiagnosed illnesses, physicians burn out, and health-care costs continue to soar in this unhealthy atmosphere. It is difficult to find satisfaction as a physician if you are rushing from patient to patient and are unable to find the time to develop a strong, heart-centered healing partnership with those who seek your care. Shifting from the head to the heart, where our compassion lies, can bring patients and physicians greater satisfaction, and it provides the essential motivation to get to the root cause of illness. This ultimately benefits the patient, the health-care system (as unnecessary and expensive tests are not performed), and the physician (as he or she experiences greater satisfaction and improved patient outcomes).

The U.S. Centers for Disease Control and Prevention recognizes that chronic illness may be a complex interplay of genetics, environmental factors, infections, and trauma. But in day-to-day practice, doctors often do not use this broad framework to understand and treat chronic illness. Usually, the HMO model encourages limited time for visits and referring patients to long lists of specialists who, if they get approval, will perform long lists of expensive tests. Yet these same insurance companies often place limits on medically necessary treatment options for economic reasons. Few physicians have the time to uncover the multifactorial causes of chronic illness. Most specialists are trained only to treat one small piece of the puzzle, one body system, or one category of causes.

I believe that the first piece of this paradigm shift must therefore be with primary care physicians. These first-line physicians must use a broader and more inclusive framework to break down chronic illness into layers by examining the mental, emotional, and physical aspects of each illness.

Then we must go even further as detectives and break these physical symptoms down into the anatomy of an illness, the biology of an illness, the biochemistry of an illness, the immunology of an illness, and the genetics behind the illness. Functional medicine and abnormalities in the biochemical pathways that drive chronic illness are a start. These often need to be examined to discover clues as to why the chronically ill patient has persistent symptoms. In medical school, doctors are not taught adequately about environmental medicine nor is the importance of what these toxins may do to the body emphasized, or how detoxification pathways work, how inflammatory cytokines (the protein molecules that are secreted by cells that can communicate with each other) cause sickness behavior, or how mental or emotional stress can negatively affect adrenal function, causing immune system dysfunction.

Physicians are trained to recognize and treat chronic infections, but many believe that the list of chronic diseases is limited to those like tuberculosis, leprosy, syphilis, chronic Q fever, or chronic viral infections, such as hepatitis B, hepatitis C, or HIV. If the medical paradigm that your doctor is working in is that other chronic infectious diseases are rare, then he or she will not look for them, nor will they find them. Yet if a doctor is smart enough to think about searching for them, the other problem he or she will face is that diagnostic tests are not necessarily reliable enough to make an accurate diagnosis.

Think of the chronic illness patient as someone with sixteen nails in his or her foot. Their physician might identify several nails in the workup, and treat those specific causes, but often, if they do not achieve a positive result by pulling out one of the nails, they believe that they have erred in the diagnosis. However, this does not mean they were wrong. If the patient still complains of pain, it means that there are fifteen nails left behind to explain the chronic foot pain. It is therefore essential to look further and find all of the nails causing the pain.

To begin with, each person's symptoms need to be considered individually, and then collected and put into likely disease categories to try and find the common denominator. This is a process doctors call "the differential diagnosis." Each chronic illness is complex, and its causes are likely interrelated. For example, a patient complains of night sweats. Let's say that the patient is a thirty- or forty-year-old female who is not in menopause. After obtaining a history and performing a physical, the medical detective would identify the most common causes of night sweats. Is it tuberculosis or non-Hodgkin's lymphoma? Is there a cough, hemoptysis (blood in the sputum), or weight loss, or has there been exposure to someone who contracted tuberculosis? A simple chest X-ray and tuberculosis test (PPD) could help rule out these two differential diagnoses while the physician checks the patient for hard, enlarged, nonmobile lymph nodes, which can be seen with a lymphoma. Has she been traveling to countries where she could have been exposed to malaria? Did the patient get a febrile illness while they were there? Examining a blood smear under the microscope (called a Giemsa stain) to rule out malaria could be helpful. Does the patient live in a tick-endemic area or has she traveled to one where she could have contracted babesiosis, which is a malaria-like illness? (Most people these days live in or have traveled to highly tick-endemic areas). Performing a *Babesia* titer (an antibody test), a Giemsa stain, a polymerase chain reaction (PCR) DNA test, or a fluorescent in situ hybridization (FISH) test of RNA, looking for *Babesia* would be helpful in this circumstance. Is the patient having hormonal issues even though they are young? Checking an FSH, LH, estradiol, progesterone, testosterone, and free-testosterone levels, as well as sex-hormone binding globulin (SHBG) would help rule out this possibility. Is she hyperthyroid? Is she suffering from weight loss, palpitations, tremors, anxiety, diarrhea, and sweats? Checking a full thyroid panel would be helpful. Has the patient undergone any recent trauma that might be triggering an anxiety disorder? By simply listing these six to seven most common differential diagnoses for night sweats and ruling out each one with a proper history, physical, and laboratory testing, answers can be found.

The three problems that I see most often that interfere with making such a diagnosis are: first, the fifteen-minute HMO model of medicine does not allow the time to think through the complexities of differential diagnoses. Second, while doctors are rushing to get to their next patient, they may not even ask the patient to tell them about all of their symptoms. Third, patients frequently don't mention symptoms that they don't think are important, or they forget to mention others. Good communication enables the treating physician to establish the proper diagnosis.

To ensure that I hear the full patient story I have a symptom questionnaire that I use with all of my patients. This questionnaire was developed years ago based on Lyme patients complaining of similar sets of symptoms. Without it I know that many important patient clues would be missing, and these are often the symptoms that are essential for the medical detective to make an accurate diagnosis.

We need to get to the source of the problems in medicine, because the world now more than ever is out of balance. The ancient adage "as above, so below" could now be applied to medicine in terms of "as without, so within." When does the illness of the world become our own personal illness? When does our own personal illness impact the balance of the world? If we identify the source of illness within us, it also informs us about what is out of balance in the world, and perhaps can teach us how to remedy it.

For example, we have an epidemic of hypertension. Is that so-called normal aging, or is it a problem with hardening of the arteries from an improper diet and exercise program, or from chronic inflammation from an imbalanced orthosympathetic and parasympathetic nervous system affected by a lifetime of stress, with elevated levels of cortisol and epinephrine, and/or from elevated levels of lead getting into our bodies from the environment? I have tested several thousand people in my medical practice with chronic illness for heavy metals, and I have found that the majority have elevated levels of lead. Most doctors do not look for elevated levels of lead in their patients, since it is not part of the standard medical screen and laboratory testing and physical and wellness exam. Yet lead is getting into people's bodies from multiple sources. We now find lead in the drinking water, there is lead glazing on plates, and there are elevated levels in seafood, and especially in shellfish. Lead is deposited in our bones during our lives and subsequently released back into the body as the bones break down with aging, osteopenia (lower bone mineral density), or osteoporosis. Lead has been linked to hypertension. So is hypertension a disease of normal aging? Or is hypertension perhaps due to a multiplicity of the above factors? If we properly diagnose and treat it, perhaps millions of people would not need blood pressure medication or suffer chronic kidney disease or kidney failure, strokes, heart attacks, or congestive heart failure. These chronic illnesses alone cost the health-care system billions of dollars and cause untold suffering for patients and their families.

Let us take another example. Is it normal to be losing your memory as you get older? Is it normal to have an Alzheimer's epidemic affecting not only the United States but also the rest of the world? Or is it possible that there are multiple etiologies at the root of these conditions? We find that the majority of our Lyme disease patients with co-infections have severe memory and concentration problems. A beginning hint of the connection between infection and dementia can be found in a report from pathologist Dr. Alan B. MacDonald, who examined brain biopsies from the McLean Hospital (an affiliate of Harvard University) data bank from patients with confirmed Alzheimer's disease (AD). His PCR analysis showed that seven out of ten of these patients had the DNA of *Borrelia burgdorferi* in their brain, the etiologic agent of Lyme disease. We also find that the majority of our chronically ill patients with Lyme disease and co-infections have been exposed to high levels of heavy metals, such as mercury and lead, and occasionally to aluminum. These also can cause memory and concentration problems, and can cause the production of elevated levels of free radicals, which can increase inflammation. Similarly, we are exposed to hundreds of environmental chemicals every day that are fat soluble and, therefore, are deposited in the brain. These can and do affect cognitive processing. We know that an inflammatory process is at work in Alzheimer's disease that helps to drive the production of amyloid (an insoluble fibrous protein that in excess can lead to neurodegenerative diseases). Are Lyme disease, co-infections, environmental toxins, and heavy metals some of the agents causing the severe memory and concentration problems currently being diagnosed as Alzheimer's disease? If we include patients who have undiagnosed B_{12} deficiency, which would be picked up by doing blood tests for B_{12} and methylmalonic acid levels, and/or patients who suffer from undiagnosed hypothyroidism, we have enough causes for an epidemic of dementia in the general population.

I have seen elderly patients with a diagnosis of dementia, with cognitive deficits, given drugs prescribed for Alzheimer's, such as Aricept and Namenda, which slow down (but do not reverse) their cognitive decline. But I have seen improvements in their cognitive functioning after treating them for chronic tick-borne infections, by detoxifying them of fat-soluble toxins with glutathione, by using oral chelating agents to remove mercury, lead, and aluminum, and by identifying and treating B_{12} deficiencies and/or hypothyroidism.

Identifying the multifactorial causes of chronic illness is the next most important paradigm shift in medicine. We cannot simply name an illness without looking into its multifactorial causes, or we will be leaving a legacy of chronic illnesses for future generations. Epidemics of autism, cancer, strokes, heart attacks, hypertension, diabetes, obesity, autoimmune diseases, mental illness, chronic fatigue syndrome, fibromyalgia, and Lyme disease with co-infections are just some of the ongoing epidemics. This should not be the normal fabric of illnesses woven through our society. We can do better.

THE ESSENTIAL TOOLS OF THE MEDICAL DETECTIVE

A wise man once said: "There are two mistakes that one can make on the road to truth: not going all the way, and not starting." When I was finishing my medical training at the Free University of Brussels medical school, I asked my spiritual teacher to tell me what he believed was the most important component for the practice of medicine. He said: "It is the quality of compassion."

When I asked what he meant, he said: "When you are building a house, you must have a proper foundation. Without a proper foundation, that house will not stand. The foundation which ensures that you will benefit yourself and others is loving kindness and compassion. Love is wanting other people to be happy. Compassion is the wish that other people be free from suffering. If you exchange yourself with others and do for them exactly that which you would want done for yourself, everything will go well."

The first most essential tool for the medical detective is therefore compassion and proper motivation. How does one develop those qualities? Most health-care providers have the wish to help others, of course. However, for many of us, on some days, we approach illness as a bother, a challenge, a duty to heal rather than as a loving, caring parent would, who does everything to relieve the pain of their suffering child. I have personally witnessed parents who have taken their children from doctor to doctor, desperate to find help for their children. A primary care doctor who approaches each patient as a parent would their own sick child will surely be more successful than one who is not as strongly invested in the outcome, or who feels that their job is as a gatekeeper for a referral to a more experienced subspecialist. Patients can feel when doctors truly care. That in itself is a healing experience.

To develop these qualities of loving kindness and compassion, we need to take some time every day to reflect upon them, so that we can integrate them into our lives. One basic skill taught in different meditative traditions is the technique of taking and sending. In this visualization one imagines that he or she breathes in the suffering and ills of others, which comes into our body through the nose as a black smoke. It goes directly into the heart and is transformed there, with love, into a white light. This then leaves through our nose and heals others, relieving them of their suffering and bringing them happiness and joy. I have been assured by those diligently practicing the technique over the years, and from my own spiritual teachers, that no harm actually comes to our bodies by doing such a visualization, and that the benefits are immense. It would appear that taking several minutes a day to meditate in this way and develop these qualities creates a strong foundation for us to help others. Wanting to be of service and help others is not only a noble philosophy but elevates us while simultaneously benefiting our patients. Compassionate self-sacrifice and putting others above ourselves allows the practice of medicine to become a spiritual path to the divine.

This technique of taking and sending is a way to exchange yourself with others and develop the important qualities of loving kindness and compassion that are necessary not only to be a healer but also to be healed.

Those of us who work with the sick have also been wounded. This practice of taking and sending can connect us with that quality of a soft open heart that joins us to our own humanity. And to the humanity of others. This moves us to practice medicine not only from the head but also from the heart, from a deep place of caring where we want the best for others. And when we do this, often the best outcomes result. Caring about others and wanting to relieve their suffering are the essential keys. According to my teachers, all the benefits seen in the practice of medicine emanate from this one source.

The next most important tool for the medical detective, which naturally follows from deep caring, is the giving of full, undivided attention to the patient. We must take the time to listen fully with empathy, or we cannot possibly discover the clues to the patient's illness. Full, undivided attention is also experienced as an act of love, and love heals. To give full attention means that we must be able to stop our own busy minds for an instant. This is not easy for most of us. We are running on the treadmill of life, with barely enough time to catch our breaths. This practice of giving full, undivided attention without letting our minds wander is one of the first foundation practices of meditation, "calm abiding." We must train our minds to stay in one place and not follow thoughts of the past, or thoughts of the present, or thoughts of the future. If we can train our minds in this way, we have the possibility of developing an inner calm. We will not be swayed by strong mental currents that frequently lead us to obsess about past failures or difficulties, nor live in fear about a future that has not yet happened. We can learn to stay in the present moment and simply be in peace. The practice is to simply listen, with full, undivided attention, to our patients' stories. This is a very challenging task for most medical providers, yet the answers to the patient's illness often emerge while sitting in a space of deep listening and deep caring. Once in this stance, the medical detective collects details of patients' illnesses and processes those facts using left-brain logical reasoning. Next he or she can calm their mind and rest in an open, undistracted meditative space, where right-brain intuitive knowledge can be accessed. I have found that combining left-brain logic with right-brain intuition can lead to better patient outcomes.

Most patients with chronic complex illnesses come into my office with a stack of medical records and a long list of complaints. By meticulously reviewing their records and using the questionnaire that I describe later to further delineate the full extent of their symptoms, I am ensuring that I am complete in obtaining a proper history. This questionnaire also provides me an opportunity to formulate the most probable differential diagnoses while interviewing the patient. Taking a proper history from patients, with these highly complex conditions, who may have been to ten to twenty doctors in the past several years, usually will take me at least one hour. It usually takes between two and three hours with each new patient to complete a social history, family history, and environmental exposure history, and to review their symptoms, conduct a complete physical examination and assessment, and devise a treatment plan. It is obvious that the HMO model of medicine (approximately one patient every fifteen minutes) is not well-suited for patients with complex chronic illnesses.

When I arrive at the final assessment and plan, I try to make sure that every symptom on the questionnaire that the patient circled has one or several potential differential diagnoses. This ensures that each symptom receives the appropriate testing, and has an appropriate plan. Often patterns emerge while I am reviewing the symptoms. Often a gestalt appears suggesting the most probable diagnoses for the patient and the most probable direction in which healing will be found.

These tools for the MD (medical detective) may seem simple, but they work. As we try and construct a new paradigm to deal with chronic illness we will see that there are several distinct advantages to this model. My health-care colleagues are experiencing burnout at high rates. I believe that the motivations and tools I review in this book can help us rediscover greater joy in helping others and in striving to help those who have not been helped in the past. Cultivating the qualities of loving kindness and compassion are not just paths using the head but also paths of the heart. The balancing of the masculine and feminine energies of both head and heart can lead us to greater joy and satisfaction in the practice of medicine, emotions so often lacking in our fast-paced medical environment. Patients seem to like this approach, too!

Finally, it turns out that this model is quite comprehensive in its scope, and it has the potential to lead to diagnosis and treatment in the shortest period of time while costing the health-care system the least amount of precious resources. Using four tools—proper motivation; listening fully with empathy; using the questionnaire to evaluate patients' complaints; and then developing differential diagnoses using the Horowitz sixteen-point chronic disease map—has the potential to offer hope to those who have suffered for a long time, and to offer them a chance for healing. I believe that these are the tools vital for every medical detective who is seeking the road to truth.

THE HOROWITZ LYME-MSIDS QUESTIONNAIRE

An Essential Tool in Determining the Probability of Lyme Disease and MSIDS

My patients typically fill out the following symptom questionnaire while in the waiting room. I then use the document to go through the thirty-eight items in Section 1 in great detail and get expanded information on each of the symptoms to develop a comprehensive set of differential diagnoses. This essential questionnaire is based on one developed by Dr. Joseph Burrascano when he started treating Lyme disease patients. He found, and other physicians have verified, that there were a number of common patient symptoms, and these complaints make up the items of the questionnaire.

You can use the following questionnaire to determine the probability of a Lyme-MSIDS diagnosis for yourself. I also highly recommend that new and experienced physicians use this as a screening tool to determine if their patients might have Lyme disease. This process ensures that no symptoms are left out and gives the provider an initial opportunity to develop a broad range of differential diagnoses while reviewing the symptom list early on in the patient visit. It provides the health-care provider with clues that point to whether the patient has a high probability of having Lyme disease, a possible case of Lyme disease, or is unlikely to have Lyme disease. It also reassures the patient that the provider will pay close attention to all of their complaints.

All of the points on the list in Section 1 are symptoms that can be seen with Lyme disease. They are not specific to Lyme disease in and of themselves, and can be found in many other illnesses. However, the gestalt that can be perceived by looking at all of the symptoms simultaneously helps the clinician reach a probability as to whether the patient may suffer from Lyme disease and associated tick-borne disorders. At the same time this list can also be used to identify simultaneous overlapping disease states, so that the true source of the patient's suffering is discovered. These multifactorial causes of illness are often at the heart of most chronic disease states, and this led me to create the MSIDS model. It can be immensely helpful in ruling out other disease processes on the MSIDS map while looking for specific symptom complexes that are frequently seen in Lyme disease (such as symptoms coming and going with good and bad days, migratory joint and muscle pain, neuralgia that comes and goes and migrates, headaches, and sleep disorders, with associated cognitive deficits).

Sections 2 and 3 of the questionnaire represent those signs and symptom complexes most associated with Lyme and MSIDS, which I have compiled after examining hundreds of our patients' charts over the last decade. Section 4 is based on two of the four questions in the Healthy Days Core Module used by the CDC to track population trends nationally and identify health-care disparities, and it helps us identify the frequency of physical and mental health problems in the preceding month.

Talk to your doctor about the results of this questionnaire. Depending on your score, you may want to follow up with blood tests for Lyme disease IFA (immunofluorescent assay), ELISA (enzyme-linked immunosorbent assay, and a Western blot, through a reliable laboratory), with confirmatory evidence of other tick-borne diseases as well. Do not just rely on the CDC criteria of using an ELISA in a two-tiered testing protocol, as this is not sensitive enough to confirm the diagnosis. You can use this questionnaire as the starting point of the decision-making detective work that will lead you to the proper diagnosis. Remember, Lyme disease is a clinical diagnosis, and blood tests only help to confirm your clinical suspicion.

Answer the following questions as honestly as possible. Think about how you have been feeling over the previous month and how often you have been bothered by any of the following problems. Score the occurrence of each symptom on the following scale: none, mild, moderate, severe.

SECTION 1: SYMPTOM FREQUENCY SCORE
0 None   **1** Mild   **2** Moderate   **3** Severe
1. Unexplained fevers, sweats, chills, or flushing
2. Unexplained weight change; loss or gain
3. Fatigue, tiredness
4. Unexplained hair loss
5. Swollen glands
6. Sore throat
7. Testicular or pelvic pain
8. Unexplained menstrual irregularity
9. Unexplained breast milk production; breast pain

10. Irritable bladder or bladder dysfunction
11. Sexual dysfunction or loss of libido
12. Upset stomach
13. Change in bowel function (constipation or diarrhea)
14. Chest pain or rib soreness
15. Shortness of breath or cough
16. Heart palpitations, pulse skips, heart block
17. History of a heart murmur or valve prolapse
18. Joint pain or swelling
19. Stiffness of the neck or back
20. Muscle pain or cramps
21. Twitching of the face or other muscles
22. Headaches
23. Neck cracks or neck stiffness
24. Tingling, numbness, burning, or stabbing sensations
25. Facial paralysis (Bell's palsy)
26. Eyes/vision: double, blurry
27. Ears/hearing: buzzing, ringing, ear pain
28. Increased motion sickness, vertigo
29. Light-headedness, poor balance, difficulty walking
30. Tremors
31. Confusion, difficulty thinking
32. Difficulty with concentration or reading
33. Forgetfulness, poor short-term memory
34. Disorientation: getting lost; going to wrong places
35. Difficulty with speech or writing
36. Mood swings, irritability, depression
37. Disturbed sleep: too much, too little, early awakening
38. Exaggerated symptoms or worse hangover from alcohol

Add up your totals from each of the four columns. This is your first score.

Score: _____

SECTION 2: MOST COMMON LYME SYMPTOMS SCORE

If you rated a 3 for each of the following in section 1, give yourself 5 additional points:

- Fatigue
- Forgetfulness, poor short-term memory

- Joint pain or swelling
- Tingling, numbness, burning, or stabbing sensations
- Disturbed sleep: too much, too little, early awakening

Score: _____

SECTION 3: LYME INCIDENCE SCORE

Now please circle the points for each of the following statements you can agree with:

1. You have had a tick bite with no rash or flulike symptoms. *3 points*
2. You have had a tick bite, an erythema migrans, or an undefined rash, followed by flulike symptoms. *5 points*
3. You live in what is considered a Lyme-endemic area. *2 points*
4. You have a family member who has been diagnosed with Lyme and/or other tick-borne infections. *1 point*
5. You experience migratory muscle pain. *4 points*
6. You experience migratory joint pain. *4 points*
7. You experience tingling/burning/numbness that migrates and/or comes and goes. *4 points*
8. You have received a prior diagnosis of chronic fatigue syndrome or fibromyalgia. *3 points*
9. You have received a prior diagnosis of a specific autoimmune disorder (lupus, MS, or rheumatoid arthritis), or of a nonspecific autoimmune disorder. *3 points*
10. You have had a positive Lyme test (IFA, ELISA, Western blot, PCR, and/or borrelia culture). *5 points*

Score: _____

SECTION 4: OVERALL HEALTH SCORE

1. Thinking about your overall physical health, for how many of the past thirty days was your physical health not good?_____days

Award yourself the following points based on the total number of days:

0–5 days=1 point

6–12 days=2 points

13–20 days=3 points

21–30 days=4 points

2. Thinking about your overall mental health, for how many days during the past thirty days was your mental health not good?_____ days

Award yourself the following points based on the total number of days:

0–5 days = 1 point

6–12 days = 2 points

13–20 days = 3 points

21–30 days = 4 points

Score: _____

SCORING:

Record your total scores for each section below and add them together to achieve your final score:

Section 1 Total: _____

Section 2 total: _____

Section 3 total: _____

Section 4 total: _____

Final Score: _____

If you scored 46 or more, you have a high probability of a tick-borne disorder and should see a health-care provider for further evaluation.

If you scored between 21 and 45, you possibly have a tick-borne disorder and should see a health-care provider for further evaluation.

If you scored under 21, you are not likely to have a tick-borne disorder.

Interpreting the Results

We see a high frequency of Section 1 symptoms in our patients, including fatigue, joint and muscle pain that often migrates, sleep disorders, as well as memory and concentration problems, and a high frequency of Section 3 symptoms, especially neuropathic pain that comes and goes and migrates (tingling, numbness, burning, etc.). These form a cluster of presenting symptoms that are characteristic of those with a high probability of having Lyme-MSIDS.

In one recent study conducted in our office of 100 consecutive patients, we found that more than 25 percent reported that the following symptoms were present most or all of the time in the month preceding their office visit. Many of these patients reported that these symptoms affected their quality of life: 71 percent reported that their physical health was not good and 47 percent reported that their mental health was not good on at least fifteen days in the previous month. The most common symptoms related to Lyme and MSIDS are:

- Fatigue, tiredness
- Headaches
- Stiffness of the neck or back
- Joint pain or swelling
- Tingling, numbness, and/or burning of the extremities
- Confusion, difficulty thinking
- Difficulty with concentration or reading
- Forgetfulness, poor short-term memory
- Disturbed sleep: too much, too little, early awakening
- Difficulty with speech or writing

I believe it is prudent that patients with these presenting symptoms be tested for tick-borne disorders. The list of most common symptoms we found in our one hundred patients also corresponds to the symptom cluster identified in Nancy Shadick's work on Lyme disease, which was published in the medical literature years ago. She examined 186 patients, each with a history of Lyme disease, and used Centers for Disease Control and Prevention (CDC) case status and 167 controls (no history of Lyme disease) in a population-based, retrospective cohort design. We have therefore identified a symptom complex that health-care providers can refer to when patients come to their offices, and if that symptom cluster is positive, they can be tested and considered for a diagnosis of Lyme disease. Using the questionnaire in that manner will help to identify chronically ill patients with undiagnosed tick-borne diseases, improving the diagnosis and treatment of these patients.

A Sample Consultation Using the Horowitz Lyme–MSIDS Questionnaire

The following is a typical initial consultation in my office. Mrs. Q is a fifty-nine-year-old white female who has suffered for the last eighteen years with a multitude of symptoms. She has been to over twenty physicians looking for answers, including visiting prestigious medical centers in the Midwest and Northeast. She has received numerous diagnoses, including chronic fatigue syndrome, fibromyalgia, and depression, labels that attempt to explain her complaints of being chronically tired, multiple musculoskeletal aches and pains, inability to get a full night's sleep, and feeling depressed over her poor, seemingly intractable state of health. She has brought medical records from the last ten years, all neatly bound in a large ring binder.

As I look through her records I note that she has had the standard battery of tests most board-certified internists and specialists would order. All of her test results are negative except for a low-level autoimmune marker (Anti-Nuclear Antibody 1:80 speckled), which is positive but not high enough to give her the diagnosis of a nonspecific autoimmune disorder. She clearly is tired of being told that it is all in her head. She looks at me with a faint smile of hope.

"Why are you here Mrs. Q? Did someone refer you to me?"

"Many friends of mine have come to you and told me that they got help."

"You know that I pay people to say that. Are you sure that these people like you and are really your friends?"

She smirks. I see that my bad medical humor is having its therapeutic effect.

"Actually, it was my specialist at the Mayo Clinic who suggested I see you. He had nothing left to offer me and thought that I might have ongoing Lyme disease."

"Well Mrs. Q, let's go over the questionnaire that you filled out in the waiting room. Let's see if we can determine your probability of having Lyme disease from a clinical standpoint."

The first thing that I notice is that she has circled almost every symptom on the list. The only one not circled is "testicular pain." I turn to Mrs. Q.

"I noticed that you have every symptom on the list except testicular pain."

"That's right Dr. H. That symptom I reserve for my husband when he doesn't give me what I want."

Uh, oh, I think, she dishes it back. I feel my legs come together ever so slightly.

"Okay, let's start at the top of the list. Fevers, day sweats, night sweats, and chills. Which of these do you have, and for how long?"

"I have had day sweats and night sweats for the last eighteen years."

"Is it primarily day sweats or night sweats?"

"Night sweats. They can be drenching."

"Did you have an early menopause? Your answer implies that the sweats started when you were forty-one years old."

"No, Dr. Horowitz. My periods had become irregular in my midforties, but all my hormonal studies were normal with my OB/GYN. She couldn't figure out why I had them. When I went through menopause at age fifty, I had hot flashes, but these feel different."

"Any travel to foreign countries? Any possibility you may have been exposed to malaria?"

"No."

"Has there been any chronic coughing, shortness of breath, or blood in the phlegm?"

"Well, I would occasionally have a cough and feel like I couldn't get enough air, but I went to see the pulmonary doctor, and he said the chest X-ray was normal and my pulmonary function tests were normal. He suspected allergies with a postnasal drip were the culprit."

"What about chills?"

"I do get chills on and off, where I feel very cold."

"And do the symptoms come and go?"

"They do, Dr. H. In fact, I just had some drenching sweats a few nights ago."

I sit up in my chair as I pose the million-dollar question. "Has anyone ever tested you for *Babesia*? It is a malaria-like organism that causes these same symptoms."

"No, Dr. Horowitz, I don't believe they have."

Actually, I see while reviewing her records that there was one physician who ordered a *Babesia* titer from one of the local laboratories, and it was negative. "Any swollen lymph nodes or weight loss?"

"I wish, Dr. H. I've gained thirty pounds over the last eight years and can't get it off. I do occasionally have a sore throat and swollen glands, but the ENT doctor told me I probably am picking up frequent viral infections."

OK, so let's stop here. How often do patients get sore throats and swollen glands one time per month for several years? She had drenching night sweats for the past eighteen years on and off, and nine years before menopause set in. There are no clinical signs of tuberculosis or lymphoma, and the chest X-rays have been negative. There's been no foreign travel, although that doesn't necessarily rule out a diagnosis of malaria. The hormonal studies ruled out hyperthyroidism, and there were no significant clinical signs of anxiety and panic attacks. I begin to think her diagnosis may include *Babesia*. Also, what is the likelihood of getting cyclical sore throats and swollen glands almost every month for the past several years? You don't usually see that with mononucleosis/Epstein-Barr Virus (EBV) or other viral infections, but Lyme disease with co-infections (*Babesia/Bartonella*) certainly can present in a cyclical manner, when symptoms come and go. In fact, it is a hallmark of Lyme-MSIDS that symptoms come and go in this fashion.

The next symptom she had circled was fatigue.

"Mrs. Q, how bad is your fatigue? Is it mild, moderate, or severe? Does it come and go? Are there good days and bad days? Do you notice if there are certain times of the day when it gets better or worse? Does food affect it at all?"

"Well, Dr. H, I have noticed that it does tend to come and go with good and bad days. In fact, some days are so bad that I can barely get out of bed, while other days I can make it out to shop."

"Okay, so the fatigue varies between moderate and severe?"

"Yes."

"And it is affected by food? Can you tell me if it is better or worse at any particular time of the day?"

"Well, I have noticed that it is especially bad at around three o'clock in the afternoon, when I feel like I could take a nap."

"Do you ever have a snack to see if it gets better?"

"Of course. I'm a nosher; I love to snack. Maybe sometimes it seems to help."

There are at least a hundred reasons why patients present with fatigue; the list is quite extensive: low blood pressure/autonomic nervous system dysfunction; sleep deprivation; reactive hypoglycemia; adrenal fatigue with abnormally low cortisol levels; or other hormonal problems, such as low thyroid hormone, low growth hormone, or low sex hormones. The list also includes: viral; parasitic; yeast; and bacterial infections, including Lyme disease and co-infections; mitochondrial dysfunction; detoxification problems, with chemical sensitivity, autoimmune issues, with elevated cytokine levels; gastrointestinal issues, including food allergies; inflammatory bowel disorders and hepatitis; functional medicine abnormalities; cardiac issues, including congestive heart failure and cardiomyopathy; and depression. The problem is that all of these etiologies also can be associated with Lyme-MSIDS and are some of the reasons that these patients continue with chronic, persistent symptomatology despite having an antibiotic treatment history. As you'll learn in the next chapter, these are some of the sixteen nails in the foot of the Lyme patient that must be removed before they can say that they no longer have pain in their foot.

Are there any clues in Mrs. Q's history to imply Lyme disease? Yes, certainly. Her fatigue comes and goes in a cyclical fashion, which is the hallmark of Lyme disease. She is also overweight and probably has metabolic syndrome, like at least half of Americans over sixty (and one third of the total population). Reviewing her laboratory results from her binder, I see an elevated triglyceride level and low HDL in a woman with central obesity and an elevated blood pressure. Her insulin resistance, with abnormally high levels of insulin, might be contributing to reactive hypoglycemia, since her fatigue is exacerbated in the midafternoon. So Lyme disease and reactive hypoglycemia are certainly some of the possible candidates we could consider so far. *Babesia* is not far behind and could be responsible for her intermittent drenching night sweats with the associated cough, shortness of breath, and air hunger that are classic symptoms seen in babesiosis.

The next symptom she circled is, loss of libido. Although Mrs. Q was fifty-nine years old and postmenopausal, I still needed to ask when it began, since 99.9 percent of all Lyme disease patients who come to my office have lost their sex drive. Even twenty-year-old men come to my office complaining of low libido, and often they have testosterone levels in the 200 to 300 range (a normal testosterone level for a twenty-year-old man is at least 700 to 800, i.e., two to three times higher).

"When did you lose your sex drive, Mrs. Q?"

"Well, Dr. H. I can't remember the last time I had sex. Of course, my memory has gotten worse over the last few years, but I'm pretty sure it's been at least in the last fifteen years."

"Does your husband still have an interest?"

"Oh, he would if I let him, but let's just say that my days of being fruitful and multiplying are done."

"Okay, you already told me about the symptoms of sore throat and swollen glands coming and going. What about the chest pain and shortness of breath that are circled on the questionnaire? Did you ever have it evaluated?"

"Oh sure, Dr. H. I've seen two cardiologists over the last eighteen years. They ran echocardiograms, EKGs, stress tests, and Holter monitors but couldn't find anything. They told me it probably was due to reflux and esophageal spasm, since the gastroenterologist found a hiatal hernia on my endoscopy."

"Does it hurt when you press on the chest wall? Does that reproduce the pain?"

I press on her sternum and both sides of her ribs laterally to see if I can elicit a response.

"It does sometimes, just not all the time," she says.

Lyme disease frequently causes costochondritis, which is inflammation in the chest wall, ribs, and intercostal muscles. Many Lyme patients complain of chest pain, shortness of breath, and palpitations and have negative cardiac workups, except for the occasional twenty-four-hour Holter monitor that shows frequent PVCs (premature ventricular contractions, or extra heartbeats). Rarely do we see first- and second-degree heart blocks, and in the last twenty-six years I've seen a patient with a third-degree heart block perhaps only three times. Fortunately, antibiotics cured the problem without the need for a permanent pacemaker.

Doctors are taught that 90 percent of all diagnoses come from listening to the patient and taking a detailed history. Internists are trained to ask patients to describe each symptom in detail. For example, with a report of pain, we ask: "Is it dull, sharp, pressure-like, or burning?" "Does it radiate anywhere, and does anything make it better or worse?" Since Mrs. Q is presenting with metabolic syndrome, she would have a higher than normal cardiovascular risk for a stroke or heart attack.

"Have you ever had a cardiac catheterization?"

"No, Dr. H."

"How about any noninvasive tests of the coronary arteries, such as a rapid CT angiogram of the heart, or CTA?"

"No, I've never had those tests."

OK, so we will store away in the memory banks consideration of a CT angiogram of the heart with a coronary calcium score at some point in the future, although she has no chest pain on exertion, and the chest pain does not radiate up into her neck or down her arms. However, her elevated cardiovascular risks bother me. Certainly, two negative cardiac evaluations make costochondritis and GERD with esophageal spasm the most likely candidates, and Lyme disease frequently causes chest pain with costochondritis, with associated palpitations and shortness of breath (which is often made worse with *Babesia*). The notes in her binder show that reactive airways disease was already ruled out by a pulmonologist who had seen her for her shortness of breath, so asthma was not high on the differential list. She had not had provoked pulmonary function testing with a methylcholine challenge, and GERD can be responsible for asthma symptoms.

"OK, how about the joint aches and muscle pains that you circled on the list. Tell me about them, Mrs. Q."

"Well, Dr. H, I hurt all over. Every joint and muscle in my body hurts."

"Do the joints ever get red and swollen or hot?"

"No, but my neck cracks a lot, and I do have a lot of neck pain and stiffness in my neck and upper back."

"Does anything make it better or worse?"

"Well, I pop a few Tylenol or Advil from time to time and that seems to help."

"Have you seen any doctors regarding these symptoms?"

"I've seen two rheumatologists and an orthopedic doctor. They took X-rays and told me for my age I had some normal osteoarthritis, but they couldn't find any other reason for the pain."

Cracking in the neck is one of those unusual symptoms that most Lyme disease patients complain of. Many doctors and integrated health practitioners, such as chiropractors, would be able to pick up on the possible diagnosis of Lyme disease simply by asking about stiffness, cracking in the neck, and migratory muscle and joint pain in their patients who also have multiple systemic symptoms. When a patient has seen several rheumatologists, I know that he or she has already been ruled out for the most common causes of arthritis, such as osteoarthritis, and has been checked for autoimmune diseases, such as lupus and rheumatoid arthritis. This is usually accomplished by taking X-rays of the affected joints and analyzing blood for an ANA and rheumatoid factor (RF). Unfortunately, Lyme disease can cause false positive ANAs and rheumatoid factors due to a patient's overstimulated immune system. This can lead to a mistaken diagnosis of lupus or rheumatoid arthritis. This is why drawing a CCP (cyclic citrullinated peptide) is so important. It is a specific marker for rheumatoid arthritis and will help determine whether the patient has true rheumatoid arthritis or not. Patients with a positive ANA or RF often are prescribed immunosuppressive drugs, such as steroids or immunomodulatory drugs, like Enbrel or Arava. These treatments can have dire consequences for the Lyme disease patient who is co-infected, since they are already immune-suppressed, and steroids can cause their underlying infections and subsequent manifestations to get much worse. These patients also usually have been checked for elevated levels of creatine phosphokinase (CPK) to rule out a myositis (inflammation and breakdown of the muscles), high uric acid levels, to rule out gout, and often they have had inflammatory markers drawn, to evaluate the amount of inflammation in their body. This is usually accomplished using the erythrocyte sedimentation rate (ESR) and C reactive protein (CRP), while checking their human leukocyte antigen status (HLA) to determine the likelihood that they have an associated autoimmune disease. On a physical examination, the rheumatologist will typically check the range of motion of the joints and press on specific areas of the body to check for areas of tenderness.

"Does it hurt when I press over these particular areas at the back of your head, neck, shoulders, spine, hips, and knees?"

All the classic fibromyalgia trigger points are tender; that is how she got the diagnosis of fibromyalgia.

"By the way, Mrs. Q, I have one important question: Does the muscle pain and joint pain migrate? Does it move around the body, so that one day it hurts in one place and two days later it hurts somewhere else? Does it tend to keep moving around, with occasional sharp, shooting pains that also come and go?"

"Yes, Dr. H. That is exactly what happens. The pain travels all over my body without rhyme or reason. They told me that I must be crazy, because of the way I keep reporting these symptoms to them."

OK, stop here! How many diseases actually cause migratory muscle and joint pain? Although it might be found in the medical literature that gonorrhea or *Mycoplasma* can cause it, there is generally only one disease that has this as one of its hallmark clinical symptoms. Yes, you guessed it. It is Lyme disease.

"Mrs. Q, did you ever notice: When you got sick with an upper respiratory infection, sore throat, or a sinus infection, and the doctor put you on antibiotics, did it make your pain better or worse?"

"It could be better or worse. Dr. H, you must be a psychic. How did you know?"

This is an easy magic trick that anyone can learn. Patients with Lyme-MSIDS often have been put on tetracyclines, quinolones, penicillins, or cephalosporin antibiotics for a variety of non-Lyme-related infections, and the patients often notice a decrease in their overall pain. Or, when they are taking these medicines for other infections, they may notice a worsening of their pain, which is caused by the release of inflammatory molecules killing off *Borrelia*, which is called a Jarisch-Herxheimer reaction.

"I also noticed that, on the questionnaire, you circled that you are having tingling, numbness, and burning sensations. Let me guess. Does that migrate around your body also, and tend to come and go?"

"That is absolutely right, Dr. Horowitz. Is that common in Lyme disease?"

"Well, Mrs. Q, one of the hallmarks of Lyme disease is migratory joint and muscle pain and neuralgia with a tingling, numbness, and/or burning that tends to come and go that we call 'migratory paresthesias.' Did they do an EMG (electromyogram, a nerve conduction test) or nerve biopsy to rule out neuropathy or diseases like carpal tunnel syndrome?"

"Yes, they did. They performed an EMG."

"Did they find anything?"

"No, they told me that it was all normal."

I notice, however, that they did not do a biopsy of the nerves to rule out a small fiber neuropathy, which is not uncommon in persistent Lyme disease.

The majority of Lyme patients I see in my practice have peripheral neuropathy. It presents as burning sensations in different parts of the body, or tingling and numbness that often comes and goes. Patients usually describe this in the upper and lower extremities, and often on their face and scalp. Many patients have gone to the emergency room for a CAT scan of the head or an MRI of the brain to rule out a transient ischemic attack (TIA) or stroke/cerebrovascular accident (CVA), since they had numbness, which was new or increased, in one part of their body.

The doctors would rule out a TIA or stroke and send them home without a diagnosis, often telling them to follow up with their primary care physician and a neurologist. Since Lyme disease can present with symptoms primarily affecting only one side of the body, it has even stymied a few neurologists along the way. They perform an ultrasound or magnetic resonance angiography (MRA) of the carotid arteries, looking for plaque that could have caused a TIA or a stroke, and come up empty-handed. They will occasionally find some unidentified bright objects (UBOs) on an MRI of the brain, but these are nonspecific and can be seen in a variety of conditions, including Lyme disease. If there are a significant amount of white spots on an MRI, the diagnosis of multiple sclerosis will usually be entertained.

"Did the neurologist ever tell you that he suspected MS?"

"Yes, he did. He said that there weren't enough white spots on the MRI, however, to make the diagnosis."

I ask her to bend her head forward and try to touch her chin to her chest. "Do you notice any increase in numbness of the extremities?"

"No, I don't feel any different."

I asked her to do this maneuver because people with MS often experience a tingling or electrical sensation in their extremities and down their spine when they touch their chin to their chest, which is known as a Lhermitte's sign.

Of course, Lyme can mimic MS. Any patient who is diagnosed with multiple sclerosis needs to rule out Lyme disease, co-infections such as chlamydia pneumonia and *Mycoplasma*, and heavy metals as possible causes for their illness. The problem is that patients with an MS presentation often try to rule out Lyme disease using an insensitive ELISA test or a Western blot conducted by local laboratories that often will not pick up Lyme disease.

"I also noticed that you circled headaches on the questionnaire. How bad are they? On a scale of zero to ten, zero being no pain and ten being the worst pain that you can imagine, how would you describe the headache?"

"It usually is a four or five on scale of one to ten, but occasionally, Dr. H, I can get to an eight or nine, when I get nauseous, vomit, and have light sensitivity."

These are classic symptoms of a migraine.

"Did the doctors ever diagnose you with migraines? Did your mother have migraines? Migraines can often be familial in nature."

"Yes, I was told that I suffer from migraines, and do have a family history. I take Imitrex from time to time, when the headaches are bad, and occasionally I also need to take a Fioricet."

Certain migraines, such as basilar ones, can increase the risk of a stroke, and she already had multiple cardiovascular risk factors. We would need to address this carefully in the future.

"Were they generally worse around your periods?"

"Oh, definitely, Dr. H. They tried me on all types of medications to try and stop them—beta-blockers, calcium channel blockers, Topamax, Depakote, Elavil—but I couldn't tolerate some of the side effects of the medications, so I didn't stay on them."

"What about the other low-level headaches that you frequently complain of. Do you ever notice that, if you don't eat, that you get a headache?"

"Yes, as a matter of fact, that does happen."

This strengthens the probable diagnosis of reactive hypoglycemia, or blood sugar swings, as one cause for her headaches. Midday fatigue accompanied by headaches, either from eating too many carbohydrates at lunch or not eating for long periods of time, are common symptoms of hypoglycemia. This is also seen in patients with metabolic syndrome and insulin resistance, which Mrs. Q complained of earlier. Another cause of hypoglycemia with associated fatigue is low adrenal function, which is commonly seen in Lyme disease and many other chronic illnesses, so that also would need to be considered in the differential diagnosis. Finally, headaches can have other causative factors, including sleep deprivation and food allergies, as well as Lyme and multiple co-infections. It is important to identify all the factors causing each symptom if the patient is to attain their greatest sense of well-being.

"I also noticed, Mrs. Q, that you circled light-headedness and vertigo on your symptom list. How often does this happen? Do you notice any light-headedness when you change positions, such as going from sitting to standing?"

As I ask this question I fit her with a blood pressure monitor. Mrs. Q's baseline blood pressure in the exam room was $^{90}/_{60}$, which is on the low side of normal.

"Yes, I usually get light-headed standing up, and then it seems to come and go for no reason."

"Have you ever seen a doctor to get it evaluated?"

"Oh sure. The neurologist sent me to an ear, nose, and throat doctor when he couldn't find the cause. They did some tests in which they squirted water in my ears and watched my eyes move, and then they moved my head into different positions, and made me stand up and close my eyes. They told me that all the tests were negative."

OK, so they tested her inner ear and cerebellum to rule out common causes for her dizziness, and all the tests were negative. No one, however, had ever conducted a tilt-table test.

"Did they ever turn you upside down in the hospital and follow your blood pressure?"

"No, Doc. It's probably the only test they didn't do."

I have Mrs. Q stand up from her chair in the examining room. The cuff showed that her blood pressure dropped to the low eighties over fifties, with an increase in her pulse rate, which means her heart rate went up in an effort to bring up the blood pressure. She probably had Lyme disease with associated autonomic nervous system dysfunction. I slowly turn to her and say:

"You probably have POTS syndrome."

She smiles. She looks at me straight in the eyes and says:

"I never did that stuff in college, Doc."

"No, no Mrs. Q. POTS (Postural orthostatic tachycardia syndrome) is a form of autonomic nervous system dysfunction. It means that you are chronically running a low blood pressure, and that is why you get dizzy when you stand up. It may be responsible in part for some of your fatigue, dizziness, and concentration problems. Did any of the other doctors ever try you on a drug like Florinef or ProAmatine, which can raise your blood pressure?"

"No, Dr. H. Those don't sound familiar."

"Moving on down the list, I noticed that you also circled light sensitivity and sound sensitivity. Do you have it all the time, occasionally, or are you getting it just when you get your migraines?"

"No, Dr. Horowitz. I have it most of the time. I have to wear sunglasses outside, and I really have a difficult time being around loud noises. That's why I tell my husband all the time to shut up. You know he's deaf as a doorknob and likes to keep the volume on the TV up, or is yelling when I can hear him perfectly."

Mrs. Q's husband was sitting in the exam room the entire time during our interview. He rolled his eyes.

"OK, and what about the symptoms of memory and concentration problems that you circled on the questionnaire? How long have you complained of this? Is it mild, moderate, or severe? Does it come and go? Are you taking any medications for it?"

"Well, Dr. Horowitz, they ran all the tests and just told me it was normal aging. It wasn't bad enough to be called Alzheimer's, but my doctor did suggest some drugs that might make it better."

No doubt those medications would've been an Aricept-Namenda combo, or something similar. In reviewing the records I noticed that they tested for B_{12} and folic acid with the routine bloods, but I did not see a methylmalonic acid (MMA) level, which is a marker for possible B_{12} deficiency. We see a small number of patients who have elevated MMA levels, and their memories improve with B_{12} supplementation. I also noticed that Mrs. Q's B_{12} level was 340. This was not below the critical level of 200, which would imply pernicious anemia, but it was still low. In fact, it was low enough that the laboratory had printed on the report that neuropsychiatric abnormalities can be seen in 5 percent to 10 percent of the population with B_{12} levels between 200 and 400. Her value at 340, therefore, put her in range for possible B_{12} deficiency.

"Have you ever taken vitamin B_{12}?"

"No. I was told my levels were normal."

OK, I make a mental note. We will be running other tests for vitamin B_{12} deficiencies and methylation defects (enzymatic reactions, where a methyl group is added to a protein, DNA, or heavy metal to modify its structure and function), specifically the MMA and methylenetetrahydrofolate reductase (MTHFR) tests, and for homocysteine levels. I would also consider a trial of methyl B_{12} shots, as they can be very helpful in a subset of Lyme disease patients, whether their B_{12} levels are abnormally low or not. This is probably due to a block in their methylation and detoxification pathways, and the extra methyl groups help them to more effectively detoxify certain chemicals and heavy metals from their bodies.

In reviewing her laboratory results from her big ring binder, I also see that her thyroid function tests, to evaluate her fatigue and memory loss, were incomplete. She was missing the tests for T3, free T3, and reverse T3. All of these tests are important markers of proper thyroid function. OK, I make a mental note to expand out the thyroid testing with the upcoming blood tests I will order. Many Lyme disease patients don't have adequate levels of active thyroid hormones and may have elevated levels of reverse T3. This can contribute to their ongoing fatigue and memory loss.

Unfortunately, the established range for low normal thyroid functions were established in healthy populations, not in a population of individuals with chronic illnesses, such as tick-borne infections. These patients also often have elevated cortisol levels due to the stress of their illness. Cortisol is a hormone that is normally produced in higher amounts by the adrenal gland during periods of stress. Elevated levels of cortisol can interfere with thyroid hormone levels and cause a sick "euthyroid" syndrome. This is a syndrome seen in patients whose thyroid does not appear to be dysfunctional, who are severely ill or malnourished, and have very low T3 and T4 levels, possibly contributing to their fatigue. Also, some of these patients have associated pituitary dysfunction, or even pituitary failure. The pituitary gland is located in the brain, and it is the master regulator of the hormones of the body. It produces hormones like thyroid stimulating hormone (TSH), which travels through the blood and goes to the thyroid, stimulating the production of thyroid hormones. If Lyme disease has affected the pituitary gland, it may not make TSH properly, lowering thyroid production. In that circumstance, a physician cannot rely on the TSH level, a test result that we learn in medical school is one of the most reliable markers for thyroid function.

"Tell me about your sleep Mrs. Q. I noticed that you circled on the questionnaire that you suffer from insomnia. Is it a problem falling asleep, frequent awakening, or both? Do you snore or have restless legs that don't allow you to sleep? Do you have to go to the toilet in the middle of the night? Do you take any medication for sleep?"

"Well, Dr. H, I have problems falling asleep, and I do frequently wake up. I went for a sleep study at the hospital a few years ago, and they told me that I only have mild sleep apnea. They said it wasn't severe enough to cause me to have this level of insomnia. They told me to take some

Ambien for sleep, but the effect doesn't seem to last. I've tried several other sleeping pills, and none of them seem to work."

"Have you ever tried Benadryl, or any herbal remedies? Some patients find that melatonin, valerian root, and green tea extracts like L-theanine will sometimes help."

"No, no one ever suggested those to me."

"How many hours do you actually sleep per night?"

"Oh, I maybe get four to five hours, tops."

Now with "normal" aging, sleep patterns do change. Lyme disease, however, can cause a severe, resistant sleep disorder in at least 80 percent to 90 percent of the patients who I see, and that includes young patients in their twenties. Without a good night's sleep it is almost impossible to reverse some of the resistant symptoms in these patients. This is because sleep deprivation leads to the production of cell-signaling molecules called cytokines, some of which are inflammatory, such as interleukin-6 (IL-6), which contribute to the symptoms of fatigue, joint and muscle pain, and memory/concentration problems in these patients. It is, therefore, essential to get to the underlying source of the patient's problem and not to just give a medication for the symptom. Patients should be evaluated for the most common causes of insomnia, such as sleep apnea, hormonal issues, restless leg syndrome, medication side effects, bladder problems, and psychiatric issues, such as depression and anxiety. MSIDS and Lyme disease can cause insomnia, but there are often overlapping factors that must be ruled out to significantly improve the quality of the patient's sleep.

"Finally Mrs. Q, I see that you circled on the questionnaire that your symptoms are worse after drinking alcohol."

"Yes, Dr. H. I never really drank a lot, but if I have a glass of red wine, I definitely feel worse."

It is very common that patients with Lyme disease report intolerance to alcohol. Red wine can exacerbate headaches as a migraine trigger, and some patients are sensitive to the sulfites in it. Beer and wine can also trigger hypoglycemic events in susceptible individuals (I always wondered why everyone in medical school could drink several Belgian beers and my head was on the table after the first one! Then I found out I had hypoglycemia).

After reviewing all of Mrs. Q's symptoms by using the questionnaire, my clinical impression was the following: There was a very strong likelihood that she suffered from Lyme disease, babesiosis, POTS with autonomic nervous system dysfunction, reactive hypoglycemia, with metabolic syndrome, and possible adrenal dysfunction, a Lyme-induced costochondritis and fibromyalgia, and a possible B_{12} deficiency. That was simply determined from taking the time to take a detailed history, reviewing the medical records and laboratory results that she had brought with her, and formulating differential diagnoses to explain her symptoms.

We can accumulate a tremendous amount of information by taking a careful history, meticulously evaluating all prior medical records and testing, and using the questionnaire. This questionnaire is an essential tool for guiding the provider in evaluating chronically ill patients and formulating differential diagnoses that were not considered in any past medical workups. Mrs. Q had seen approximately twenty physicians over the previous eighteen years who were unable to help her. Knowing that, I already knew that I needed to consider diseases and conditions that might have been missed or overlooked by my colleagues. These include: Lyme disease; babesiosis and co-infections; heavy metal burden; mitochondrial dysfunction; functional medicine abnormalities in the biochemistry of the body; certain vitamin and mineral deficiencies; environmental illness, with chemical sensitivity and associated detoxification problems; hormonal abnormalities, such as adrenal dysfunction and growth hormone deficiency; and reactive hypoglycemia, with or without Candida and food allergies.

In the following chapters we will be looking at a list of sixteen differential diagnoses that I have found to be essential in the evaluation of patients with chronic persistent illness. This list can be of immense value in understanding previously unexplained symptoms and in helping you get to the source of your illness.

Lyme disease is a complex illness. In the next chapter we'll begin to look at the first point on the sixteen-point MSIDS map as we explore the science behind Lyme disease and associated co-infections found in ticks. We will then explore treatment options that are based on the results of taking a history using the questionnaire and performing a complete physical examination. We will also learn how to order targeted laboratory testing based on the history and physical, and then how to apply the Horowitz sixteen-point differential diagnostic map to determine if there are overlapping etiologies responsible for the present illness.

This model is not just theoretical; it works in clinical practice. This model has been meticulously developed after personally seeing and treating over twelve thousand chronically ill individuals. These patients had remained ill despite the best efforts of our present-day medical system, yet when the MSIDS model was applied to them, it helped solve their medical mysteries, and they often achieved greater health than they had thought possible. The MSIDS model offers hope to those with chronic diseases who have been unable to find answers for their symptoms.

TWO

The Horowitz Sixteen-Point Differential Diagnostic Map

One of the most important axioms in medicine is: "First do no harm." The second most important axiom is: "An open mind doesn't mean that your brain will fall out." The information in this chapter may nudge some readers out of their diagnostic comfort zones. However, if you have a strong motivation to feel better, or to help sick and suffering patients, leaving your comfort zone can be rewarding.

Let's start with the basics. Naming an illness and prescribing a drug for it does not necessarily mean that you have properly understood the illness or adequately treated it. When it comes to Lyme disease in particular, and chronic illness in general, we can no longer practice medicine in that fashion. We must now accept a new truth: Most chronic illnesses are the result of complex, multifactorial processes, and therefore require dissecting each illness piece by piece into its component parts.

In the last chapter we began the process by using the Horowitz MSIDS questionnaire to identify the many different symptoms that can accompany Lyme disease. The next step to successful treatment is to divide these symptoms into component parts to discover their source. In some instances we'll find that they stem from one disease process. However, it is much more likely that, if you or your patient is suffering from a chronic disease, there may be many interconnected and overlapping illnesses responsible for the chronic symptoms.

One of the essential problems with the current medical model is that doctors are taught in medical school that there is generally only one etiology for each illness. As I mentioned earlier, this model originated from the brilliant researcher Louis Pasteur, and it has been passed down to doctors since the late 1800s without a significant paradigm shift. Because of this, many patients who have been diagnosed with Lyme disease end up traveling from doctor to doctor, specialist to specialist, receiving treatment for one of their symptoms at a time, often without positive results. Or they are forced to suffer silently with a multiplicity of seemingly unrelated symptoms because they have been told that they are suffering from other, equally "mysterious" diseases, including chronic fatigue syndrome, fibromyalgia, MS, ALS, an unexplained nonspecific autoimmune disease, or a stigmatizing psychiatric disorder.

One implication of this model is that if a doctor can't find a single answer to your host of problems, then they assert that the problem must be in your head, since the sophisticated laboratory tests and imaging studies in modern-day clinics and hospitals surely are reliable and comprehensive. Worse still is the enduring notion that psychological distress does not affect the body in real ways.

The second implication from this outdated model is financial. If we do not change the way we perceive disease, we will continue to see healthcare costs rise. A 2006 study by scientists affiliated with the U.S. Centers for Disease Control and Prevention showed that for patients who were accurately diagnosed with Lyme disease and treated early in the course of infection, the annual "burden of disease" (BOD) was less than $1,500, usually for only one year. But for patients who were not diagnosed early, and who became progressively sicker, the annual BOD was over $16,000 per year, year after year. This higher cost of unresolved Lyme disease is much more than direct medical costs. The study showed that 88 percent of the average annual cost of $16,199 for Lyme disease consisted of indirect medical costs, nonmedical costs, and productivity loss.

Instead of looking for one answer, I believe that we should be looking for many. The majority of my Lyme patients, as well as others suffering from persistent chronic illness, generally do not have one sole cause for their symptoms. They often have an overlapping set of medical problems, as in the analogy I introduced earlier: having sixteen nails in their foot.

We must proceed with a new, multifactorial approach of pulling out each nail that may be causing you or your patient pain, one by one.

My approach has identified sixteen likely categories of illnesses that can occur simultaneously with Lyme disease Lyme-MSIDS, or exacerbate the symptoms of other diseases that occur without Lyme disease (non–Lyme-MSIDS). The difficulty in establishing a diagnosis is that Lyme disease can cause symptoms that are seen with each of these sixteen separate medical conditions. Lyme disease, like its cousin syphilis, can mimic many illnesses commonly seen in a modern-day medical practice and exacerbate previously existing medical problems: For example, if you were always prone to headaches, you may begin to have migraines. The medical literature provides abundant evidence on this subject, even though it is not entirely clear why the disease manifests in different ways for each particular individual. It may be influenced by your genetic code and unique bioindividuality, as well as by the number of tick bites you received, other co-infections, your present immune status, your environmental toxin load and detoxification ability, your underlying psychological status, and the particular strain or species of *Borrelia* you were infected with. The term "species" refers to the classification of living things, including plants, animals, and bacteria, while a strain is a genetic variant or subtype of the species.

Because of all of these disparate factors, each person can present with Lyme disease in his own unique way. For example, although many of my patients were diagnosed with a primary psychiatric disorder before they first came to see me, Lyme disease has been known to cause a host of neuropsychiatric abnormalities. In fact, virtually every psychiatric diagnosis listed in the Diagnostic and Statistical Manual (DSM), the bible of mental health diagnoses, can be caused by Lyme disease and associated co-infections. Similarly, Lyme disease can mimic a whole host of neurological syndromes: It can cause neurocognitive deficits in both children and adults, and it has even been associated with Tourette's and neurological syndromes such as Alzheimer's disease. The same problem exists with chronic fatigue syndrome (CFS has also been renamed as myalgic encephalomyelitis, or ME) and fibromyalgia (FM). Lyme disease can also mimic autoimmune disorders such as rheumatoid arthritis, lupus, and multiple sclerosis. The patient's resistant symptoms are therefore possibly the result of failing to diagnose and treat the underlying infections correctly and from not having addressed enough of the abnormalities present on the MSIDS map.

I believe that the persistent symptoms of Lyme disease are more than simply one infection that will not go away. Of the twelve thousand patients seen in our medical center, almost none of them had "pure" Lyme disease, which explains the discrepancies reported in the medical literature. In fact, most Lyme disease patients have a clinically recognizable "syndrome," an association of several symptoms that are occurring together. Some typical Lyme symptoms are worsened by co-infections, as well as by the presence of multiple overlapping factors, some caused by the Lyme disease and co-infections, and some unrelated but nevertheless affecting their clinical course.

I call this condition MSIDS: multiple systemic infectious disease syndrome, and I believe that it better defines those patients for whom these treatments have not worked. MSIDS is a symptom complex of Lyme disease and multiple associated tick-borne co-infections that encompasses not only infections with *Borrelia burgdorferi*, the etiologic agent of Lyme disease, but also other bacterial infections, viral infections, parasitic infections, and fungal infections. It also includes: immune dysfunction; inflammation; environmental toxicity; allergies; nutritional and enzyme deficiencies, with functional medicine abnormalities in biochemical pathways; mitochondrial dysfunction; neuropsychological issues; autonomic nervous system dysfunction; endocrine abnormalities; sleep disorders; gastrointestinal abnormalities, with abnormal liver functions; and issues with pain, drug use, and physical deconditioning. By using this definition I can treat my patients more effectively, because these patients are unable to recover their prior state of health unless *all* of these factors are addressed, simultaneously.

This may be the reason why so many people don't improve with the standard Lyme treatments, such as one month of doxycycline or Rocephin. The design of many of the double-blind placebo-controlled studies on the best treatments for Lyme disease do not take into account these potential multifactorial causes, so giving only one or two antibiotics for a short period of time only addresses a small piece of the complex puzzle. The answers lie in a more holistic diagnostic approach.

I have developed this new definition over the past twenty-six years, and it has constantly evolved based on the feedback I received from seeing over 12,000 patients. As a medical detective, each time I found another piece of the puzzle, I added it and expanded the list of possible diagnoses, so the list has become increasingly comprehensive over time.

The MSIDS model explains in part the differences between the IDSA and ILADS approach. These are currently the two divergent standards of care for the diagnosis and treatment of Lyme disease: IDSA guidelines and ILADS guidelines. The ILADS guidelines stress the importance of a doctor's clinical judgment in making the diagnosis, because the scientific literature has found that the existing testing is unreliable. The IDSA narrowly restricts the diagnosis to include just the CDC criteria. However, many doctors in the United States do not follow IDSA guidelines. Instead, my model allows Lyme to be redefined as MSIDS: a clinical syndrome that encompasses multiple overlapping factors that keep patients chronically ill. Some doctors have adopted the model, based on my having presented the MSIDS map at scientific conferences, and have validated its utility in clinical practice.

UNDERSTANDING LABORATORY TESTING
TO DIAGNOSE LYME DISEASE

Various guidelines and case definitions are used to diagnose Lyme disease: The IDSA guidelines are based on the CDC's strict surveillance definition, which was developed for national reporting of Lyme disease and is primarily used by health departments for epidemiological purposes. The CDC surveillance case definition is narrow, meaning that only a minority of actual cases will meet its strict criteria. The definition can be satisfied in the following two ways:

A. a case with an EM rash 5 centimeters or larger
B. a case with at least one late, objective manifestation, such as meningitis (inflammation occurring in the membranes covering the brain and spinal cord), cranial neuropathy (nerve damage of the cranial nerves), brief attacks of arthritis, or AV block (an electrical conduction defect in the heart) that is laboratory confirmed

Health-care providers following the IDSA guidelines use these criteria.

According to this CDC surveillance case definition, late manifestations require laboratory confirmation. This may involve obtaining a positive culture for *Borrelia burgdorferi* from blood, skin, a joint, or cerebral spinal fluid (CSF), or by identifying antibodies to the bacterium in the cerebrospinal fluid; the most common method, however, known as the two-tier testing algorithm, uses a specific sequence of blood tests. The first is an ELISA, the second is a Western blot. These are indirect tests of infection, because instead of identifying the organism itself, they look for antibodies to *Borrelia burgdorferi* that were made by the immune system. ELISA tests measure the total amount of anti-*Borrelia burgdorferi* antibodies present, while Western blots identify individual antibodies and look for specific protein patterns that are unique to *Borrelia*. If enough of these *Borrelia* proteins are present, the test is considered to be positive. Although the surveillance case definition does firmly establish a Lyme disease diagnosis, many patients unfortunately do not meet these criteria because these tests are often inaccurate. That is why the CDC has publicly stated on their Web site: "This surveillance case definition was developed for national reporting of Lyme disease; it is not intended to be used in clinical diagnosis."

No one test or combinations of tests are perfect in establishing a laboratory diagnosis, and there are extensive scientific references in the medical literature documenting false negative blood tests. The CDC points out that there are problems with testing, and that a patient with Lyme disease may not be diagnosed using these criteria. This has been confirmed in many studies. The first was a New York State Department of Health study conducted in 1996, which was reported to the CDC. Among the 1,535 patients studied, 81 percent of non-EM cases were not confirmed with the present two-tiered testing algorithms. In other words, the presently used two-tiered testing missed 81 percent of the Lyme cases, especially when the patient did not have a bull's-eye rash.

One of the most comprehensive reviews of the standard Lyme tests comes from a 2005 study at John's Hopkins University, confirming the poor sensitivity of the ELISA. Working with early diagnosed Lyme disease patients from Pennsylvania and Maryland, the Hopkins scientists studied state-of-the-art blood and DNA tests (PCR testing) for Lyme and found serious flaws: Most tellingly, when the standard two-step method recommended by the CDC was used on patients with other laboratory evidence of Lyme disease, it was positive between 45 percent and 77 percent of the time. As for the DNA tests, the Hopkins researchers reported that these rarely pick up otherwise confirmed Lyme disease at all. In another study, published in the *Journal of Medical Microbiology* in 2005, Dr. Antonella Marangoni reported that three different commercial ELISA tests showed discrepant results. The sensitivity for the same blood tested varied between 36.8 percent and 70.5 percent. A study by Ang in 2011 confirmed that not only was the ELISA an insensitive test, but that various Western blot kits often gave discordant results on the same specimen. He concluded that the likelihood of a patient being diagnosed with Lyme disease was highly influenced by which ELISA–Western blot combination was used. This confirmed the results of a prior study done by Lori L. Bakken published in the *Journal of the Clinical Microbiology* years before. Another study, published in 2007 in the *British Medical Journal* by Ray Stricker, MD, and Lorraine Johnson, found that the overall sensitivity of the combined ELISA–Western blot was only 56 percent. These findings mirror what I have found in my own practice: Many of my patients do have Lyme disease, but testing protocols were not sensitive enough to pick it up, and those patients who fail the ELISA may never go on to be tested with a confirmatory Western blot.

Another set of guidelines, developed by ILADS, states that Lyme disease is a clinical diagnosis. Cases meeting the CDC definition qualify under the ILADS definition, as do patients who have symptoms consistent with Lyme disease and a history of potential exposure to the ticks that transmit the illness, particularly if symptoms cannot be rightfully attributed to other illnesses. Positive two-tier testing is not required, because they hold the view that the present available testing is unreliable. Patients may have some Lyme-specific bands on the Western blot (e.g., 23 kDa, 31 kDa, 34 kDa, 39 kDa, 83–93 kDa) but not have the same exact pattern required to be considered positive by the CDC—and yet have a clinical presentation and treatment response consistent with the illness when other disease processes have been ruled out. The CDC criterion also demands looking for Lyme disease without testing for multiple strains: They recommend trying to find 5 out of 10 positive bands on an

IgG Western blot, or two out of three specific bands on an IgM Western blot (23 kDa, 39 kDa, 41 kDa) to confirm the diagnosis, and only if the ELISA is positive. Yet in clinical practice, patients with persistent Lyme disease symptoms rarely meet CDC criteria. The magnitude of real Lyme patients eluding the standard tests could be vast, as suggested by screening conducted to confirm the diagnosis in a study for the National Institutes of Health (NIH). When Dr. Brian Fallon, an internationally recognized expert in the neuropsychiatric aspects of Lyme disease, screened patients known to have been exposed to Lyme in a NIH double-blind study, only approximately one out of one hundred patients actually met the CDC criteria, although they clearly had been exposed to *Borrelia*, and remained ill.

These opposing views have confused many health-care providers as to the best way to diagnose and treat Lyme disease. I have found nine basic standards that help me establish a clear diagnosis:

1. Lyme disease is a clinical diagnosis, and lab results serve to support the clinical diagnosis.

2. An EM rash is definitive evidence of Lyme disease, and does not require laboratory confirmation to make a diagnosis.

3. Patients are often seronegative (have negative blood tests) if tested too early, or if antibiotics have been used early in the course of the disease, since this may prevent antibodies from being produced.

4. The two-tiered protocol of using a Lyme ELISA followed by a Western blot will miss the majority of Lyme patients, due to the insensitivity of the tests.

5. The Western blot may provide us with more useful information, but it also has its limitations. There are multiple strains of *Borrelia* present in the United States (approximately one hundred), and there are over three hundred strains worldwide. Blood tests often do not cross react between these strains, and consequently can lead to false negative results. The utility of the Western blot is therefore based on the expertise of the laboratory performing the test, which strain(s) of *Borrelia* the patient was exposed to, and identifying the specific bands on the Western blot that reflect exposure to *Borrelia burgdorferi*.

Borrelia-specific bands reflect outer surface proteins (Osp) on the surface of the organism that are seen more often in Lyme disease than in other infections. These bands include the following five proteins, each with different molecular weights (in kDa): 23 kDa (Osp C, e.g., outer surface protein C), 31 kDa (Osp A), 34 kDa (Osp B), 39 kDa, and 83–93 kDa. If any of these bands are present on a Western blot, there is a high likelihood that the patient has been exposed to Lyme disease, especially with the right clinical symptomatology. If two or more of these specific bands are present, the likelihood increases even further. We have found that a specialty lab, such as IGeneX, has a better chance of finding more *Borrelia*-specific bands on the Western blot, because it uses different strains of *Borrelia burgdorferi* for its testing (both the B31 and 297 strains). While use of this laboratory often has been considered controversial among some IDSA physicians, many ILADS physicians find it to be a reliable resource. IGeneX has passed the strict testing guidelines of New York State and California, and is certified by the U.S. government via the Centers for Medicare & Medicaid Services (CMS). I perform a Western blot only through highly qualified laboratories, as there may be discrepancies in the testing, similar to the problems we face with the ELISA test.

6. Other tests: Polymerase chain reaction (PCR), a DNA test, is an important diagnostic tool for patients who have negative blood tests, but many require multiple samples over time, using specimens from different body compartments (such as serum, aspirated joint fluid, synovial tissue, urine, cord blood, placenta, and/or spinal fluid), and it must be performed at a reliable laboratory. The PCR has an overall sensitivity of around 30 percent on any individual specimen, with a specificity of over 99 percent (it is highly specific for the disease, with few false positive results). Recent advances in more sensitive PCR tests were reported by researchers in 2012; newer tests for the direct molecular detection and genotyping of *Borrelia* (identifying the specific species) increased the sensitivity to 62 percent in early Lyme disease. I may need to send off several sets of PCRs on blood or urine before getting back a positive result.

Since the ELISA, Western blot, and PCR tests may not always pick up evidence of an infection, other tests are occasionally used to help confirm a clinical diagnosis: the lymphocyte transformation test (LTT, *Borrelia* ELISpot) and a commercial culture of *Borrelia* (Advanced Laboratories).

The LTT was not used for years in the United States because of questions about its reliability. A newer version called the *Borrelia* ELISpot test is now being used in Europe. The *Borrelia* ELISpot test was formally evaluated in 2012, and the results were published in the journal *Clinical and Developmental Immunology*. It was found to have a very high specificity, and is currently used by European physicians to help with the diagnosis of Lyme disease. The LTT had been used years ago by American physicians, based on extensive scientific literature showing specific T-cell responses to *Borrelia*. The T cells are a type of white blood cell, some of which can retain the memory of a prior infection, reactivating and expanding their numbers when they are reintroduced to the infecting agent. Several laboratories in the United States are now starting to make the LTT available to physicians again, and it may be part of the laboratory panel used to confirm a clinical diagnosis. Further studies need to be done in the United States to confirm the sensitivity and specificity of the newer LTT tests.

Another test that became commercially available, in 2012, is the *Borrelia* culture, through Advanced Laboratories. They have been certified by various state agencies. Culture of *Borrelia* is the gold standard for testing, and is universally accepted by the IDSA, ILADS, and the CDC. The successful culture of *Borrelia* isolates in the laboratory, but using *Borrelia*-specific Barbour-Stoenner-Kelly (BSK) media, however, even from confirmed Lyme disease cases, has been a challenging task. The very slow growth of this organism in culture has complicated its cultivation. In the last two decades there have been several attempts to develop a more successful *Borrelia* culture. Unfortunately, results from those studies, from different clinical specimens (peripheral blood, cerebrospinal and joint fluids, and skin biopsies), have been very disappointing. The reported sensitivities ranged from as low as 5 percent to a maximum of 71 percent in skin samples but register only 40 percent to 44 percent with peripheral blood samples. Dr. Joseph Burrascano worked closely with Advanced Laboratories to help them mimic in vitro the conditions that exist in a living host to support growth in culture, and preliminary results are encouraging (a sensitivity of 94 percent at sixteen weeks, with a specificity of over 95 percent). The accuracy of the *Borrelia* culture was confirmed in a 2013 peer-reviewed study by Eva Sapi, PhD, but the CDC is challenging the validity of the culture test, as recently reported in the online *Jour-*

nal of Clinical Microbiology. The laboratory is working on other lines of proof, and we await more research to see how it holds up.

7. In the Northeast, 10 percent to 20 percent of the *Borrelia* presently in ticks are not *Borrelia burgdorferi*, the causative agent of Lyme disease, but are genetically related to *Borrelia miyamotoi*, the agent of relapsing fever in Japan. These organisms will not test positive by ELISA, Western blot, or PCR assays for Lyme disease. A patient with a Lyme-like illness may actually have been exposed to other strains of *Borrelia*, explaining seronegative test results for Lyme disease.

8. Other tick-borne diseases, such as *Babesia* (a malaria-like parasite) and *Bartonella* (cat scratch disease) can be transmitted with the same tick bite that transmits Lyme disease. These diseases complicate the clinical presentation, often making the symptoms of Lyme disease much worse. They are similarly difficult to diagnose reliably using standard screening procedures, e.g., *Babesia* smear (Giemsa stain) and *Bartonella* titer (immunofluorescent assay, IFA), and testing must not only include antibody titers, but may need to include PCR assays as well.

9. Any positive titer for one tick-borne disease (TBD) suggests that other TBDs may be present, since ticks are multiply co-infected. This is especially true for patients failing treatment regimens for any one specific disease process.

IDENTIFYING MULTIPLE SYSTEMIC INFECTIOUS DISEASE SYNDROME

I created the Horowitz differential diagnostic system as a road map for identifying the multiple components of MSIDS. For every patient who comes into my office, I review the potential sixteen differential diagnoses against the results of the questionnaire and patient history. By doing so I can gather the most complete assessment of my patient's current health and what needs to be done regarding testing and treatment going forward.

Most of the disease processes that I am about to discuss are not new. But when health-care providers can look at them together, the strength of using this system is that they will finally have a single tool that organizes the list of seemingly unrelated symptoms that a chronically ill patient brings to the doctor.

Although the diagnostic process began with searching for answers for Lyme disease patients, I believe the MSIDS model is applicable to all patients with chronic illness. All patients with chronic diseases may have elements of MSIDS, and all patients with a chronic illness may benefit from using the sixteen-point differential diagnostic map described below. Chronic inflammation lies at the heart of most chronic illnesses, and addressing the underlying causes of inflammation, using the MSIDS map, has the potential to decrease inflammation and improve health. The initial inflammation may have developed as a direct effect of Lyme disease and associated co-infections, or it could be a response to an overstimulated immune system, environmental toxins, food allergies, or an associated sleep disorder.

Another benefit of the MSIDS model is that even if patients are having a positive response to medications, they may have untoward long-term side effects, and there may be ways of mitigating those side effects by finding other treatable causes for their disease.

This diagnostic tool can therefore serve as a map for clinicians evaluating not just a patient with Lyme disease and co-infections but any patient with a chronic, unexplained illness. There may be disease processes that we still don't completely understand, but the patients will benefit clinically from using this model. Understanding this syndrome is the key to gaining a better understanding of chronic disease states, as we uncover hidden underlying factors driving their illness.

The MSIDS model and the laboratory testing standards described above offer an intelligent and sensible path to help diminish the cost and the burden of disease for Lyme and associated co-infections. By *not* driving Lyme patients (and their insurance companies) to search relentlessly and fruitlessly, year after year, for other diseases that might be responsible for symptoms, it provides a methodology for processing diagnosis and treatment options that can save millions of dollars annually.

MSIDS: OVERLAPPING FACTORS CONTRIBUTING TO CHRONIC ILLNESS

1. Lyme disease and co-infections
2. Immune dysfunction
3. Inflammation
4. Environmental toxins

5. Functional medicine abnormalities with nutritional deficiencies
6. Mitochondrial dysfunction
7. Endocrine abnormalities
8. Neurodegenerative disorders
9. Neuropsychiatric disorders
10. Sleep disorders
11. Autonomic nervous system dysfunction and POTS
12. Allergies
13. Gastrointestinal disorders
14. Liver dysfunction
15. Pain disorders/addiction
16. Lack of exercise/deconditioning

USING THE HOROWITZ SIXTEEN-POINT DIFFERENTIAL DIAGNOSTIC MAP

You can begin to use this system to determine if you are suffering from more than just Lyme disease. You may quickly find that you have MSIDS, and you will be able to use this tool with your doctor to begin to improve your symptoms and overall health.

The first step is to get copies of all of your medical records. This may be difficult if you have been seeing many different doctors. However, it is your right as a patient to have access to your medical information. This information is essential so your current health-care provider can review the scope of your testing and treatment and determine how best to proceed.

Once you have gathered your documentation, the next thing you want to determine is whether you have been appropriately and comprehensively tested for all of the conditions that comprise the sixteen-point differential diagnostic map. The following table can help you determine which tests to ask for, based on the results of your questionnaire.

This list includes some of the most common differential diagnoses and medical conditions responsible for the associated symptoms. It is not intended to be a comprehensive differential diagnostic list nor a comprehensive list of laboratory testing to consider for an individual patient. The laboratory testing that evaluates fatigue is part of a full initial workup for MSIDS.

Table 2.1: Symptoms and Associated Medical Conditions on the Sixteen-Point MSIDS Map

Symptoms	Possible Related Medical Conditions	Laboratory Testing to Consider
Unexplained fevers, sweats, chills, or flushing	• Lyme disease (chronic and other bacterial, viral, parasitic, and fungal infections) • Babesiosis • Malaria • Brucellosis • Hyperthyroidism • Hormonal failure (early menopause) • Tuberculosis* • Non-Hodgkin's lymphoma* • Panic disorders • Autoimmune disorders • Inflammation	• CBC with a white cell count • CMP with liver functions • Giemsa stain and malarial smears • *Babesia* IFA • *Babesia* WA-1/*duncani* titers • *Babesia* FISH • *Babesia* PCR • Thyroid function tests (TFTs) • Sex hormone levels • Chest X-ray/PPD • Antinuclear antibody (ANA) • Rheumatoid factor (RF) • Erythrocyte sedimentation rate (ESR) • C-reactive protein (CRP) • Cytokine panel
Unexplained weight change, either loss or gain	• Lyme disease • Certain co-infections (brucellosis, among others) • Hormonal disorders (thyroid, adrenal, low sex hormones) • Metabolic syndrome with increased insulin secretion • Malignancy*	• Lyme ELISA • IgM/IgG Western blot • *Brucella* antibodies/agglutination test • TFTs • Sex hormones • DHEA/cortisol • HbA1c with insulin levels • Lipid profile • Appropriate cancer screening
Fatigue, tiredness	• Lyme disease and associated co-infections • Immune dysfunction • Inflammation • Environmental toxins and mold • Functional medicine abnormalities with nutritional deficiencies • Mitochondrial dysfunction • Endocrine abnormalities • Neurodegenerative disorders	• Lyme test, including IgM/IgG Western blots (IGeneX/specialty labs preferable; evaluate for Lyme specific bands, 23 [OspC], 31 [OspA], 34 [Osp B], 39, 83–93) • *Babesia microti* IFA • *Babesia duncani*/WA1 • *Babesia* FISH • *Babesia* PCR • *Borrelia hermsii*

Symptoms	Possible Related Medical Conditions	Laboratory Testing to Consider
Fatigue, tiredness *(continued)*	• Neuropsychiatric disorders • Sleep disorders • Autonomic nervous system dysfunction and POTS • Allergies • Gastrointestinal disorders • Liver dysfunction • Pain disorders/addiction • Lack of exercise/deconditioning	• *Ehrlichia* and *Anaplasma* titers • *Bartonella* IFA, PCR +/− FISH • *Mycoplasma* (including *M. fermentans*) • Chlamydia pneumonia • RMSF, Q-fever, typhus • Tularemia • *Brucella* • Viruses (HHV6, EBV, CMV, West Nile) • CBC, CMP • ANA, RF • ESR, CRP • Ganglioside antibodies • Complement studies • CPK • HLA testing (DR2, DR4, B27) • GM1AB IgM/IgG, Mag IgM/IgG ABs, ASI GM AB IgM/IgG • Immunoglobulin levels (IgM, IgA, IgG) • Cytokine panels • Six-hour urine DMSA challenge for heavy metals • Mineral levels (serum magnesium, RBC mag++, iodine, zinc) • Parasite studies (stool CDSA, blood) • Food allergy panel (IgE and IgG) • Antigliadin AB/TTG • Hormonal studies (thyroid: T3, free T3, T4, reverse T3, TSH, DHEA/cortisol salivary testing, sex hormone levels: estradiol, progesterone, testosterone, both total and free, DHT, SHBG, pregnenolone, IgF1) • Five-hour glucose tolerance, with insulin levels • Tilt table with ANS evaluation • B_{12}, folate • MMA and HC levels

Symptoms	Possible Related Medical Conditions	Laboratory Testing to Consider
Fatigue, tiredness *(continued)*		• MTHFR (methylenetetra-hydrofolate reductase), genetic • Mold (*Stachybotrys* titers, mold plates) and ERMI (Environmental Relative Moldiness Index) testing • Organix test (Metametrix Labs) for EI • Lipid oxidation: thiobarbituric acid reactive substances assay (TBARS) and lipid peroxides • DNA oxidation (8-OhdG, autoanti-bodies to oxidized DNA, modified Comet assay) • Protein oxidation (protein carbonyls) • Sleep studies • Neuropsychiatric evaluation with SPECT scans • MRI brain scan
Unexplained hair loss	• Lyme disease and co-infections • Stress • Inflammation • Dermatological disorders* • Autoimmune disorders • Pregnancy* • Mineral deficiencies • Hormonal disorders	• Infections • Mineral levels • Iron deficiency • Thyroid deficiency • ANA • ESR, CRP • Cytokine panel • Dermatological evaluation
Swollen glands	• Lyme disease and co-infections, especially *Bartonella* and tularemia if lymph nodes are significantly enlarged • Viruses such as mononucleosis/ Epstein-Barr virus • Malignancy*	• Lyme and co-infections • Appropriate cancer screening
Sore throat	• Lyme disease (if symptom comes and goes in monthly cycles) • Strep* • Viral infections • Allergies	• Throat swab and/or culture for strep • Test for viruses • Lyme and co-infections • Allergy testing

Symptoms	Possible Related Medical Conditions	Laboratory Testing to Consider
Testicular pain (men), pelvic pain (women)	• Lyme disease • Epididymitis with or without orchitis* • Testicular torsion* • Endometriosis/ovarian cysts* • Urinary tract infection (UTI)*	• Lyme • Physical examination with urethral swabs • Abdominal/pelvic ultrasounds • Urinalysis and culture
Unexplained menstrual irregularity	• Lyme disease • Hormonal dysregulation • Stress	• Female hormones and prolactin levels • Lyme
Unexplained milk production, breast pain	• Lyme disease • Hormonal dysregulation • Fibrocystic breast disease*	• Female hormones and prolactin levels • Serum iodine levels • Significant caffeine use? • Lyme testing
Irritable bladder or bladder dysfunction	• Interstitial cystitis, with or without Lyme disease and *Bartonella* • Dropped bladder* • BPH (benign prostatic hypertrophy with outlet obstruction)* • UTI (bacterial)* • Fungal infections • MS and diseases that affect nerve function	• Urinalysis (UA) • Culture and sensitivity (C+S) • Urological examination with scope and cystometric studies • Lyme and co-infection • Testing for MS (VEP, AEP, MRI, spinal tap checking for oligoclonal bands and MBP)
Sexual dysfunction or loss of libido	• Lyme with overlapping co-infections • Low sex hormones (testosterone, estrogen) • Psychological factors	• Lyme and co-infections • Hormone evaluations: testosterone, free T, DHT, DHEA-S, SHBG, estradiol, pregnenolone and progesterone (women) • Check thyroid and adrenal if sex hormones normal • Psychological evaluation
Upset stomach	• GERD with reflux* • *H. pylori* • Gallbladder dysfunction* • Food allergies	• GI testing: serum antibodies for *H. pylori* +/− breath test • Upper endoscopy • Food allergy testing

Symptoms	Possible Related Medical Conditions	Laboratory Testing to Consider
Upset stomach *(continued)*	• Stress • Medications* • Lyme disease	• Evaluation of side effects of medications • Lyme
Change in bowel function (constipation or diarrhea)	• Irritable bowel syndrome (IBS) • Small intestinal bowel overgrowth (SIBO) • Inflammatory bowel disease (IBD) • Celiac disease • Food allergies and intolerances • Stress • Dehydration* • Infections (*E. coli* 0:157, *Salmonella, Shigella, Campylobacter, Yersinia, Clostridium difficile*, rotaviruses, parasites) • Magnesium deficiency • Lyme disease • *Candida*	• CBC • CMP with electrolytes, BUN/creatinine, liver functions (LFTs) • Mineral levels • Antigliadin and TTG levels • Food allergy panel • Breath test for small intestinal bowel overgrowth (SIBO) • Stool cultures: bacteria, parasites, *Candida* • Stool for *Clostridium difficile* toxin A and B • Stool CDSA (comprehensive digestive stool analysis) • GI evaluation with colonoscopy • Lyme
Chest pain or rib soreness	• Lyme disease • Costochondritis (inflammation in the ribs) • Coronary artery disease* • Fractures*	• Lyme • EKG and cardiac evaluation, if necessary • Physical examination (pushing on the ribs is usually painful with costochondritis) • X-ray if suspecting fractures (pain, rub on auscultation)
Shortness of breath, cough	• Over 90 percent of coughs are due to allergic rhinitis with a postnasal drip, with or without asthma with reactive airway disease, and GERD with reflux* • *Babesia* presents with an atypical cough and "air hunger" • COPD* • Interstitial lung disease • Malignancy in smokers* • Inflammation	• *Babesia microti* and *duncani* IFA, FISH, PCR, Giemsa stain • Allergy evaluation • Pulmonary function tests (PFTs) • Arterial Blood Gas (ABG)/oximetry • Diffusing capacity (Dlco) • Chest X-ray • Rapid CT scan chest • Ongoing cough should be evaluated by a pulmonologist, with bronchoscopy if a cough persists without an obvious etiology • Cytokine panel

Symptoms	Possible Related Medical Conditions	Laboratory Testing to Consider
Heart palpitations, pulse skips, heart block	• Lyme disease, co-infections • Inflammation • Stress • Anxiety • Reactive hypoglycemia • POTS • Caffeine* • Medications* • Heart disease with arrhythmias*	• Lyme disease and co-infections • Cytokine panel • EKG • Holter monitor and stress testing in appropriate clinical settings • Five-hour GTT, with insulin levels • Tilt table with ANS evaluation • Evaluate side effects of medications
Any history of a heart murmur or valve prolapse	• Q-fever endocarditis • Brucella endocarditis • Bacterial endocarditis* • Mitral valve prolapse* • Heart valve abnormalities* • History of rheumatic fever* • PFO (patent foramen ovale)* • Lyme disease	• EKG • Echocardiogram +/− transesophageal echocardiogram (TEE) • Cardiac evaluation • Lyme disease and co-infections • Q-fever with phase I and phase II antibody titers • Brucella titers/agglutinating antibodies
Joint pain or swelling	• Lyme disease and co-infections • Autoimmune diseases • Inflammation • Osteoarthritis (OA)* • Gout* • Acute bacterial infections (joint sepsis)* • Acute trauma*	• Lyme disease and co-infections • ANA, RF • CCP • ESR, CRP • Autoimmune markers if appropriate (ss and ds-DNA, anti-RNP, etc.) • Cytokine panel • Uric acid levels • X-rays • MRI of the joint, if appropriate • Tap of joint to check for infection
Stiffness of the joints, neck, or back	• Lyme disease and co-infections • OA • Autoimmune diseases • Muscle strain* • Trauma*	• Lyme disease and co-infections • X-rays • Autoimmune markers

Symptoms	Possible Related Medical Conditions	Laboratory Testing to Consider
Muscle pain or cramps	• Lyme disease and co-infections • Inflammation • Myositis • Trichinosis • Potassium and magnesium deficiencies • Dehydration*	• Lyme disease and co-infections • Cytokine panel • CPK • Aldolase and LDH levels • Eosinophil count with *Trichinella* ELISA • Serum and RBC magnesium levels • K+ level • BUN/creatinine on CMP
Twitching of the face or other muscles	• Lyme disease • *Bartonella* • Magnesium deficiency • Stress • Caffeine* • Sleep deprivation • Motor neuron diseases (ALS causes characteristic twitching in the extremities, tongue with loss of the muscles in the thenar eminence)	• Lyme disease and co-infections • *Bartonella*: IFA, PCR • RBC and serum magnesium levels • EMG to rule out ALS and motor neuron diseases
Headaches	• Lyme disease and co-infections • Food allergies • Reactive hypoglycemia • Migraines • Mineral deficiencies with environmental toxins • Mold • Tension headaches with stress • Inflammation • Caffeine withdrawal* • Medications* • Trauma* • CNS infections • Tumor*	• Food allergy • Five-hour glucose tolerance, with insulin levels • Serum and RBC mineral levels • Six-hour urine DMSA testing for heavy metals, and Organix, if environmental toxin exposure • *Stachybotrys*/mold toxins, ERMI • Lyme disease and co-infections • Cytokine panel • Psychological evaluation if history of trauma and PTSD • CT scan/MRI brain
Neck cracks, neck stiffness	• Lyme disease • OA*	• Lyme disease • X-rays or MRI, if severe

Symptoms	Possible Related Medical Conditions	Laboratory Testing to Consider
Neck cracks, neck stiffness *(continued)*	• Muscle strain* • Bacterial and viral meningitis (stiff neck, often with associated light and sound sensitivity, headaches, occasional vomiting, if meningitis. Meningococcal and other bacterial meningitis are often clinically more severe than the presentation with acute neurological Lyme disease)*	• Neurological evaluation with spinal tap, if clinically appropriate
Tingling numbness, burning or stabbing sensations	• Lyme disease • *Bartonella* • Autoimmune disorders • Carpal and cubital tunnel or any nerve entrapment syndrome (thoracic outlet)* • Diabetes* • Hypothyroidism* • Pregnancy* • Heavy metal toxicity (Hg, Pb, As) or other environmental toxins (TCE) • Vitamin deficiencies • Immune deficiency • Mitochondrial dysfunction • MS • Strokes or TIAs* • Anxiety, with hyperventilation	• Lyme disease and co-infections • GM1 AB IgM/IgG, Mag IgM/IgG ABs, ASI GM AB IgM/IgG • EMG • Small fiber nerve biopsy +/− ANS evaluation • Hypothyroidism (T3, T4, free T3, TSH) • B-HCG • Blood sugar and HbA1c levels • B_{12} • Folate • MMA and HC levels • Immunoglobulin levels with subclasses • Six-hour urine DMSA challenge for heavy metal burdens • Accuchem laboratory evaluation for environmental toxin exposure, if appropriate (blood, fat biopsy) • Lipid peroxide levels and other markers of oxidative stress • MS (MRI, VEP, AEP, spinal tap for MBP, oligoclonal bands) • CT head or MRI, if suspecting acute stroke or TIA • Neuropsychiatric evaluation

Symptoms	Possible Related Medical Conditions	Laboratory Testing to Consider
Facial paralysis (Bell's palsy)	• CNS Lyme disease • CNS viral infections (herpes viruses) • Stroke* • Sarcoidosis* • Trauma*	• Brain CT scan or MRI • Lyme disease with lumbar puncture (LPs can be negative in early and late Lyme) • Spinal tap, rule out lymphocytic meningitis • Viral titers • Kveim test with ACE level and chest X-ray, if ruling out sarcoid
Eyes/vision: double, blurry, floaters	• Lyme disease • Co-infections, especially *Bartonella* • Inflammation • Environmental toxins • Functional medicine abnormalities • Concussion* • Trauma* • Stroke* • Brain tumor compressing the optic nerve* • Accommodation problems with aging*	• Lyme disease and co-infections • Eye examination • Cytokine panel • Brain CT scan or MRI • Organix/ION, with functional medicine workup
Ears/hearing: buzzing, ringing, ear pain	• Lyme disease • Co-infections • Heavy metal burdens (Hg) • Medications*	• Lyme and co-infections • Six-hour urine DMSA challenge for heavy metals • Evaluate medication side effects (macrolides)
Increased motion sickness, vertigo	• Lyme disease and co-infections • Viral infections (acute labyrinthitis) • Environmental toxicity, including heavy metal burdens • Eighth nerve or cerebellar disorders	• Lyme disease and co-infections • Six-hour urine DMSA challenge for heavy metals • Organix/ION • Brain CT Scan or MRI • ENT evaluation with ENG
Light-headedness, wooziness, poor balance, difficulty walking	• Lyme disease and co-infections • Metabolic disorders • Environmental toxin exposure • Functional medicine abnormalities	• Lyme disease and co-infections • Blood alcohol and ammonia levels • Six-hour urine DMSA challenge • Organix/ION

Symptoms	Possible Related Medical Conditions	Laboratory Testing to Consider
Light-headedness, wooziness, poor balance, difficulty walking *(continued)*	• Reactive hypoglycemia • POTS • Inflammation • Neurological diseases (MS, ALS) • Strokes*	• Five-hour GTT with insulin levels • Tilt table, with ANS evaluation • Cytokine panel • Brain CT Scan or MRI • Neurological evaluation
Tremor	• Lyme disease and co-infections • Mercury toxicity • Environmental toxins (pesticides) • Functional medicine abnormalities • Hyperthyroidism • Hypoglycemia • Anxiety • Caffeine* • Medication*	• Lyme disease and co-infections • Six-hour urine DMSA challenge • Organix/ION • Blood sugar (5-hour GTT) • Thyroid functions (T3, free T3, T4, TSH) • Evaluate medication side effects
Confusion, difficulty thinking	• Lyme disease and co-infections • Viral encephalitis • Metabolic abnormalities • Inflammation • Reactive hypoglycemia • POTS • Strokes and neurological injury* • Hypothyroidism • Heavy metal burdens and other environmental toxins • Mold • Functional medicine abnormalities • Alzheimer's disease • Jacob-Creutzfeldt (prion disease)* • Vitamin deficiencies	• Lyme disease and co-infections • Blood alcohol and ammonia levels • Cytokine panel • Five-hour GTT, with insulin levels • Tilt table • Thyroid (T3, free T3, T4, TSH) • Six-hour urine DMSA challenge for heavy metals • Mold (*Stachybotrys* titers, mold plates, ERMI) • Organix/ION testing, (Metametrix/Accuchem) • Lumbar puncture with CT or MRI, with neurological consultation if appropriate for severe cases • Apo E positive • B_{12}/folic acid
Difficulty with concentration or reading	• Lyme disease and co-infections • Inflammation • ADD/ADHD* • Reactive hypoglycemia • POTS • Food allergies and intolerances • Heavy metals or environmental toxins (TCE, mold)	• Lyme disease and co-infections • Cytokine panel • Five-hour GTT, with insulin levels • Tilt table, with ANS evaluation • Food allergies • Six-hour urine DMSA challenge • Organix/ION testing

Symptoms	Possible Related Medical Conditions	Laboratory Testing to Consider
Difficulty with concentration or reading *(continued)*	• Functional medicine abnormalities • Sleep deprivation • Hypothyroidism • Metabolic abnormalities • Depression/anxiety • Vitamin deficiencies	• Testing for environmental toxin exposure • Mold (*Stachybotrys* titers, mold plates, ERMI) • Sleep studies • Thyroid function (T3, free T3, T4, TSH) • Blood alcohol and ammonia levels • Neuropsychiatric evaluation • B_{12}/folic acid
Forgetfulness, poor short-term memory	• Lyme disease and co-infections • Inflammation • Viral encephalitis • Metabolic abnormalities • Reactive hypoglycemia • POTS • Strokes and neurological injury* • Hypothyroidism • Heavy metal burdens and other environmental toxins • Mold • Functional medicine abnormalities • Alzheimer's disease • Jacob-Creutzfeldt (prion disease)* • Vitamin deficiencies	• Lyme disease and co-infections • Cytokine panel • Blood alcohol and ammonia levels • Five-hour GTT, with insulin levels • Tilt table, with ANS evaluation • Thyroid (T3, free T3, T4, TSH) • Six-hour urine DMSA challenge • Organix/ION • Testing for environmental toxin exposure (Metametrix/Accuchem) • Mold (*Stachybotrys* titers, mold plates, ERMI) • Lumbar puncture with CT or MRI, with neurological consultation if appropriate for severe cases • Apo E positive • B_{12}/folic acid
Disorientation: getting lost, going to wrong places	• Lyme disease and co-infections • Inflammation • Viral encephalitis • Metabolic abnormalities • Strokes and neurological injury* • Hypothyroidism • Heavy metals; environmental toxins • Mold exposure • Functional medicine abnormalities • Alzheimer's disease • Jacob-Creutzfeldt (prion disease)*	• Lyme disease and co-infections • Cytokine panel • Blood alcohol and ammonia levels • Thyroid (T3, free T3, T4, TSH) • Six-hour urine DMSA challenge for heavy metals • Organix/ION • Environmental toxin exposure • Mold (*Stachybotrys* titers, mold plates, ERMI) • Lumbar puncture with CT or MRI, with neurological consultation, if appropriate for severe cases • Apo E positive

Symptoms	Possible Related Medical Conditions	Laboratory Testing to Consider
Difficulty with speech or writing	• Lyme disease and co-infections • Inflammation • Viral encephalitis • Metabolic abnormalities • Reactive hypoglycemia • Strokes and neurological injury* • Parkinson's disease • Hypothyroidism • Heavy metals and other environmental toxins • Mold exposure • Functional medicine abnormalities • Alzheimer's disease • Jacob-Creutzfeldt (prion disease)*	• Lyme disease and co-infections • Cytokine panel • Blood alcohol and ammonia levels • Five-hour GTT with insulin levels • Thyroid (T3, free T3, T4, TSH) • Six-hour urine DMSA challenge for heavy metals • Organix/ION • Environmental toxin exposure • Mold (Stachybotrys titers, mold plates, ERMI) • Lumbar puncture with CT or MRI, with neurological consultation if appropriate, for severe cases • Apo E positive
Mood swings, irritability, depression	• Lyme disease and co-infections • Inflammation • Heavy metal burdens • Environmental toxins • Mineral deficiencies • Functional medicine abnormalities • Mold • Sleep deprivation • Trauma* • PTSD • Depression • Medication* • Food allergies and intolerances • Reactive hypoglycemia	• Lyme disease and co-infections • Cytokine panel • Neurotransmitter levels • Six-hour urine DMSA challenge for heavy metals • Serum mineral levels • Organix • Environmental toxins • Mold (Stachybotrys titers and mold plates, ERMI) • Sleep evaluation • Food allergy profile • Five-hour GTT, with insulin levels • Evaluate medication side effects
Disturbed sleep: too much or too little or early awakening	• Lyme disease and co-infections • Inflammation with pain • Nocturia (urination several times per night secondary to bladder problems, BPH)* • Depression or anxiety • Medication* • Caffeine use late in the day*	• Sleep study • Lyme disease and co-infections, • Cytokine panel • Neurotransmitter levels • Urological evaluation, with urinalysis/culture and sensitivity • Medication evaluation

Symptoms	Possible Related Medical Conditions	Laboratory Testing to Consider
Disturbed sleep: too much or too little or early awakening *(continued)*	• Reactive hypoglycemia • Obstructive sleep apnea (OSA)* • Restless leg syndrome (RLS)*	• Five-hour GTT with insulin levels • Neuropsychiatric evaluation
Exaggerated symptoms or worse hangover from alcohol	• Lyme disease and co-infections • Nutritional deficiencies • Functional medicine abnormalities	• Lyme disease and co-infection • Serum and RBC mineral levels • Organix/ION

*These medical conditions are not generally part of the MSIDS map but are part of a differential diagnostic list that should be considered in a patient with those symptoms.

Health-care providers can also refer to this list while interviewing patients who have failed multiple interventions. You can include a copy of this list in your patients' charts to remind you of which approaches you have tried and where your successes and failures have been. I might use the sixteen-point map to decide when to stop antibiotics if my patient has been through several rounds of medications and has not had adequate benefit, leading me to look at other approaches and see which points on the map have not adequately been addressed. This approach also allows us to combine different intracellular medications simultaneously to maximize the effect but reduce possible side effects.

The sixteen-point differential diagnostic map is therefore an essential blueprint for your health and clearly shows why certain treatment regimens may not have worked. If a patient remains ill despite my last treatment regimen, I can look at the list and see which tests have not been performed and those treatments we have not yet tried. Perhaps the patient has not gotten well because he/she suffers from adrenal fatigue with low cortisol levels. This condition is quite commonly seen in patients with MSIDS. If the antibiotics are not working, it is essential that patients send their DHEA/cortisol adrenal test to the lab. The results will then indicate whether they need adrenal supplements and/or hydrocortisone. Often we will see clinical improvements once a patient's adrenal function is normalized. Similarly, patients may have a B_{12} deficiency or methylation block and require methylcobalamin to help their neuropathy, or a positive heavy metal test for mercury and lead, and the reason their neuropathy is not improving is because we have not adequately detoxified them via chelation to remove their heavy metals, which also can cause neuropathy. Heavy metals also create oxidative stress (free radicals) and inflammation in some cases causing the Lyme-induced neuropathy to worsen. Or perhaps we are giving the correct antibiotics, the patient's cortisol levels are balanced, and heavy metals have been adequately removed, but the patient's sleep patterns are still poor, which is driving chronic inflammation and increasing IL-6 levels. IL-6 is part of a group of molecules in the body called cytokines that increase inflammation. The patient may require a medication that helps promote sleep, such as Lyrica, trazodone, Seroquel, Gabitril, or Xyrem, since they have failed standard sleep medications, such as Ambien or Lunesta. Their poor sleep can be the reason their fatigue and memory and concentration problems persist. Or perhaps they have nutritional deficiencies in magnesium, iodine, or zinc, which are needed for proper hormone production, detoxification, and immune function, and we have not run the appropriate blood and urine tests to check their detoxification pathways (such as an Organix test, through Metametrix laboratories). Other possibilities include mitochondrial dysfunction from oxidative stress (free radical damage to cells of the body, in this case, the mitochondrial membranes responsible for energy production in the body), which has not been corrected, or perhaps they have a parasite that has not yet been discovered on a CDSA (comprehensive digestive stool analysis) and are deconditioned from a lack of exercise, which could account for their ongoing fatigue.

It is essential to keep returning to the Horowitz sixteen-point differential diagnostic map and use it as a simple method for tracking which tests have been performed and those that must still be completed.

TESTING: THE NEXT STEP IN DIAGNOSTICS

The patient with MSIDS can be extremely complex, and some of these tests and interventions may hold the key to helping someone who previously has traveled from doctor to doctor without finding answers. I can now use the sixteen-point differential diagnostic map to take the final step: ordering the necessary testing to validate my hypothesis. It guides me in terms of which diagnoses are the most likely and which should be prioritized in the patient's evaluation and treatment. It allows me to maneuver through the maze of patients' complex symptomatology and guide my laboratory and imaging studies as I look for bacterial, viral, parasitic, or fungal infections. It reminds me to evaluate the patient for autoimmune diseases and to look for inflammation and inflammatory markers in the body. It helps me determine which hormonal studies to complete, which mineral deficiencies to look for, and which functional medicine biochemical abnormalities may be present. It reminds me to look for possible food allergies, mitochondrial dysfunction with heavy metals, and to evaluate the possibilities of heavy metals underlying psychiatric issues and etiologies for their sleep disorder.

MRS. Q AND THE HOROWITZ SIXTEEN-POINT DIFFERENTIAL DIAGNOSTIC MAP

After I collected all of the information from Mrs. Q's questionnaire, I began to cross-reference her symptoms against the most likely diagnoses. I thought about some of her answers and realized that before I could prescribe a treatment regimen, I needed to have her take several other tests, in order to fully evaluate her symptoms.

First, I ordered a test for heavy metal burdens. Heavy metals such as mercury can cause fatigue, headaches, paresthesias (tingling, numbness, and/or burning sensations), joint and muscle pain, and mood disorders. Mrs. Q had several mercury amalgam fillings in her mouth, and often enjoyed eating fish several times per week. We would send her home with a six-hour urine Dimercaptosuccinic acid (DMSA) challenge to check her level of exposure to heavy metals.

She also had never had a twenty-four-hour DHEA/cortisol test to check for adrenal dysfunction. Low adrenal function could be responsible for her ongoing fatigue and inability to properly fight infections, and high cortisol levels at night could be interfering with her sleep. She would also go home with a test kit from Aeron labs or Labrix services to check her adrenal function.

Others we would run, in our office, include looking for nutritional deficiencies, such as checking serum and red blood cell magnesium, iodine, and zinc levels. Magnesium deficiency could exacerbate her muscle spasms and affect her detoxification pathways, since magnesium is necessary in over three hundred enzymes in the body that are essential for the detoxification of environmental chemicals. Many Lyme-MSIDS patients do not detoxify well based on their symptoms, laboratory testing, and excellent response to glutathione, which removes fat-soluble toxins from the body.

We would also check for iodine deficiency, since iodine is a trace mineral essential for thyroid hormone production, and, finally, we would check for zinc deficiency, which is needed for proper immune function. Low levels may drive cytokine production, leading to sickness behavior in patients. Zinc is also a necessary component of phase 1 enzymes, which are part of the liver's detoxification process. A zinc deficiency could cause a backup of phase 1 enzymes, leading to excess production of aldehydes; these are the by-products of chemical reactions involving alcohol, which are part of the sugar molecules contained within the body. One aldehyde is chloral hydrate, which acts as a sedative. Chloral hydrate is affectionately known by seasoned physicians as the old "Mickey Finn," and was used to get people to sleep in the olden days of medical pharmacology. Zinc deficiency with subsequent chloral hydrate production could therefore exacerbate the brain fog commonly seen in these patients, and it should be considered in a differential diagnosis of cognitive deficits. I would also check for food allergies. This might be helpful with Mrs. Q's history of fatigue, headaches, and joint pain.

Other tests that I would order include checking for elevated immunoglobulin levels. There are five different types of immunoglobulins produced in the body, known as IgA, IgM, IgG, IgD, and IgE antibodies. These have different functions, such as fighting infections and helping the body with foreign allergies. In Mrs. Q's case, I would check her for elevated immunoglobulin levels (IgM) to see if she had a disease such as Waldenström's macroglobulinemia, which could account for her TIA-like symptoms. A TIA is a transient ischemic attack, and it mimics the symptoms of a stroke. It is due to a temporary loss of blood flow to the brain or spinal cord, and can be caused by Waldenström's macroglobulinemia, in which excess amounts of IgM antibody thicken the blood. Immunoglobulin levels would also show if she was immunodeficient and unable to properly fight chronic infections. Several Lyme disease patients present with common variable immune deficiency (CVID) and require intravenous immunoglobulin (IVIG) therapy to boost deficient immunoglobulin levels, and also to treat their resistant neuropathy. We also frequently find IgG subclass deficiencies, IgA deficiency, and IgM deficiencies, which may also contribute to an inability to properly deal with chronic infections. I often find low IgM levels in patients with persistent Lyme-MSIDS. According to immunologists we have spoken with, low IgM levels are generally only seen with unresolved Lyme disease. Although it is not a specific marker for Lyme disease, it is not uncommon to find it in this subset of patients and may be one of several clues that points to the existence of Lyme, and helps explain persistent symptoms in Lyme-MSIDS patients.

Finally, we would, of course, check Mrs. Q for a broad range of bacterial and viral co-infections not tested for by the other physicians. These would include different strains of babesiosis, including: *Babesia microti* and *Babesia* WA-1 (*Babesia duncani*) by IFA, *Babesia* FISH, and *Babesia* PCR; *Ehrlichia* or *Anaplasma*; *Bartonella*; rickettsial infections such as Rocky Mountain spotted fever, Q fever, and typhus; tularemia; *Brucella*; chlamydia pneumonia; *Mycoplasma* species, including *Mycoplasma fermentans*; viruses such as EBV, CMV, HHV 6; and parasites such as toxoplasmosis. We have been finding many individuals with significantly elevated toxoplasmosis titers, which can be problematic in the immunocompromised individual.

MOVING FORWARD

The testing and approaches that I will be describing throughout this book have been used in thousands of patients without ill effects, and where the benefit is outweighed by any possible risk. Although there are no double-blind placebo-controlled trials to test this method, I have had enough clinical success over the years without causing any significant patient harm that I believe the following diagnostic and treatment approaches are warranted in treating sick patients for whom the traditional medical diagnostic model has not worked.

I will attempt in each of the following chapters to give the most important and relevant scientific data that support each approach. These will be broad brushstrokes that will give the reader a foundation for understanding each aspect of MSIDS. This book is not intended to be a textbook of medicine. But it is my hope that this book, and each chapter, can serve nevertheless as a road map of healing for health-care providers and patients who have not found answers in the approach that modern medicine often uses in diagnosing and treating chronic illness.

THREE

Detecting and Treating Lyme Disease

he next challenge to solving the mystery of Lyme disease and chronic illness is determining the appropriate treatments. In the early years I would attend Lyme conferences and sit and discuss cases late into the evening as we tried to figure out the pieces of the puzzle: Why did some of our patients not get better? We now know that *Borrelia burgdorferi*, the etiologic agent of Lyme disease, can occur in different forms in order to evade the immune system, the body's primary method of attacking intruding bacteria. Each occurs as the organism changes shape or moves into different tissues and compartments and adapts to its environment.

The three major forms, or locations, are:

- the cell wall
- cystic (also called cell wall deficient, S-forms, or L-forms, as defined by their shape)
- intracellular locations, where the mobile spirochete and/or cystic forms can be found within a host cell

Ticks carrying Lyme disease are commonly found on mice, deers, foxes, raccoons, songbirds, chipmunks, and squirrels. It is transmitted in a zoonotic cycle. This means that it is transmitted to humans by ticks, which initially acquire the infection after feeding on an infected host (such as rodents and deer). One notable exception to this rule is another *Borrelia* spirochete, *Borrelia miyamotoi*, related to the relapsing fever group of spirochetes. Recent scientific evidence published in 2013 by Rollend and colleagues demonstrated that there is transovarial transmission of *B. miyamotoi* directly from infected eggs to larvae, without the ticks needing to feed on an infected host. According to Dr. Richard Ostfeld, senior scientist and disease ecologist at the Cary Institute of Ecosystem Studies, 6 to 73 percent of larval ticks are now infected with *Borrelia miyamotoi*. This is particularly worrisome because numbers of larval ticks are ten to fifty times higher than nymphs and adults that infect humans, and larvae are so small that they are literally impossible to detect. This significantly increases the risk of transmission of this borrelial species and, since there is no available diagnostic test, it could explain "Lyme-like" relapsing symptoms in individuals who test negative for Lyme disease.

The Lyme bacteria first enter the body during a tick bite in the classical corkscrew shape, which is the cell wall form. There are anywhere from three to six flagella attached to either end, allowing the bacterium to have bidirectional motility, and the tails propel the organism to move through the body's tissues. In hostile environments of extreme temperature (heat or cold) or high or low acidity, the *Borrelia* changes form, and a circular structure, or cyst, is created. This protects it from being killed off by the immune system and allows the organism to survive dormant for long periods of time; from there it can reactivate later, when circumstances are more favorable for its survival. The organism can also penetrate varied cells and enter the intracellular compartment, the area inside the cell wall that includes the nucleus and cytoplasm and contains all of the organelles that allow the cell to function metabolically. Like the cystic form, it allows the bacteria to hide from the immune system. These varied bacterial forms and locations occur as a dynamic process that is constantly going on in the body, and it is the basis for the therapeutic approaches for Lyme disease treatment that I have developed.

Regardless of the form, the disease can spread throughout the body from the site of the initial bite, and even within twenty-four hours can invade the central nervous system. The *Borrelia* bacteria has a preference for certain areas, such as the eye, brain tissue and glial cells, the heart, collagen and skeletal muscle fibers, and the synovial membrane that sur-

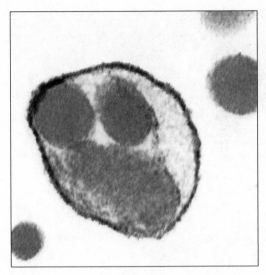

Cyst form of Borrelia burgdorferi *under the microscope.*

Electron micrograph: Cystic Borrelia *form from a culture of human blood in BSK 1987. Electron Microscopy at Stony Brook School of Medicine. Bernard P. Lane, Professor of Pathology. Photo final magnification 135,000x.*

FROM THE PERSONAL COLLECTION OF ALAN B. MACDONALD, M.D., REPRINTED WITH HIS PERMISSION.

rounds the joints. This explains why the most common Lyme-related inflammation occurs in those tissues, causing optic neuritis (inflammation in the optic nerve), iritis (inflammation in the anterior chamber of the eye), meningitis, encephalitis (inflammation in the sac surrounding the brain and in the brain tissue itself), carditis (inflammation of the heart), and arthritis.

Some physicians may only prescribe a cephalosporin drug such as Ceftin when a patient presents with an EM rash. However, Ceftin or amoxicillin only treat the cell wall forms and are therefore not routinely effective in treating all cases of Lyme disease. Dr. Gary Wormser published a study in the 1990s that compared doxycycline (a tetracycline) and Ceftin in treating early Lyme disease that demonstrated that up to 20 percent of patients did not adequately respond to this treatment and went on to develop chronic symptomatology despite both medications. Doxycycline will primarily treat the intracellular forms (and is also useful for multiple intracellular co-infections). Neither of these two drug families treats the cystic forms. Dr. Eva Sapi at the University of New Haven was the first to show that doxycycline with or without Plaquenil can cause the organism to transform into its cystic form. This would explain why some patients treated with doxycycline alone go on to develop chronic symptomatology.

There are now four separate treatment options to kill the cystic forms

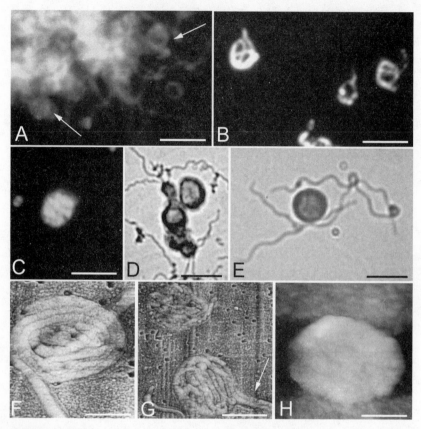

Persisting atypical and cystic forms of Borrelia burgdorferi *in neurological Lyme disease.*

Rolled and cystic forms of Borrelia burgdoferi *spirochetes observed after one week of culture in medium to which Thioflavin S had been added.* **A:** *Observation by Thioflavin S fluorescence. Arrows point to rolled cystic forms at the periphery of an agglomerated mass of spirochetes from strain B31. Rolled* **(B)** *and cystic* **(C)** *forms observed by dark field microscopy (strain B31).* **D** *and* **E:** *Cyst forms of* Borrelia burgdorferi *(strains ADB1 and B31, respectively), following immunostaining with the monoclonal anti-OspA antibody.* **F–H:** *Atomic force microscopy (AFM) images of* Borrelia *cysts. Rolled spirochetes are clearly visible in F (strain B31) and G (strain ADB1). Arrow in G shows that the cyst is formed by two spirochetes rolled together. H: The cystic form is entirely covered by a thickened external membrane masking the content of the cyst.*

REPRINTED WITH PERMISSION FROM DR. JUDITH MIKLOSSY. INITIALLY PUBLISHED IN "PERSIST-ING ATYPICAL AND CYSTIC FORMS OF BORRELIA BURGDORFERI AND LOCAL INFLAMMATION IN LYME NEUROBORRELIOSIS," J. MIKLOSSY ET AL. *JOURNAL OF NEUROINFLAMMATION.* 2008, 25:40.

of Lyme disease, all of which have been published in the scientific literature. These include the use of three drugs: Plaquenil, Flagyl, and Tindamax, as well as the nutraceutical grapefruit seed extract. Dr. O. Brorson
has shown the effectiveness of grapefruit seed extract against the cystic
forms in the scientific literature. Since patients can have strong reactions
to cystic drugs, we will often pulse these medications (use them several
days in a row, then take a break for several days) to keep down flares and
the worsening of symptoms. These drugs (especially Flagyl and Tindamax)
have the potential to cause increased yeast problems, as well as the unwanted side effect of neuropathy (increased tingling, numbness, or burning sensations). These side effects can be minimized through pulse therapy
and giving high doses of B vitamins, enabling the patient to better tolerate the treatment. Despite possible side effects and Herxheimer reactions
(primarily with Flagyl and Tindamax), many patients improve resistant
symptoms after their use, and the use of cystic drugs may help to lower
the bacterial load of *Borrelia* in the body.

The ability to cure early Lyme disease and prevent it from progressing
is essential in trying to control many of the extreme clinical manifestations that I unfortunately witness daily. In my medical practice we treat
the cell wall, cystic, and forms located in the intracellular compartment
simultaneously, or rotate among the different drugs to treat the different
forms and locations of *Borrelia burgdorferi*. We change antibiotics when
patients do not improve and use IV antibiotics if central nervous system
symptoms continue despite oral treatments or intramuscular shots. I've
also found that I need to keep my patients on sugar-free, yeast-free diets,
to keep down yeast infections that can often accompany antibiotic use,
and load them up with lots of probiotics to prevent diarrhea. Beneficial
probiotics include different strains of acidophilus (found in yogurt) and
saccharomyces boulardii, a yeast that helps prevent antibiotic-associated
diarrhea.

Apart from the cell wall, cystic, and intracellular locations of Lyme
disease, the spirochete has also been found to survive in biofilm forms.
Biofilms are aggregates of bacteria in which the cells adhere to each other
and are frequently embedded in a slimy substance that protects them
from antibiotics. *Borrelia* in biofilm colonies have been found in various
areas of the body, including the skin. My colleague Dr. Steven Fry has also
found biofilms using microscopic analysis of blood. Biofilms may protect

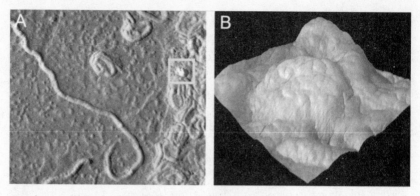

Cyst forms of **Borrelia burgdorferi** *embedded in* **Borrelia** *biofilms.*

Atomic Force Microscopy images of Borrelia burgdorferi B31 *strain at the edge of a biofilm (***A***), with a small round body (cyst form) indicated (in the box), and a higher magnification of a small round body/cyst form (***B***).*

PHOTO COURTESY OF DAVID LUECKE AND DR. EVA SAPI, UNIVERSITY OF NEW HAVEN, LYME DISEASE RESEARCH GROUP (UNPUBLISHED DATA, 2013).

the organism from the effects of antibiotics, which may be another reason why *Borrelia* can still survive after seemingly adequate antibiotic therapy. There are several mechanisms to prevent the formation of *Borrelia* biofilm, as well as aiding its destruction. Doxycycline, as well as natural enzymes such as nattokinase, lumbrokinase, and serrapeptase have all been shown to affect *Borrelia* biofilms, decreasing their formation.

If the patient has adequately responded to a tetracycline (like doxycycline) with Plaquenil, with or without pulse Flagyl or Tindamax, for the treatment of acute Lyme disease, then after one month we will often rotate the patient to a cell wall, cystic, and intracellular protocol for an additional month. This protocol would include a combination of:

- cell wall drugs: cephalosporins such as Omnicef, Ceftin, or penicillins such as amoxicillin;
- cystic drugs: Plaquenil, and/or grapefruit seed extract (GSE), occasionally combined with Flagyl or Tindamax;
- intracellular drugs: Zithromax or Biaxin; and
- Nystatin: to prevent yeast infections associated with antibiotics.

Typically, acute Lyme disease without any other co-infections will resolve in approximately 75 percent of patients with this treatment. Yet

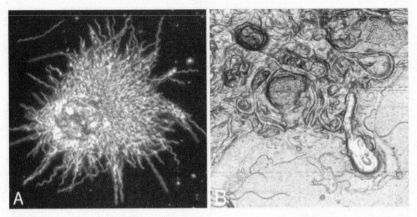

Dark field image of a small developing in vitro Borrelia burgdorferi *B31 strain biofilm* (**A**); *spirochetes at the edge of the biofilm can be easily identified but not the other alternative forms such as the cystic forms. Atomic Force microscopy image of a similar biofilm* (**B**); *several alternative forms, such as the cystic forms, become readily apparent.*

PHOTO COURTESY OF DAVID LUECKE AND DR. EVA SAPI, UNIVERSITY OF NEW HAVEN, LYME DISEASE RESEARCH GROUP (UNPUBLISHED DATA, 2013).

I have also found that many of my patients need a longer course of antibiotics than simply the two-month regimen described above, especially if they are presenting with a stiff neck, headache, and/or tingling and numbness of the extremities or with multiple EM rashes. If a patient has one of these presentations, this implies that they have disseminated Lyme disease: It has spread throughout the body. A single EM rash does not necessarily imply dissemination, but multiple EM rashes means that the organism has spread, and the patient will require longer and more aggressive treatment to try and prevent chronic illness. A stiff neck and headache with an EM rash implies that the organism has effectively penetrated into the central nervous system early on in the disease, where antibiotics may not penetrate well. Tingling, numbness, and/or burning of the extremities with an EM rash imply that the organism has penetrated into the peripheral nervous system (PNS). In these cases, thirty to sixty days of antibiotics may not cure the disease.

Table 3.1: Designing Combination Treatment Therapies		
Cell Wall Form	**Cystic Forms**	**Intracellular Location**
Penicillins: • Amoxicillin • Augmentin • Bicillin (intramuscular)	Plaquenil	Macrolides: • Zithromax • Biaxin
Cephalosporins: • Ceftin • Omnicef • Cedax • Suprax	GSE	Quinolones: • Cipro • Levaquin • Avelox • Factive
IV Cephalosporins: • IV Rocephin • IV Claforan	Flagyl Tindamax	Rifampin tetracyclines: • Doxycycline • Minocycline • Tetracycline HCL
Other IV Medication: • IV vancomycin • IV Primaxin		Other IV medication: • IV doxycycline • IV Zithromax • IV Levaquin/Avelox • IV rifampin

Drug regimens usually include several antibiotic combinations to help hit the different forms of Lyme disease, and also to help prevent antibiotic resistance that could arise from single-drug therapy. Although we have not seen antibiotic resistance clinically in our practice, it is a theoretical concern and should always be on the minds of health-care practitioners prescribing long-term antibiotics.

Lastly, I make sure that my patients get enough sleep by giving them either herbal and natural remedies or mainstream medications for insomnia. Often Lyme patients suffer from terrible insomnia, and it is a challenge to differentiate whether some of their chronic symptoms, such as fatigue, muscle aches, and brain fog, are from chronic sleep deprivation with associated fibromyalgia or from the spirochete itself.

Mary Required Longer Treatment

My patient Mary exemplifies the thousands of my patients who were not adequately diagnosed early. When she first came to see me, she was beside herself. Mary sat across from me at my desk in my office. "Dr. H, what else can we do?" she asked. "I really want another child."

Mary had been my patient for two years and initially presented with symptoms of constant fatigue, migratory joint pain, intermittent tingling and numbness of her extremities, headaches, chest pain, palpitations, and memory and concentration problems. Her prior physicians had given her multiple diagnoses for her illness, including chronic fatigue syndrome, fibromyalgia, and even something called "stressed mommy syndrome." She had a two-year-old child who was still keeping her up at night, and Mary's doctor suggested that her active child may be one of the main causes for her symptoms.

Her initial history and physical were unremarkable, but her Western blot was positive. Her clinical course was fairly typical for most Lyme patients. Her symptoms would come and go, and some symptoms would flare up temporarily with Jarisch-Herxheimer flares (a worsening of symptoms as the spirochetes died off), requiring either stopping the antibiotics or rotating the regimen. She improved month after month, and after two years of treatment she reported being back to 100 percent normal. This was a tremendous improvement from her baseline functioning of 50 percent normal.

I decided to continue her treatment for two more months to prevent a relapse. She then told me she wanted to have another child. Mary seemed well enough to get pregnant once she finished the antibiotic regimen. She returned six weeks later, feeling great, although she was complaining of fleeting joint pain in her hands. "Let's take you off the antibiotics and see how you do," I told her, and six weeks later she returned and announced that she was pregnant, and feeling "great."

"Excellent," I said. "Let's follow up in several months and see how you are doing."

Mary came back six weeks later, brokenhearted. She had just miscarried. I ordered polymerase chain reaction (PCR) tests on the fetus and placenta just to be sure that Lyme disease wasn't involved in the miscarriage. Unfortunately, the results came back positive: *Borrelia* was found in both the placenta and the fetus. It appeared that Mary was still infected with Lyme disease, which she had passed onto her unborn child.

The next time I saw her, Mary told me again that she wanted another child more than anything in the world. I turned to her slowly and said, "OK, Mary. Let's put you back on antibiotics." Although she still couldn't pinpoint any active symptoms, the Lyme was clearly present. I reviewed the ob-gyn literature, which did show evidence of occasional maternal-fetal transmission of Lyme. Dr. Alan McDonald and other researchers, including Dr. Alan Steere, had published on it, but it didn't seem to be a common phenomenon, based on a review of the literature. I placed Mary on Ceftin and Zithromax with meals. These antibiotics were both category B drugs for pregnancy (safe for the fetus). The Ceftin would cover the cell wall forms of *Borrelia*, and the Zithromax would cover the intracellular forms (although Zithromax doesn't cross the placenta readily). I also ordered a low carbohydrate diet with lots of healthy fruits and vegetables and told her to take frequent doses of acidophilus, a probiotic used to replace the good bacteria killed by the antibiotic treatment, and which helps to prevent diarrhea. I really hoped that this treatment course would allow her to carry her next pregnancy to term.

Mary was doing fine at her six-week follow-up. She had no Lyme symptoms, and her complete blood count and liver-function tests were normal while she was on the antibiotics. However, the same dreaded scenario played out sixteen weeks later. We again sent off PCR testing on the placenta and fetus. Both were PCR positive for Lyme disease.

Mary had gone back to her ob-gyn in between our appointments and reported that he could not find any other cause for her miscarriages. All of her hormone levels were normal, and there were no antiphospholipid/antilupus antibodies. It had to be the Lyme disease that kept showing up in her unborn baby that was causing the miscarriage.

When she came back to my office, tears were flowing down her cheeks. Mary and I had a long discussion of the pros and cons of her continuing to get pregnant, including the psychological burden it was placing on her and her family.

"I'm up for it, Dr. H," she said. "Just tell me what to do."

After extensive discussions, we decided that we needed to be as aggressive as we could be to prevent this organism from being transmitted again to the fetus. I decided on using IV Rocephin during the first tri-

mester of her pregnancy, when the baby was most at risk. Mary understood the possible gallbladder complications that are already inherent in
pregnancy due to normally high estrogen levels and the fact that there
are reports of patients having gallbladder problems while on Rocephin.
She understood the possible complications of IV access, including phlebitis and infection, since the drug is given by a peripherally inserted
central catheter (a PICC line, which is a stationary IV line that remains in
the arm).

Once she knew she was pregnant, we would begin treatment. Eight
weeks later, Mary started on IV Rocephin, for the cell wall forms of *Borrelia*, and Zithromax, for the intracellular forms. We scheduled monthly
follow-ups, and she also saw her high-risk obstetrician on a regular basis.

There were no problems at month one. No problems, month two. No
problems, month three. A sonogram was scheduled for week sixteen. We
held our breath waiting for the results. I got a call from her after the
sonogram.

"So far, so good, Dr. H. All is well."

Once we got past the sixteen- to twenty-week mark, I removed the IV
line and put her back on oral antibiotics. I prayed that she would have a
continued healthy pregnancy. I didn't know if her family or I could take
another fetal loss. Fortunately, the rest of the pregnancy was uneventful.
She gave birth to a healthy eight-pound baby boy that June. I received a
letter in the mail from her with a picture of her new baby. It said, "If it
wasn't for you, Dr. Horowitz, none of this would have been possible."

When my wife, Lee, read this card, she wanted to know just how
much of a role I actually played in this pregnancy! You learn over time
not to push the limits of comedy with a potentially jealous Sicilian wife.
"Oh, honey, come on. He barely looks like me. Except for maybe that
nose. Does his nose look a little big to you?"

How is it possible that after years of antibiotics the *Borrelia* could persist, and even be transmitted to a developing fetus? The answer lies in the
types of antibiotics used. At the 12th International Conference on Lyme
Disease in 1999, I presented original scientific data on the use of a specific antibiotic, Flagyl, for Lyme disease. I had noticed early on in my
treatment of Lyme patients that when patients were treated with tetracyclines, Flagyl, and bismuth for *Helicobacter pylori*, the organism that Drs.
Marshall and Warren had identified as the cause of peptic ulcer disease,

patients often had severe Jarisch-Herxheimer flares. These were worse flares than when they took tetracyclines alone for Lyme disease.

As fate would have it, one of my patients knew about some research being done in California by Dr. Martin Atkinson-Barr, who described strong positive reactions to Flagyl in patients treated for *Helicobacter pylori*. Some of these patients complained of fatigue, joint aches, and memory problems but had not been diagnosed as having Lyme disease, and when treated with Flagyl they seemed to get better. Was Flagyl a possible treatment for Lyme disease?

I called Dr. Atkinson-Barr, and we discussed our results. I decided that it was worth doing a scientific study in my medical office on the use of Flagyl in Lyme disease. Flagyl is an anaerobic antibiotic that is generally used for infections in the gastrointestinal tract such as diverticulitis, parasitic infections, such as trichomonas, or parasites such as amebiasis and giardiasis, which cause travelers' diarrhea. I could not find evidence that it had been used for Lyme disease, and it was not on the list of commonly used and approved drugs.

I had patients sign an informed consent and gave them Flagyl alone for several months. They were instructed to avoid alcohol, as the combination could cause severe nausea or vomiting, and to let me know if they had any unusual tingling or numbness, as Flagyl has been associated with a peripheral neuropathy (painful nerve involvement in the peripheral extremities). The problem with that particular side effect is that up to 70 percent of Lyme patients with ongoing symptoms present with a chronic peripheral neuropathy, complaining of tingling, numbness, and burning sensations in the extremities, which often comes and goes and migrates to different parts of their body. It would, therefore, be difficult to differentiate a symptom flare from a true side effect of Flagyl. Nevertheless, the patients understood the protocol and were given 50 mg of vitamin B_6 three times per day to try and keep down any untoward side effects. I also suggested that they take the drug with potato chips: It appears that salt takes away the bitter taste of the drug (and since I love potato chips, I suggested this source of salt).

The Flagyl results were astonishing. Patients with fatigue, headaches, joint and muscle pain, tingling and numbness, and cognitive deficits with memory and concentration problems showed quick improvement, and over time more and more of their symptoms improved. The Jarisch-

Herxheimer flares, however, were severe in certain patients, and we did need to stop the drug intermittently to let the flares die down.

Flagyl was clearly effective in the treatment of Lyme disease. But how did it work? As early as 1967 *The British Journal of Venereal Diseases* had published a study showing Flagyl to be effective in certain cases of syphilis, and that it had an effect on bacterial DNA and RNA irrespective of bacterial replication. Could this be the mechanism of Flagyl's action against *Burrelia burgdorferi*?

The key to Flagyl's effectiveness on Lyme, however, was not reported until several months after my study was presented. Dr. O. Brorson, a Norwegian researcher, published a paper on Flagyl and its effect on the cystic forms of Lyme disease six months after I presented my research. The cystic form of Lyme disease, it turns out, is one mechanism that *Borrelia burgdorferi* utilizes to persist in the body. Dr. Brorson reported that Flagyl would cause *Borrelia* cysts to rupture, and he went on to publish that he could see under the microscope the cell wall forms of *Borrelia burgdorferi* (helical/spiral–shaped organisms) transform into cystic forms, and under proper conditions convert back into mobile spirochetes.

A review of the medical literature revealed that these cystic forms had, in fact, been reported in syphilis. No one had clearly made the link between *Borrelia* and a cystic form of the organism that could persist for long periods of time in a dormant state. It was a highly evolved survival mechanism that would allow the organism to reemerge when conditions were optimal.

My patient, Mary, had been treated initially with Plaquenil, which according to Dr. Brorson's research also affects the cystic forms, yet it appeared that it was not powerful enough to destroy the dormant forms and prevent a relapse, or to prevent her from passing it on to her fetus. She had also been treated with drugs that addressed the cell wall and intracellular forms of Lyme. Although Plaquenil has some effect on cystic forms, it is often primarily used in antibiotic regimens with Lyme disease to alkalize the intracellular compartment, modulate autoimmune reactions, and affect essential enzymes necessary for bacterial replication. Clearly, however, it is not powerful enough to destroy enough of the dormant forms of *Borrelia burgdorferi*, since relapses are the rule when patients are on Plaquenil in combination drug regimens, especially if Lyme disease is not caught early in its acute phase. Mary's case clearly illustrates that point.

But what of all the women who never saw a tick bite or rash and had miscarriages? Might some of these losses be related to Lyme? What about the millions of women with children with active Lyme disease but don't know it? Might these children have Bb (*Borrelia burgdorferi*) and associated tick-borne disorders and be misdiagnosed with ADD, autism, or a neuropsychological disorder later in life?

I have now treated approximately one hundred pregnant women with antibiotics classified as safe for the fetus. We have found that the women with active Lyme symptoms had an easier time during their pregnancy on antibiotics, and the babies were all healthy at birth. A few of the babies were, however, PCR positive for *Borrelia* in the placenta or cord blood despite maternal therapy. They are being followed carefully by their pediatricians to determine if further therapy is needed. Hopefully, these children will not turn into future patients with persistent Lyme disease. Fortunately, even years later, Mary's story turned out with a happy ending. Armed with the appropriate diagnostic and treatment protocols, we can have more happy endings like this one for patients suffering from Lyme disease.

RECOGNIZING JARISCH-HERXHEIMER REACTIONS

Jarisch-Herxheimer (JH) flares are a temporary worsening of the symptoms of Lyme disease that occur when the Lyme spirochete is being killed off by antibiotics or by the body's own immune defenses. This common reaction was first described in the medical literature in relation to syphilis—a spirochetal cousin of Lyme disease. JH reactions produce inflammatory molecules called cytokines, such as TNF-alpha, IL-1, and IL-6. These inflammatory molecules then create inflammatory symptoms, including increased fever, muscle and joint pain, headaches, cognitive impairment, and a general worsening of the patient's underlying symptomatology. This is a major hidden reason why so many people with Lyme disease seem to get worse—and not better—when they are taking antibiotics.

Unfortunately, when I take my patients experiencing JH reactions off of the antibiotics, although their symptoms may temporarily subside, they often return. This creates a difficult situation: The antibiotics are making the patient better while they temporarily make them feel worse.

The only way to break the cycle is to either hold off using the antibiotics for a period of time until the symptoms die down, or to use intermittent flare protocols with glutathione, which help relieve the symptoms in the majority of patients. For example, in my office we sometimes hold back on the use of antibiotics during JH flares, and then place them back on the antibiotics, or a different combination of antibiotics, when the symptoms have subsided. This can sometimes mean that treatments take much longer than thirty to sixty days.

Chris Had an Ongoing JH Reaction

Chris is a twenty-eight-year-old white male who came to see me for the first time in 2009. He had a past medical history significant for food allergies, exercise-induced asthma, temporal mandibular joint (TMJ) dysfunction, peptic ulcer disease, hypoglycemia, and Lyme disease. Chris had possibly been exposed to Lyme five years before a diagnosis had been made. He was asymptomatic until he sustained a concussion in the tenth grade, and then developed forgetfulness, joint pain, headaches, light sensitivity, dizziness, and significant insomnia. He suffered for the next five years without getting relief from his symptoms until he was correctly diagnosed with Lyme disease. His blood tests came back with a positive ELISA and IgM Western blot, and he was treated for the next three years with oral antibiotics. These included antibiotic rotations of amoxicillin, Zithromax, Biaxin, doxycycline, tetracycline, and Flagyl. He had gradual improvement in his symptoms, and treatment was therefore stopped. He contracted the Epstein-Barr virus the next spring, which led to a diagnosis of chronic fatigue syndrome.

By the time he came to see me he had been without any treatment for eight to nine years. He complained of: moderate to severe fatigue; joint pain in his toes, knees, ankles, and fingers that migrated around his body; mid- to low-back pain; tingling and numbness of his extremities; muscle pains; drenching night sweats several times per month; temperature dysregulation, with low-grade fevers; weight loss; decreased libido; testicular pain; constipation alternating with loose stools; occasional shortness of breath; twitching of his eyes; blurry vision; ringing in his ears; light-headedness and balance problems; tremors in his hands; mild to moderate memory, concentration, and word-finding problems; and irritability, anxiety, and depression, all of which would come and go, with good and bad days. Chris was very discouraged by these symptoms, which were severely interfering with his ability to work. Due to his declining health and work-related stress, he had to quit his job.

Chris had an essentially normal history and physical, except for: swollen mucosa inside the nasal passages consistent with his allergies; a small axillary lymph node, approximately half a centimeter in size, which was mobile and slightly tender; decreased vibratory sensation in his extremities; and some stretch marks across his lower back. These stretch marks were suggestive of the skin lesions that I often have seen in patients suffering from Lyme disease and *Bartonella*, and the lack of perceived vibration in his extremities was consistent with Lyme neuropathy, when the nerves are often affected.

I reviewed the extensive medical records that he brought in with him. He had normal blood tests, including a CBC and a biochemistry profile; tests of his sedimentation rate and thyroid function (TSH) had been done and found to be normal; and he'd been checked for an autoimmune disorder with an antinuclear antibody, as well as for markers for celiac disease (antigliadin/TTG) and for sex hormone levels. Tests for other tick-borne disorders, including ehrlichiosis/anaplasmosis, babesiosis, and *Bartonella* had also been done. For his muscle and joint pain and neurological problems, he had normal MRIs of his cervical and thoracic spine, normal MRIs of his brain, and a normal SPECT scan (a test that checks for abnormal blood flow in the brain). His prior physician had done a good job of ruling out many different diseases to explain his symptoms, but there were still several tests that had not yet been done. These included: a more extensive endocrine evaluation, with different tests for thyroid function for his severe fatigue (free T3, T3, T4, and reverse T3); a DHEA/cortisol test, to rule out adrenal fatigue; and an insulin-like growth factor 1 (IgF1) level to rule out growth hormone deficiency. We also sent off for vitamin D levels, a MTHFR test, to check for methylation/detoxification problems with methylmalonic acid; folate and homocysteine levels; immunoglobulin levels, to evaluate his immunity, as well as a six-hour urine DMSA challenge for heavy metals, to try and explain his severe memory problems at twenty-eight years old. DMSA is a FDA-approved drug that binds heavy metals (chelates) and removes them from the body. We can give this drug and collect urine over the subsequent six hours to evaluate a patient's burden of heavy metals. I also ordered an expanded food allergy panel, given his history of allergies and asthma; an *H. pylori* test, given his history of peptic ulcer disease; and an expanded tick-borne co-infection panel, including testing for viruses (HHV, Epstein-Barr Virus, or EBV, Cytomegalovirus, or CMV, and West Nile), *Mycoplasma*, chlamydia, Rocky Mountain spotted fever, *Brucella*, and Q fever, as well as a repeat testing for Lyme disease and *Bartonella*. He was also sent for a neurological evaluation for his peripheral neuropathy, with an EMG, a small-fiber biopsy, and an autonomic nervous system evaluation. Lyme disease can cause a small fiber peripheral neuropathy, which affects the skin, peripheral nerves, and autonomic nervous system, leading to paresthesias, temperature dysregulation, and abnormal sweating. A small fiber skin biopsy helps establish the diagnosis.

Chris's testing came back positive for Lyme disease and for another type of *Babesia* (*Babesia* WA-1/*duncani*) that he had not been tested for previously, and that titer (serum antibody) returned significantly elevated at 1:2048 through Quest Diagnostics. A normal *Babesia* titer is less than 1:64, so this implied that he had a significant infection with *Babesia duncani*. The babesiosis would explain in part the temperature dysregulation with drenching night sweats and the severity of his symptoms, since babesiosis usually makes Lyme patients much sicker. His adrenal testing showed very low cortisol at 8:00 A.M. (1.2; the normal range is between 3 and 6 ng/ml) and high levels at night (5.7; normal range is 0.15 to 0.5 ng/ml), which would explain in part the severe fatigue in the morning and problems falling asleep at night. His food allergy panel returned positive for dairy, wheat, and eggs, with a low serum IgA, often seen in patients with multiple food allergies. These could have contributed to his allergic symptoms, as well as his fatigue and muscle and joint pain. His MTHFR testing showed that he was homozygous (had both genes), causing methylation defects, which could interfere with his detoxification of heavy metals. This was important, because his heavy metal test came back positive for elevated levels of mercury (9.7; the normal reference range is less than 3 mcg/g creatinine) and lead (9.8; the normal range is less than 5 mcg/g creatinine), and his EMG (electromyelogram, a nerve conduction test) showed a sensory polyneuropathy (abnormal nerve conduction), with a small-fiber biopsy confirming a small-fiber neuropathy. The combination of the heavy metals, adrenal problems, food allergies, detoxification problems, *Babesia*, and Lyme disease could have been responsible for the neuropathy, fatigue, sweats, joint and muscle pain, insomnia, and cognitive difficulties that he was complaining of. The testing of his autonomic nervous system, which controls temperature regulation, was also abnormal, showing moderate effects of the Lyme disease on his sympathetic nervous system. All in all, Chris had MSIDS: multiple abnormalities responsible for his chronic symptoms, which explained his resistance to simple Lyme treatment.

We gave Chris IV glutathione for his resistant fatigue and neurocognitive deficits. Glutathione is a protein made in the liver that helps detoxify chemicals in the body, and it can be given orally or intravenously to help patients with resistant Lyme symptoms. Chris noticed an improvement in his symptoms almost immediately, before leaving the office; his energy and concentration improved significantly. We therefore suggested he take N-Acetylcysteine (NAC) and alpha lipoic acid (ALA), supplements that support glutathione production, as glutathione also helps detoxify heavy metals and neurotoxins from the body. We also gave him DMSA to pull mercury and lead out of his body, as well as adrenal support with a hypoglycemic diet for his fatigue and difficulty sleeping. He took B vitamins for his methylation defect and was told to avoid his allergic foods. Finally, we started treating him for *Babesia*, a co-infection that he had never been treated for during his previous several years of treatment.

Over the subsequent two years of treatment Chris was rotated through multiple Lyme and *Babesia* regimens. These included ones to treat the *Babesia*, which included rotations of Mepron and Zithromax, Malarone, Lariam, Coartem, clindamycin (oral), as well as herbal therapies, including *Artemisia*, liposomal artemisinin, neem, and *Cryptolepis*, antimalarial herbal therapies which have been used effectively in our practice to help control resistant *Babesia* symptoms. He would improve temporarily on these regimens, with a decrease in his night sweats, shortness of breath, and fatigue, but would often relapse each time he was taken off of these drugs and herbs. He was rotated through multiple oral antibiotics for the Lyme, including different cell wall drugs such as amoxicillin, Omnicef, cystic drugs, such as Plaquenil, grapefruit seed extract, and Tindamax (pulsed with his history of neuropathy to avoid an increase in symptoms) and intracellular drugs like Zithromax (macrolide antibiotics), doxycycline and minocycline (tetracycline antibiotics), rifampin and Levaquin or Factive, which are quinolone antibiotics.

However, each time he was given any cystic or intracellular drug, he had extremely severe Jarisch-Herxheimer reactions. His fatigue, muscle and joint pain, cognitive difficulties, depression, anxiety, and sleep problem would worsen. We would therefore have to stop the drugs to let the Jarisch-Herxheimer reaction die down. Yet every time we stopped the drugs, although his symptoms had temporarily gotten better, he would relapse and feel worse again within days. What else could be done to control the severity of his Lyme flares and get Chris better?

Sleep disorders increase inflammation in the body, and some of the same inflammatory molecules produced from sleep deprivation (interleukin-6, or IL-6), are also produced during Jarisch-Herxheimer reactions. We therefore gave him several sleep medications and herbs to help him go to sleep and stay asleep, since sleep deprivation makes all of the Lyme symptoms worse. We tried Ambien, Lunesta, Flexeril, Remeron, Restoril, Gabitril, Trazodone, as well as nutraceuticals, including valerian root, melatonin, and phosphatidylserine. He was only able to tolerate Remeron (an antidepressant, with sedating effects at the lowest dose), as it did not cause side effects and helped him to stay asleep. This helped decrease the severity of the flares.

He was also given low-dose naltrexone (LDN) with herbs such as curcumin and green tea extract to decrease inflammation. He took oral liposomal glutathione every day, since he had had a positive response to IV glutathione, and this was used in higher doses with Alka-Seltzer Gold when he had a Herxheimer flare. This would also give him some relief from his symptoms. Yet every time we tried to reintroduce any of his cystic drugs or intracellular medications for the Lyme disease, he had severe reactions, with a worsening of his symptoms. We therefore switched him over to intramuscular shots of Bicillin, a long-acting penicillin that is particularly effective in patients with persistent Lyme disease and MSIDS. He did notice marked improvement with the addition of Bicillin, and with pulsing the intracellular medications.

However, after months of trying these different regimens, although he was better, he still was not well enough to return to work. We therefore discussed starting subcutaneous B_{12} injections, for his ongoing fatigue and neuropathy, and IV therapy with intravenous Rocephin (ceftriaxone), rotating eventually through IV *Babesia* medications, such as IV Cleocin (clindamycin) for his ongoing night sweats. Chris was also started on mitochondrial support for his resistant fatigue, with nutritional supplements, including NT factor, acetyl-L-carnitine, and D-ribose. These are nutritional supplements that help to support energy production in the body.

Chris returned the next month after starting IV Rocephin. His Lyme disease symptoms were definitely starting to improve, and he felt that the mitochondrial support with NT factor was also helping: Whenever he stopped the mitochondrial support, his fatigue worsened. He had also been placed on Biaxin and doxycycline as a double intracellular regimen, along with pulsed Tindamax three days a week and Malarone for the babesiosis. This treated the cell wall, cystic, and intracellular forms of the Lyme disease, while simultaneously treating the *Babesia*. This also significantly helped; he said he felt "awesome" after four weeks, the best he had felt in the previous two years. The combination of the IV medication and years of attacking the Lyme disease were finally showing considerable progress.

Yet his *Babesia* symptoms persisted. The resistant night sweats, temperature dysregulation, and shortness of breath were intense, and he still had some ongoing symptoms of fatigue, brain fog, and joint pain. We therefore rotated his IV Rocephin after a month to IV Cleocin, a drug that is frequently used to treat babesiosis, and changed the doxycycline to Septra DS, a sulfa drug that is also useful in the treatment of resistant babesiosis and *Bartonella*.

Chris returned a month later. He had had an amazing response to the new regimen. His energy was improving, the temperature dysregulation was better, there were less frequent night sweats, his libido was finally improving (his wife, sitting next to him in the room, gave out a shout of joy with this one), the dizziness was better, and there was less peripheral nerve pain. These symptoms all improved within several days on the new regimen. Yet Chris still had an occasional significant Herxheimer flare while on these drugs. We therefore stopped all of his antibiotics and placed him on a traditional Chinese herbal protocol from Dr. Zhang instead (*Coptis*, HH, Circulation P, and AI#3).

At the follow-up visit, Chris felt the best he had in the last fifteen years. His only residual symptoms were a headache, which he attributed to his TMJ, and his good days were up to 90 percent of normal, with only occasional, mild fatigue. He no longer had any of his severe Herxheimer reactions when he was off of the antibiotics. We therefore discussed his diet and exercise program in order to build him back up, and we kept him on his adrenal and detox supplements, mitochondrial support, sleep medication, and the traditional Chinese herbal protocol, which was clearly helping him.

The keys to getting Chris better were aggressive treatment for the Lyme disease and babesiosis, getting him to sleep, treating his low adrenal function, avoiding the food allergens, stopping blood sugar swings with a hypoglycemic diet, chelating his heavy metals, mitochondrial support, detoxing him properly, and shutting down the production of inflammatory cytokines responsible for the Jarisch-Herxheimer flares. These were the essential components that led to his successful treatment. The MSIDS approach, treating multifactorial causes for his illness and simultaneously treating the three I's of Lyme disease—infection, inflammation, and immune dysfunction—was the key for getting clinical improvement and helping Chris get his life back.

TICKS CAN CARRY MORE THAN LYME

Many people who have received treatment for Lyme disease do not feel well either during treatment or once the courses of antibiotics are completed. For these patients, the Horowitz sixteen-point differential diagnostic map is the best way to determine if they are suffering from MSIDS. From there I can determine what other factors are causing my patients to remain chronically ill.

In the following chapters you will learn exactly how other illnesses can impact Lyme disease, and how Lyme bacteria can affect other medical problems you may have. First, we will explore bacterial infections that can occur simultaneously with Lyme disease, as we are finding that many ticks are carrying more than Lyme bacterial spirochetes. You'll also learn about other types of bacterial, parasitic, viral, and fungal infections that may be dormant in your system and then reawaken with Lyme exposure.

PART II

Lyme and MSIDS

FOUR

Lyme and Common Tick-Borne Bacterial Infections

The first category in the differential diagnostic map is infections. Ticks are often carrying multiple infections inside of them, which can all be transmitted simultaneously to a host—you or your patient—at the time of the tick bite. These include a broad range of bacterial, parasitic, and viral infections.

You may also unknowingly be carrying other bacterial, parasitic, viral, and fungal infections that are completely unrelated to the tick bite. These infections may be so minute that they don't affect your daily life. However, they can be reactivated or exacerbated by the Lyme bacteria. I have found that the sickest patients are usually the ones who have Lyme along with multiple other infections. Co-infections may increase the severity of symptoms in Lyme-MSIDS, in part through suppressing the immune system and preventing the body from properly fighting off these and other unrelated infections.

Patients with MSIDS are often co-infected with multiple organisms simultaneously, and the treatment approaches vary significantly for each organism. Making sure that patients are properly screened and treated for all of the co-infections, including bacterial, parasitic, viral, and fungal infections, is essential, which is why the Lyme-MSIDS questionnaire, in combination with the Horowitz sixteen-point differential diagnostic map, is crucial for creating both a testing as well as a treatment plan.

The following is a list of the most common bacterial co-infections we find with Lyme disease.

EHRLICHIA/ANAPLASMA

Many of my patients test positive for *Ehrlichia* or *Anaplasma*. These bacteria, along with babesiosis (which we will discuss in the next chapter), are some of the most common tick-borne co-infections.

Ehrlichiosis comes in many forms, including human sennetsu ehrlichiosis (HSE), human granulocytic anaplasmosis (HGA), human monocytic ehrlichiosis (HME), human ewingii ehrlichiosis (HEE), and the recently discovered human ehrlichiosis Wisconsin-Minnesota (HWME). Most of these organisms are transmitted by a specific species of hard-bodied insects called *Ixodes scapularis* ticks, but other tick-borne infections, such as HME, are transmitted by the lone star tick, *Amblyomma americanum*. This tick has also been associated with other bacterial infections such Tularemia, and Southern tick associated rash illness (STARI), and as per the Centers for Disease Control and Prevention (CDC), it is also now thought to carry a novel viral infection known as the Heartland virus. In a 2012 article published in the *New England Journal of Medicine*, the Heartland virus was found to cause an illness nearly identical to ehrlichiosis, but was unresponsive to antibiotics.

The most common symptoms for ehrlichiosis are a high fever accompanied by severe headaches, flulike symptoms, muscle pains, and fatigue in the spring, summer, or fall. It is important to clinically suspect and treat for *Ehrlichia* and *Anaplasma* in the very young and in the elderly since, like Rocky Mountain spotted fever and *Babesia*, they can be fatal in individuals who are immunocompromised.

Most patients who tested positive for *Ehrlichia* or *Anaplasma* when we tested for Lyme disease were completely unaware that they had ever had a tick bite. When properly diagnosed and treated, *Ehrlichia* or *Anaplasma* do not appear to cause the same severe chronic clinical manifestations that we see with other organisms such as *Bartonella*, *Mycoplasma*, or *Babesia*.

Ehrlichia or *Anaplasma* can be diagnosed through a combination of blood tests, including antibody titers, a complete blood count (CBC), and liver functions. The HME and HGA titers are antibodies that can be seen early on (IgM) and later in the illness (IgG). A CBC is especially useful in diagnosing *Ehrlichia/Anaplasma*, as there are specific abnormalities that can alert the clinician to the presence of *Ehrlichia* species, including a low white cell count (leukopenia), low platelet counts (thrombocytopenia), as well as elevated liver functions (AST, ALT). Intracellular colonies, called "morulae," can also be visualized under the microscope when examining white blood cells, bone marrow, and the cerebral spinal fluid (CSF) of cells infected with *Ehrlichia*.

If *Ehrlichia* is suspected, it is best to treat immediately with a tetracycline, such as doxycycline, until the blood tests return. Patients who are very young (less than eight years old) with whom tetracyclines may be ill advised, to avoid staining the teeth (some pediatricians will evaluate the risk/benefit to the patient and give a very short course of tetracyclines if necessary), or patients who are allergic to tetracyclines can use rifampin instead.

Jennifer's Walk in the Woods

Jennifer was seventeen years old, with no significant past medical history, and went to camp for the first time to work as a counselor. I received a panicked call from her parents three days after she left. Jennifer was complaining of the worst headache of her life, had flulike symptoms, severe muscle aches all over her body, overwhelming fatigue, and a fever of 102. She had not noticed a tick bite or thought to look for a rash, but she was working in wooded areas.

I advised Jennifer's parents to take her to the local emergency room and have them specifically check a CBC, to see if she had a low white cell count and platelet count, as well as check her liver functions, to see if they were elevated. I also advised them to test her for tick-borne diseases, such as Lyme disease and babesiosis, but explained to the family that these tests might return negative because she was early in the course of her illness and may not have mounted an antibody response yet. It takes time for antibodies fighting against bacterial organisms to be produced. Jennifer was experiencing symptoms after being in a wooded area for only three days, which is typically shorter than the usual time it takes to mount an antibody response.

Because of the wooded location of the camp, along with her very severe headache, severe muscle and joint pains, and high fever—flulike symptoms that are uncommon in the summertime—I strongly suspected a tick-borne bacterial illness, such as ehrlichiosis, and suggested a course of doxycycline if any of the laboratory values were abnormal, even if no other immediate cause could be found. *Ehrlichia*, like Rocky Mountain spotted fever, can be dangerous in certain individuals if not caught early.

I got a phone call from the parents the next day. They were amazed when the blood tests came back exactly as I had predicted. The ER doctor was also surprised that Jennifer had a low white cell count (2.9; normal falls between 4 and 10), low platelet count (113,000; normal is 145,000 or higher), and elevated liver functions (AST 62, ALT 76; the normal range is below 40). Jennifer had ehrlichiosis. The ER doc agreed with my suggestion and placed her on doxycycline, and within twenty-four hours her fever broke, and she was feeling much better. Jennifer has remained well, without any evidence of any other chronic tick-borne illness. *Ehrlichia* and Lyme disease can both be cured if caught early.

BARTONELLA

Bartonella henselae, or cat scratch disease, is relatively easy to diagnose and treat. It usually presents as a rash or papule (a small, red, raised bump on the skin) that progresses to a vesicular, or blistery, crusty stage, and within one to two weeks causes the regional lymph nodes to swell. Seventy-five percent of cases are thought to be mild and self-limiting. Several other species of *Bartonella*, such as *Bartonella quintana*, are caused by human lice, which are responsible for trench fever. *Bartonella bacilliformis*, which is transmitted by sand flies, causes Carrion's disease.

Doctors used to think that *Bartonella* could only be transmitted to humans through the bite or scratch of a cat. It was not until the late 1990s that *Bartonella* was considered to be a tick-borne co-infection associated with symptoms in persistent Lyme disease. Medical journal articles started to appear in 1998 and 1999 reporting on investigations of several species of *Bartonella*. One paper, published in the *Journal of Clinical Microbiology*, showed a high percentage of ticks with three simultaneous infections: *Borrelia burgdorferi*, *Ehrlichia*, and *Bartonella*. European journals were reporting that ticks in Europe were infected with *Bartonella*. But no one was certain if these findings had clinical implications.

In 1998 the *Journal of Infectious Diseases* published a report on a novel *Bartonella* species showing up not in Europe but in the midwestern United States. *Bartonella* was now being found in the white-footed mouse. In the study, 46 percent of the mice were positive for Bb by culture, 12 percent were positive for *Babesia* by PCR, and 5 percent to 10 percent were positive for *Bartonella* by culture. By 2000 and 2001, *Bartonella* was now being discussed at the yearly international lyme conferences. In 2001 an article appeared in the *Archives of Neurology*, by Eugene Eskow, demonstrating concurrent infection of the central nervous system by *Borrelia burgdorferi* and *Bartonella henselae* both in ticks and in the cerebral spinal fluid of patients presenting with neurological symptoms.

The typical manifestations of *Bartonella* taught in medical school are not the same as we usually see in patients with MSIDS. Patients with Lyme disease and overlapping *Bartonella* infections can have unusually severe neurological manifestations, including new episodes of seizures and ophthalmological problems, and they may even resemble other medical illnesses, such as sarcoidosis (inflammation of the lymph nodes). One unusual presentation is stretch marks found on the abdomen, flanks, thighs, breasts, and upper shoulders, which are often mistaken for stretch marks due to weight loss. This presentation was originally described by Dr. Martin Fried at a Lyme Disease Association conference: He reported that the rash was found in patients who tested positive for *Bartonella*. I tried biopsying the same lesions on my own patients but have never been able to get back positive PCR results for *Bartonella* or *Borrelia burgdorferi*. Regardless of whether they are due to Lyme disease itself, with *Borrelia* burrowing through the subcutaneous fat, or to *Bartonella*, they appear to be indicative of tick-borne infections. Pharyngeal crescents (red crescent–shaped lesions in the back of the throat) and pain in the soles of the feet, with an occasional positive VEGF (vascular endothelial growth factor) blood test, have also been reported in Lyme disease patients co-infected with *Bartonella*.

Bartonella can also be transmitted from a mother to a fetus. This just adds one more organism to the long, growing list of infections that we must pay attention to in women of childbearing age. By becoming cognizant of these infections, we have the opportunity to prevent miscarriages and possible disabilities.

Based on this new scientific evidence making its way into the medical literature, my office assistants Dylan and Lauren, and I, started to test my patients for *Bartonella henselae*. The problem was that the serological testing for *Bartonella* was unreliable, just as it can be for Lyme disease. Our literature review showed that the diagnosis could not be made on the basis of an IFA (immunofluorescent antibody) test alone. So we began to conduct serial PCR analyses and our own laboratory study on our very ill, treatment-resistant Lyme disease patients to determine how often *Bartonella* was present.

The two questions that we set out to answer early on in our investigations were: How accurate were the blood tests for *Bartonella*? And could we demonstrate an effective treatment regimen to treat it if we found it in our patients? I asked these questions, because as we started to do our initial studies, the basic serological tests were often negative (antibody titers, i.e., IFA/ELISA), yet patients were testing positive for *Bartonella* by DNA testing (PCR). Also, patients who were being sent to me after seeing other Lyme-literate physicians would occasionally test positive for *Bartonella* by PCR even after having undergone an extensive course of tetracyclines, antibiotics that should have been effective in killing *Bartonella*. Perhaps this organism was still alive despite an extensive course of antibiotics, just as we had seen with persistent Lyme infections. Perhaps *Bartonella* was evading the immune system and was not being killed by antibiotics that should have been effective against it.

We discovered that *Bartonella henselae* IFA and ELISA testing was positive in less than half of the patients who had evidence of Lyme disease. PCR testing was able to detect *Bartonella* in 53 percent of the patients who were seronegative in our office, and several patients had positive PCR results despite months of classical *Bartonella* antibiotic treatment regimens. This included medication courses of tetracyclines (doxycycline and minocycline), macrolides (Zithromax and Biaxin), IV cephalosporins, such as Rocephin, and quinolones (Cipro, Levaquin, or Avelox).

Therefore, several things became immediately clear. First, we couldn't rely on antibody testing but needed to do PCR testing in multiple sets for patients failing treatment. Second, we couldn't rely on a single-drug regimen to treat *Bartonella*. The one remaining mystery was: Which specific patient symptoms were indicative of *Bartonella*? Going back to the medical literature, a medical detective could use several clinical clues to try and ferret out whether *Bartonella* was present:

- Did patients have an atypical manifestation of Lyme disease?

- Had they failed classical courses of antibiotics?

- Were there resistant neurological symptoms, such as headaches, encephalopathy with severe cognitive dysfunction, a new episode of seizures, or a radiculitis, myelitis, or vasculitis (inflammation in the nerves coming out of the spine, or spinal cord, or inflammation in the blood vessels)?

- Were there unusual ophthalmological manifestations, such as a neuroretinitis (inflammation of the retina) and vision loss, branch retinal artery occlusions, an oculoglandular syndrome with pre-auricular lymph nodes (inflammation of the eyes and lymph nodes in front of the ears), and/or conjunctivitis (pink eye)?

- Was there a systemic inflammatory disorder resembling sarcoidosis with associated painful red nodules (erythema nodosum), arthritis, osteolytic lesions (destruction of the bones), and a lymphomalike pathology (hard, swollen lymph nodes)?

Based on this list of possible symptoms, we began screening patients for *Bartonella* as part of their co-infection workup. I designed a study using two intracellular antibiotics simultaneously, as it became apparent that one antibiotic was insufficient to treat it. We screened fifty Lyme patients for co-infections with *Ehrlichia*, *Babesia microti*, *Mycoplasma*, and *Bartonella henselae*. The patients then were divided into two groups: one of which had a *Bartonella* titer and/or a PCR that was positive, with evidence of Lyme disease and other co-infections, and one group whose *Bartonella* titer and PCR were negative, with Lyme disease alone or with other co-infections. Each of these groups were further divided into two groups: one took a low-dose tetracycline regimen, and the other was assigned a higher-dose tetracycline regimen, with hydroxychloroquine and a quinolone. The dependent variables to evaluate symptoms both before and after treatment were scored, and patients reported improvement, on a scale ranging from 0 percent to 100 percent.

Our results, which we presented at the 16th International Scientific

Conference on Lyme Disease, in June 2003 in Hartford, Connecticut, demonstrated that patients who had serological evidence of *Bartonella* by titer and/or PCR had a 25 percent greater improvement on quality of life measures such as their Karnofsky score and self-reported scores with combination intracellular therapy than patients with no prior evidence of *Bartonella* exposure. The study also showed that several patients who had previously not responded to classical regimens for Lyme disease had a remarkable improvement in their symptoms with the addition of a quinolone drug such as Cipro. Bottom line: Two drugs are better than one, especially where intracellular bugs are concerned.

John Had *Bartonella*

John was a sixty-one-year-old male with a past medical history of benign prostatic hyperplasia (enlarged prostate), and he had had a growth removed from his right eye. In January 2001, he began developing progressive bilateral weakness of his lower extremities with stiffness in his legs. He subsequently was unable to walk and came to our office several months later in a wheelchair. He'd been diagnosed by a local neurologist as having transverse myelitis (an inflammation of the spinal cord). His brain MRI was normal and did not show any evidence of demyelinating lesions, which would typically appear in a patient who had MS. A spinal tap revealed a slight increase in total protein, one oligoclonal band, and a slight increase in myelin basic proteins (proteins found in the spinal fluid in increased amounts in diseases such as MS and Lyme disease). In other words, John didn't present with any evidence linking his symptoms to an autoimmune disorder. His white blood cell count from his spinal fluid was normal, as was his glucose and Gram stain. The Gram stain uses special dyes to look under the microscope and identify any evidence of bacterial infection. All these tests were negative, ruling out an apparent infection in his central nervous system.

We ruled out a B_{12} deficiency, syphilis, Lupus, and MS. A serum Lyme antibody test was negative. John said that he couldn't feel any sensations in his lower extremities, and this was confirmed by a neurological test (the somatosensory evoked potential), which measures nerve conduction of the peripheral nerves.

His neurologist gave him IV Medrol to decrease the inflammation in the spinal cord, along with oral steroids with Zanaflex for muscle spasms, but John had no improvement. He did not report any other significant symptoms, including fevers, sweats, chills, joint pain, or cognitive difficulties. John's social and family histories were unremarkable. His physical exam was significant only for his neurological symptoms. He was alert and oriented, and his cranial nerves were intact, but he was paraplegic and unable to elicit any movements from his lower extremities.

We sent off labs to evaluate him for Lyme disease and co-infections. His Lyme IgM Western blot was CDC positive, his IgG Western blot was CDC positive, and he had positive titers for HME and babesiosis, a negative *Bartonella* IFA, and a *Bartonella* PCR that was positive through Medical Diagnostic Laboratories.

John had come into our practice at a time when I had just recently expanded my complementary medical staff. I had a chiropractor, massage therapist, yoga teacher, psychologist, and acupuncturist on staff. We had recently employed a Chinese medical doctor, Dr. Lin, who had practiced as a surgeon in China. She was now practicing Chinese medicine in the United States and, specifically, was using a different form of acupuncture/acupressure and Qi Gong than most acupuncturists were used to employing. My spiritual teacher had let me know that it would be good to have her work at our center, so I gave her a room in the complementary wing. When we first met, and we discussed referring patients who would be appropriate, she said: "Oh, I fix everything."

I asked, "You fix everything?"

She said, "Yes, I fix everything."

Now that is a pretty bold statement for any health-care practitioner. Here was John, a paraplegic who had been unable to walk for the previous six months. Classical medical treatment with the local neurologist had failed, and I was seeing him for the first time for a history and physical and blood tests. I asked him whether he would be open to doing a trial of acupuncture, and he agreed. As I wheeled him down the hallway, I thought to myself: "Okay, let's see her fix this!!!"

Dr. Lin knocked on my door a half hour later. "Come see," she said.

I walked into her room, and there was John, lying on her acupuncture table. She said, "Okay, you can lift your legs now." He had about sixty acupuncture needles sticking out of both legs. On command, John lifted his right leg six inches off the exam table. Then John lifted his left leg. I shook my head in disbelief. She fixed everything, I thought. Dr. Lin provided one more example of how complementary and alternative medicine techniques can sometimes be very effective medicine. Acupuncture and Chinese medicine are clearly useful adjuncts in certain treatment-resistant patients, even though we may not fully understand why it works.

John was started on doxycycline with a traditional Chinese herbal regimen of allicin, *Artemisia*, Circulation P, and *Cordyceps* that would address his Lyme disease and *Bartonella*. He returned one month later. He still had complaints of heaviness in his legs, but he was now able to evoke a slight movement bilaterally in his lower extremities. He had no complaints of Jarisch-Herxheimer flares on the antibiotics. I added Cipro to the doxycycline to cover *Bartonella*. The doxy would have covered his *Ehrlichia*, and he didn't complain of any active day or night sweats, so we just left him on *Artemisia* to cover the low-level *Babesia* titer. I set him up to get a PICC line placed and started him on IV Rocephin therapy. By the time the line was in, he was already feeling stronger with the *Bartonella* treatment. Within three days of IV Rocephin as a cell wall drug and doxycycline with Cipro as a double intracellular regimen, he started to increase the movement of his toes and was now able to lift his legs two to three inches off of the bed. Then I ordered active physical therapy. By September 2002, he had been on six weeks of the IV Rocephin. He now had increased strength in his lower extremities and was able to transfer from his bed to his wheelchair on his own, and even stand in place for five minutes. He also walked a few steps with a walker for the first time since the beginning of his illness.

We rotated the doxycycline and Cipro to Mepron with Zithromax plus Septra DS, since his progress was still slow. The Mepron would cover the *Babesia*, and the Zithromax and Septra combination is an excellent regimen that helps with *Babesia* and *Bartonella*. After one month, John was up to walking ten feet with a walker. His chief complaint was stiffness in his right hip and the ongoing weakness of his lower extremities. We therefore changed back to the doxy/Cipro combination and added Plaquenil, which helps to alkalize the intracellular compartment and may help intracellular drugs to be more effective.

By the fifth month of treatment, John was able to walk forty-five feet with a walker, and on one occasion, he walked sixty-four feet uninterrupted. He still had balance problems and bladder irritability, but his physical examination showed significant increase in strength in his lower extremities. He was now up to a motor strength of two to three out of five of the lower extremities bilaterally. Repeat *Bartonella* PCRs were negative. The IV line was removed, and John continued to improve on oral medication.

MYCOPLASMA

Thanks to the work of Dr. Eva Sapi at the University of New Haven, there are now many species of *Mycoplasma* identified in the same ticks carrying Lyme. We are now finding ticks carrying *Mycoplasma pneumoniae*, *Mycoplasma genitalium*, and *Mycoplasma fermentans*, the latter organism the one responsible for Gulf War syndrome, and occasionally these organisms are also found in patients with Lyme-MSIDS. It is difficult to know the exact role that *Mycoplasma* species are playing in these patients with Lyme disease, since the blood tests are unreliable and the signs and symptoms overlap other diseases. Therefore, we often perform both Immunofluorescent Antibodies (IFA) and Serial PCRs (polymerase chain reaction) blood tests to check for different *Mycoplasma* species.

It is possible that *Mycoplasma* species are exacerbating the symptoms of patients with MSIDS, especially for those who present with autoimmune manifestations. *Mycoplasmas* have been shown to interact with B-lymphocytes, one of the primary immune cells in the body, which secretes antibodies in response to infection. There are five different types of immunoglobulin-antibody molecules produced by plasma cells and B-cells: IgA, IgM, IgG, IgD, and IgE antibodies. *Mycoplasma* species may cause these B-cells to be overstimulated, promoting autoimmune reactions and rheumatoid diseases. This subsequently leads to symptoms of increased fatigue and joint and muscle pain, and in part is due to *Mycoplasma*'s ability to increase the production of proinflammatory cytokines such as Il-1, Il-2, and Il-6, which cause those symptoms. Since *Mycoplasma* has been found in the joint tissues of patients with rheumatological diseases, this strongly suggests their pathogenic involvement. It is therefore interesting to speculate about whether the disease-modifying drug regimens given by rheumatologists to treat rheumatoid arthritis (DMARD, which stands for disease modifying antirheumatic drugs), such as Plaquenil and minocycline to decrease inflammation, are in fact having their primary mechanism of action by treating Lyme disease, *Mycoplasma*, and other intracellular co-infections, all of which may be increasing inflammation and cytokine production.

We did a retrospective study in our medical office years ago, looking at the prevalence and role of *Mycoplasma fermentans* in our MSIDS patients, since this organism has been associated with Gulf War syndrome, and its symptoms overlap those of Lyme-MSIDS. The study demonstrated that *Mycoplasma* may be a chronic persistent infection in some patients, just like Lyme disease, *Babesia*, and *Bartonella*. Using a PCR analysis in our patient population, we found that despite long-term treatment for *Mycoplasma* (up to almost one year), using either macrolides, tetracyclines, or quinolones, which should have been effective against *Mycoplasma*, all twenty-seven patients analyzed showed evidence of persistent *Mycoplasma fermentans* infection by PCR analysis after an average length of antibiotic treatment of 10¾ months. The average patient received 6½ months of macrolide therapy, ¼ month of quinolone therapy, and four months of doxycycline therapy. No significant difference was found among the different antibiotic regimens (Zithromax, Biaxin, Dynabac, Cipro, Avelox, and doxycycline). Ongoing symptoms at the end of the study included fatigue (96 percent), joint pain (93 percent), cognitive difficulties (78 percent), and headaches (33 percent).

Mycoplasmas are intracellular infections that can persist despite long-term therapy. This organism could explain in part why patients who are infected with Lyme disease and tested positive for *Mycoplasma* continue to complain of persistent symptoms. *Mycoplasma* has also been shown to drive autoimmune reactions and increase cytokine production, just as Lyme disease can. The major histocompatibility complex (MHC) are genes and gene products that have a strong association with certain disease processes, especially autoimmune diseases. MHC molecules, located on the surface of cells, help the immune system differentiate between its own cells and that of invaders. These surface molecules resemble, in part, the molecules of invasive pathogens like *Mycoplasma*, and under certain circumstances the immune system gets confused and attacks itself, the classic autoimmune response. We see this in some Lyme patients who test positive for human leukocyte antigen (HLA) DR 4 on blood tests. These HLA markers are part of the MHC complex. Lyme patients who are HLA DR 4 positive have particularly strong autoimmune reactions when they are coinfected with *Mycoplasma*. Any patient with an atypical autoimmune disorder should therefore be checked for the presence of *Borrelia* and *Mycoplasma*.

CHLAMYDIA

Chlamydia is an intracellular infection like *Mycoplasma* and is treated with similar intracellular drugs. Ticks aren't known to carry chlamydia, and not all chlamydia is sexually transmitted. There are other forms of chlamydia, such as chlamydia TWAR, that causes upper respiratory infections, and dormant chlamydial infections can be reactivated when Lyme and other tick-borne co-infections are present. Chlamydia is important to keep in mind because of its association with oligoarthritis (arthritis in multiple joints), and because it can exacerbate Lyme symptoms. There are several scientific references implying a causative role for chlamydia in Lyme disease patients with arthritis who are coinfected, so chlamydia joins the list of bacteria which might be causing overlapping symptoms in our Lyme disease patients.

There is also fascinating research showing that the combination of heavy metals with intracellular bacteria, such as chlamydia, may also be contributing to the severe arthritis seen in MSIDS patients. Heavy metals such as mercury have already been reported in the scientific literature to cause arthritis, drive autoimmune reactions, and create free radicals and oxidative stress that can turn on nuclear factor kappa b (NFKappaB), a switch in the nucleus of the cell that creates cytokines, the inflammatory molecules. Heavy metals can also increase arthritis in patients co-infected with chlamydia. Both our own clinical experience and the scientific literature support testing and treating Lyme patients for multiple intracellular co-infections such as chlamydia and detoxing them for heavy metals.

RICKETTSIAL INFECTIONS

Rickettsia are bacteria that live within host cells like chlamydia and *Mycoplasma*, but some rickettsial organisms (*R. typhi* and *C. burnetii*) can also survive for extended periods of time outside the host and remain extremely infectious. The most common rickettsial infections that we see in our clinical practice are Rocky Mountain spotted fever (RMSF, *R. rickettsii*), typhus (*R. typhi*), and Q fever (*Coxiella burnetii*). Rickettsia such as RMSF are transmitted by several different species of ticks, including the lone star tick (*Amblyomma americanum*), the wood tick (*Dermatocenter andersoni*), and the dog tick (*Dermatocenter variabilis*). It is rare that we see an acute case of RMSF due to *Rickettsia rickettsii* where we live in New York, but quite often we pick up antibody titers in patients who have been exposed. RMSF can be fatal in the very young or the very elderly, who are immunocompromised. It is therefore essential to place the patients immediately on a tetracycline, such as doxycycline, if there is any clinical suspicion of acute exposure to rickettsia.

Unfortunately, the early clinical presentations of this bacterial infection can be nonspecific. Patients may have fever, nausea, vomiting, severe headaches, and muscle pains, which can be commonly mistaken for a flulike syndrome. The classic red spotted petechial rash—tiny red hemorrhagic spots from blood vessels that have broken—that can appear on the palms and soles of the feet are only present 50 percent to 80 percent of the time, and may not be present until after the sixth day of exposure. Therefore, finding the rash as a means to diagnose Rocky Mountain spotted fever is not a reliable clinical sign. The CBC may present with some of the same abnormalities seen in ehrlichiosis, such as low white cell counts, low platelet counts, and elevated liver function, which is fortunate, since both bacterial infections, although caused by different organisms, are treated effectively with tetracyclines.

Q fever is another rickettsial infection; it's caused by *Coxiella burnetii*. It can similarly present with nonspecific symptoms, and in 50 percent of the cases there are no signs of an acute clinical illness. Patients can present with symptoms that could be confused with an acute viral illness, such as high fevers, chills and sweats, severe headaches, and muscle pains. However, Q fever can also present with a myriad of diverse symptoms, and therefore could be considered as one of the great imitators, like Lyme disease and syphilis. Coxiella can present as: hepatitis, with associated nausea, vomiting, and diarrhea; pneumonia, with a nonproductive cough; meningoencephalitis, with confusion; myelitis, with an inflammation of the spinal cord; and even as Guillain-Barré syndrome (GBS). One of the most troubling symptoms is that it can cause a chronic endocarditis, an infection of the heart valves, which can occur one to twenty years after the initial infection. Any patient with unresolved Lyme disease who presents with any of the above symptoms and has associated elevations in liver functions and/or a heart murmur must be checked for Q fever. We have occasionally had to send patients for echocardiograms and/or transesophageal echocardiograms to rule out a coxiella-induced endocarditis. It is reasonable to seek opinions by both an infectious disease consultant and a cardiologist regarding the possible diagnosis and treatment, since this can be an especially serious manifestation of a tick-borne illness.

Q fever is commonly transmitted from domestic animals, especially cattle, sheep, and goats. Coxiella can produce a mild infection in these animals, and the organisms can infect their placenta and mammary glands, transmitting the organism in infected milk and meat products. Coxiella can also survive in the environment in dust and soils on animal farms, so that a highly infectious aerosol can be found around infected animals. To make matters worse, Q fever is also a bioterrorist agent. I have had many conversations with various state and local health departments regarding Q fever titers that have come back positive for my patients: We needed to quickly determine whether these results were the first sign of an impending bioterrorist threat, or if the patient had been on an animal farm and/or drank unpasteurized goat milk, or simply received a tick bite. The implications are obviously quite different!

The diagnosis of Q fever is made using blood antibody testing, called phase I and phase II titers. These are compared in a ratio. High phase I : phase II titers indicate an acute infection; high phase II : phase I titers indicate a chronic infection, and this is seen in patients with chronic Q fever, and especially in chronic Q fever endocarditis, where coxiella has infected the heart valves. Over the years we have had at least forty to fifty positive Q fever titers, and several of them did show a fourfold rise in the phase II titers consistent with possible chronic Q fever and a chronic endocarditis. Therefore, rickettsial infections such as Q fever join the ranks of intracellular co-infections that can persist chronically in the body and may require long-term double intracellular antibiotic therapy.

The treatment for chronic Q fever endocarditis is several years of doxycycline and quinolone or doxycycline and rifampin with Plaquenil to alkalize the intracellular compartment and make these antibiotics more effective. In fact, one of first the scientific articles that supported the use of Plaquenil for treating intracellular infections, published in 1992, was regarding Q fever.

TICK-BORNE RELAPSING FEVER:
BORRELIA HERMSII AND *BORRELIA MIYAMOTOI*

Up until now we have been discussing tick-borne diseases transmitted by hard-bodied ticks (family: Ixodidae), but there are also tick-borne infections in the United States that can be caused by soft-bodied ticks (family: Argasidae). Tick-borne relapsing fever (TBRF) is caused by the bite of the fast-feeding soft tick, *Ornithodoros hermsii*, and the organism responsible for TBRF is *Borrelia hermsii*, a cousin of the Lyme disease spirochete, *Borrelia burgdorferi*. Since soft ticks remain attached for only fifteen to twenty minutes while feeding, and the bites are usually painless, most people are unaware of ever having been bitten. Infection can also take place from contamination of the wound or skin by tick secretions or from exposure to body lice that carry the organism (then known as louse-borne relapsing fever). Tick-borne relapsing fever is found throughout most of the world but is endemic in Colorado, California, and the Pacific Northwest, as well as in parts of Central and South America, Asia, and most of Africa. These soft ticks may survive for twenty years without feeding, and they remain infectious for up to ten years following infection. Infected ticks pass the spirochetal organism onto their offspring.

Just as one of the hallmarks of Lyme disease is that the symptoms tend to come and go, the natural course of TBRF is that there are periods of high fevers (101.3 degrees Fahrenheit to 104 degrees Fahrenheit), with drenching sweats and shaking chills and an associated headache, fatigue, and joint and muscle pains that can last for several days (with associated large numbers of spirochetes found in the blood), and then resolve, only to return in a relapsing fashion every several days. Associated symptoms can include a loss of appetite, dry cough, abdominal pains, nausea, vomiting, neck stiffness (meningismus), light sensitivity (photophobia), and neurological complications, including confusion with an encephalitis, facial nerve palsy, unilateral hearing loss, iritis (inflammation in the iris of the eye), peripheral neuropathy, and neuropsychiatric disturbances. These symptoms will relapse as *B. hermsii* rearranges its DNA on its outer surface. This creates different antigenic markers known as "variable major proteins," which allows it to evade recognition by the immune system. This antigenic variation allows it to hide in different organs of the body, during periods without a fever, and relapse occurs in a cyclic fashion when the new serotype (bacteria with new cell surface antigens) reenters the bloodstream and causes bacteremia (bacteria in the bloodstream).

Clinical signs that accompany the infections with relapsing fevers (which may last from twelve hours to seventeen days) may include a variety of skin rashes. These can include a flat reddish rash (macular eruption), diffuse petechiae throughout the body (small red spots due to minor hemorrhaging in the skin), or erythema multiforme (target-shaped lesions, not to be confused with the bull's-eye rash in Lyme disease). The liver can be enlarged, as well as the spleen, and liver functions could be elevated, including signs of obstruction with jaundice secondary to liver congestion. Severe complications include potentially fatal disseminated intravascular coagulation (DIC), when blood coagulation factors and platelets are used up, occasionally causing the patient to hemorrhage (including strokes with cerebral hemorrhage) and become hypotensive (low blood pressure), with cardiac dysfunction and arrhythmias secondary to injury to the myocardium (myocarditis). In rare cases, acute respiratory distress syndrome (ARDS) has been reported, which also can be fatal.

Like Lyme disease, TBRF can also affect pregnant women, and it can result in fetal death and spontaneous abortion, or premature birth with perinatal sickness. Fetal death is probably caused by DIC, due to the low platelet counts and hemorrhage in the uterus that can result from it.

The diagnosis of TBRF is confirmed by a Wright-Giemsa stain, with paired acute and convalescent antibody titers by EIA and IFA (we compare the enzyme immunoassay/indirect immunofluorescent antibodies in early and late stages of the disease). Western immunoblots, culture, and PCRs as well as monoclonal antibodies may also help in establishing the diagnosis.

We have had many patients in our practice with Lyme disease from *Borrelia burgdorferi* test positive for antibodies against *Borrelia hermsii*. Since many patients recover from the illness either with or without antibiotic treatment, this may indicate either a larger spread of the illness than has been recognized or false positive titers for relapsing fever, as these patients often do not present with the appropriate clinical picture.

Patients with symptoms of a meningitis or encephalitis should also use IV Rocephin (ceftriaxone), as the brain may serve as a reservoir for *Borrelia*.

Other relapsing fever spirochetes, such as *Borrelia miyamotoi*, that are found in hard-bodied ticks can also present with similar signs and symptoms (high fevers and relapsing febrile illness). *Borrelia miyamotoi* has been reported to cause relapsing fever and Lyme disease–like symptoms in Russia, Western Europe, and the United States: a meningoencephalitis (inflammation in the brain and meningeal sac surrounding the brain and spinal cord), possibly with an erythema migrans–type rash in up to 9 percent of patients. Since *B. miyamotoi* infection is now found in 1 percent to 16 percent of ticks worldwide (*Ixodes persulcatus* in Russia, *Ixodes ricinus* in Western Europe, and *Ixodes scapularis* in the United States), patients with the appropriate clinical picture need to be considered for relapsing fever from either *Borrelia hermsii* or *Borrelia miyamotoi* as well.

Since there is no standard diagnostic test for *B. miyamotoi* at this time, and the organism is transmitted transovarially to larvae (6 percent to 73 percent), increasing its prevalence, many patients with presumed Lyme disease who test negative on standard tests are probably infected with either *B. miyamotoi* alone, or are co-infected with both species.

TICK PARALYSIS

Tick paralysis (TP) is a potentially lethal tick-borne bacterial infection. It can be caused by some four hundred different tick species, including the same ticks that transmit Rocky Mountain spotted fever, such as the Rocky Mountain wood tick, the American dog tick, and occasionally the lone star tick, the Eastern black-legged tick, and the Western black-legged tick.

Symptoms can include a nonspecific viral-like illness with malaise and weakness, followed by a neurotoxic phase in which the one who is affected will be unable to sit up and walk without help (an acute ataxia, the lack of coordination of muscular movements), with the paralysis progressing upward from the lower extremities, causing the muscles to lose function. These symptoms are caused by salivary neurotoxins secreted by the ticks leading to a paralysis of the muscles that starts with the lower extremities yet leaves sensory functioning (feeling) intact.

Unfortunately, this clinical presentation is most often confused with Guillain-Barré syndrome, which presents in a similar fashion. This confusion may lead to unnecessary therapies, such as plasmapheresis (a plasma exchange, which removes the patient's plasma from their blood, treats it, and returns it to the circulation) that is commonly used in GBS. However, this will not be effective in tick paralysis.

Instead, the first line of treatment is to remove the tick from the body (often found in children on the head and scalp). If the tick is not removed, the patient may die from respiratory complications. Proper and prompt tick removal is therefore necessary, as the fatality rate for TP has been reported to be up to 6 percent in retrospective case studies. When properly diagnosed and treated by prompt tick removal, full neurological recovery can take place within one to two days.

STARI (SOUTHERN TICK-ASSOCIATED RASH ILLNESS)

Although most EM and bull's-eye-type rashes are due to Lyme disease, there are other rashes that resemble Lyme disease but are not caused by *Borrelia burgdorferi*, as we saw with *Borrelia miyamotoi*. Southern tick-associated rash illness (STARI), also known as Master's disease (named after Dr. Ed Masters, a physician in Missouri who first described this clinical presentation), is another one of them. They are indistinguishable from the ones seen in early Lyme disease but have not been proven to lead to the same long-term arthritic and neurological complications in most patients. Long-term follow-up of patients is lacking in some of the published scientific studies, however, and there are patients who do complain of long-term symptoms after getting the diagnosis of STARI. This has led some patients in the southern United States to disagree with the CDC, so further research is desperately needed to determine the cause of their chronic symptoms.

The cause of STARI has not yet been identified, but it can be transmitted by the bite of one of the ticks occasionally responsible for Rocky Mountain spotted fever (the lone star tick, *Amblyomma americanum*). Many patients, as those with RMSF, similarly improve with a tetracycline antibiotic treatment. There is no reliable blood test for STARI to aid in the diagnosis, so patients should be treated as if they have contracted early Lyme disease to prevent any possible long-term complications.

TULAREMIA

This tick-borne illness has classically been associated with living in the country and/or being exposed to rabbits. It can also be acquired through several other means: the bite of a deerfly; inhaling aerosolized bacteria; or exposure to infected rabbits or ingesting contaminated rabbit meat. Of course, close contacts with rabbits are rare for most of us, unless one is a hunter, a chef, or enjoys eating specialty Belgian and French food (*lievre à la bière* is one of my favorites!).

Tularemia is caused by an intracellular bacteria, *Francisella tularensis*. The symptoms may vary in severity and presentation, based on the virulence, dose, and site of contact. Nonspecific initial symptoms are reminiscent of a viral-type illness, as with other tick-borne infections, such as fevers, chills, body aches, runny nose, sore throat, and headache. As with Q fever, it also can present with atypical symptoms reminiscent of pneumonia, or mimic a gastrointestinal infection (the typhoidal form), with nausea, vomiting, and diarrhea. It can even occasionally present with sepsis, a potentially fatal blood-borne infection. Some of the most classical presentations of tularemia, however, are the ulceroglandular form (ulcers on the skin, with enlarged lymph nodes) and oculoglandular presentations (eye symptoms such as conjunctivitis with enlarged lymph nodes). The ulceroglandular form may happen when tularemia is contracted handling an infected animal, and an ulcer forms on the hands where the animal was touched, also causing regional lymph nodes to enlarge. The oculoglandular form can occur when the patient touches their eye with a contaminated finger. These are the most classic clinical presentations.

Steven Had Tularemia

Steven was a forty-year-old male who recently came to my medical office from Georgia. He had been sick for the previous four years; his history included hypertension, hyperlipidemia (elevated cholesterol), and weight gain, and he complained of severe fatigue, headaches, loss of libido, joint and muscle pains, and memory and concentration problems. He was so severely ill that he was unable to work at his profession as a chef. He also recently had been diagnosed with retroperitoneal fibrosis of unknown cause, a disease in which his internal organs were being compressed by an inflammatory process, causing him to go into temporary renal failure that required a stent placed in his ureters (the connection between the kidneys and the bladder) to keep the flow of urine open. This was associated with significantly enlarged lymph nodes in his groin as well as ulcers all over his lower extremities that were extremely painful. Once one ulcer would heal up another one would appear. The doctors at a nearby prestigious university hospital had been unable to identify a cause for his symptoms. He had been seen by his primary care doctor as well as multiple subspecialists, including a rheumatologist, a dermatologist, and a gastroenterologist, and the biopsy of his lymph nodes and ulcers, the cultures of the ulcers, and a GI evaluation failed to reveal a cause for his multiple symptoms. He was initially diagnosed with inflammatory bowel disease, with the ulcers ostensibly representing a case of pyoderma gangrenosum, a painful skin lesion characteristic of ulcerative colitis. However, no inflammation could be found on a colonoscopy, so his ulcers and severe symptomatology remained a mystery.

I spent four hours in our initial consultation going through the Horowitz Lyme-MSIDS questionnaire as well as the voluminous records that he brought in from his prior doctors. They had been quite complete in their evaluations, and I was not sure that I was going to be able to solve his mystery. His symptoms of severe fatigue, headaches, and memory difficulties at forty years old, with migratory joint pain, sounded like Lyme disease, and his unusual night sweats could certainly have been babesiosis. However, neither would account for his enlarged lymph nodes and ulcers. I reviewed his social history in detail again. Not only was he a chef, but he regularly prepared rabbit, and one of the steps for making this dish was skinning them. It was possible that Steven had handled an infected rabbit and/or was bit by a tick carrying Lyme and babesiosis, and then by a tick carrying tularemia, although a single tick could have been carrying all three organisms. I hurriedly called in my support staff to look at their first classic case of tularemia!

Steven also tested positive for Lyme disease, babesiosis, low adrenal function, and had a very low testosterone level, below 200 (hormonal disorders that would contribute to his fatigue); he also had metabolic syndrome, which was indicated by a slightly elevated HbA1c of 5.7 (elevated blood sugars and cholesterol, which increased his cardiovascular risk). He started a course of antibiotics that included Plaquenil, doxycycline, and rifampin, with intramuscular (IM) bicillin injections for his bacterial infections and high-dose Malarone with artemisia for his babesiosis (although the rifampin is helpful for the tularemia, it can lower the drug levels of Malarone, so higher doses were used). He was then switched to IV Rocephin with Plaquenil, Mepron, Zithromax, and Septra and noticed significant improvement in his symptoms. His ulcers completely cleared up, his retroperitoneal fibrosis improved, and his lymph nodes came down in size.

I have only had three patients test positive for tularemia over the years, and it presents a significant clinical dilemma when the test returns positive, since IV gentamicin and IV streptomycin are some of the drugs of choice, which can have significant side effects, such as ototoxicity (hearing loss), if not used correctly.

BRUCELLOSIS

Human brucellosis is an intracellular bacterial infection caused by various strains of Brucella (Brucella melitensis, Brucella abortus, Brucella suis, and Brucella canis), although most human disease is due to B. melitensis. It is a rare infectious disease that can present with nonspecific clinical symptomatology in patients, such as fever, sweats, headaches, cough, and arthralgias (joint pain), and GI symptoms that include diarrhea and constipation. It can be transmitted by a tick, but human infection most commonly results from the ingestion of infected animal tissue or milk products, or through skin wounds during contact with freshly killed animal tissues, which meat-packing workers can experience, or with ingestion of infected milk, as with Q fever. Over 90 percent of patients will experience chills, drenching sweats and fevers, along with weakness and general malaise. The most distinguishing characteristic is that over half the patients experience significant weight loss, usually averaging up to fifteen to twenty pounds. The most common signs, apart from high fevers, are lymphadenopathy (swollen lymph nodes) and hepatosplenomegaly (an enlarged liver and spleen), which we can also see in severe cases of babesiosis.

Brucella can present as one of the great imitators, as it can also cause multiple pulmonary complications, osteomyelitis (infections of the bones), urinary tract infections, optic neuritis (inflammation of the optic nerve) with a host of eye complications, including keratitis, uveitis, and retinopathy (inflammation of the cornea iris/uvea and retina) and can even present with a meningitis or encephalitis, or an endocarditis, as we have seen with Q fever. According to Dr. Garth Nicolson's 2005 research, which was published in the *Journal of Chronic Fatigue Syndrome*, *Brucella* infections have also been found to occur in up to 10 percent of chronic fatigue syndrome patients, especially those living in rural areas, and in some patients *Brucella* infections occur simultaneously with *Mycoplasma* infections, increasing the severity of the illness.

Treatment is similar to the treatment for tularemia, using gentamicin, tetracyclines with or without streptomycin, and tetracyclines with rifampin, especially in cases with meningoencephalitis. All antimicrobial regimens need to be continued for at least six weeks' time, and relapses are common, as with many of the other tick-borne illnesses we have been discussing, if treatment does not begin early in the course of the illness.

Linda's Night Sweats Were Not Menopausal

Linda came to my medical office in January 2007, when she was thirty years old, with the chief complaint of several years of fatigue, intermittent joint and muscle pain, headaches, memory and concentration problems, occasional chills, and drenching night sweats. She had been diagnosed with Lyme disease by another physician and came to see me for a second opinion regarding her symptoms, which had persisted despite one year of antibiotics. Her past medical history was significant for frequent foreign travel, and she had lived in Mexico for several years as a child before her family moved to the United States, having had several "nonspecific infections" while she was there.

I reviewed the laboratory work done by her prior physicians. They had done a chest X-ray, to rule out tuberculosis and lymphoma, but no one had ordered a *Babesia* or *Brucella* titer for her occasional drenching sweats and resistant fatigue. Her thyroid functions were normal, and she was having normal menstrual cycles, ruling out other common hormonal causes of sweats. I sent off both *Babesia* IFA and *Babesia* FISH tests to IGeneX laboratory in California, and a *Brucella* IFA to Quest laboratories. Both tests came back positive. Linda had both infections, explaining her resistant symptoms.

I treated her babesiosis with Mepron, Zithromax, Septra DS, Plaquenil, and nystatin for the first month. When Linda returned, some of her symptoms had clearly improved. The sweats were less frequent and intense, and her fatigue, muscle and joint pain, and memory problems were beginning to show signs of improvement. We then tried her on a classic cell wall, cystic, and intracellular drug regimen to treat her Lyme disease and babesiosis, with Omnicef, Plaquenil, and Zithromax, and rotated Mepron to Malarone, since the sweats had decreased.

She had only minimal improvement, however, when she came in the following month. We discussed putting her on a classic double intracellular drug regimen that would treat her Lyme disease and brucellosis. We rotated her to doxycycline and Plaquenil, with rifampin, and left her on this regimen for the next six months, since every month she was feeling better and better. After one year of treatment, in total, and several rotations of antibiotics, she was almost 100 percent back to normal. We stopped the antibiotics and rotated her onto Samento and Banderol, an herbal regimen we have found effective in treating Lyme disease. She has remained well now for the last several years, with intermittent flare-ups of her symptoms which are manageable with natural therapies.

TREATING LYME DISEASE WITH BACTERIAL CO-INFECTIONS

When patients come to see me complaining of the symptoms associated with Lyme disease, the medical detective in me assumes from years of experience that there is another underlying problem, or several problems, and that they all have to be treated. If testing confirms that these patients have *Borrelia* as well as one or multiple bacterial co-infections, there are certain basic rules I keep in mind regarding treatment. First, I must design regimens that hit as many of these organisms simultaneously as possible. If you are under attack from multiple sources, it is always best to have multiple defensive strategies.

Second, I must monitor the patient's clinical response to determine the direction of the treatment. I have found that thirty days of treatment is adequate in up to 80 percent of cases in determining whether or not the patient will respond to a specific regimen. Therefore, I consider rotating the regimen after one month if a particular treatment does not appear to be working. The only exception would be severe Jarisch-Herxheimer flares with a specific therapy, which will confound the clinical presentation and make it seem as if the therapy is not working. Often when the patient stops taking antibiotics, and the classic Jarisch-Herxheimer reactions resolve, their symptoms will improve.

There is no one treatment regimen that is universally effective in patients with Lyme-MSIDS. Examples of possible combinations are listed in the following table, with more details, including dosages, listed in the appendix. These combinations work on a variety of intracellular organisms, including *Ehrlichia*, *Mycoplasma*, chlamydia, and rickettsial infections such as Rocky Mountain spotted fever, Q-fever, *Brucella*, and others.

COMBINATION ANTIBIOTIC REGIMENS FOR TREATING INTRACELLULAR BACTERIAL INFECTIONS IN MSIDS

- Plaquenil/ doxycycline/rifampin/nystatin
- Plaquenil/doxycycline/Zithromax/nystatin
- Plaquenil/doxycycline/Levaquin/nystatin
- Plaquenil/Zithromax/Septra/nystatin
- Plaquenil/Zithromax/rifampin/nystatin
- Plaquenil/rifampin/Factive/nystatin
- Plaquenil/rifampin/Factive/tetracyclines (doxycycline) /nystatin

Single antibiotic therapies are often insufficient in patients who are multiply co-infected. Patients will often still test positive for many of these bacterial co-infections and remain ill, despite months of single antibiotic treatment. We have had tremendous success in MSIDS patients with chronic resistant symptoms using these types of combination therapies.

FIVE

Lyme and Other Co-infections: Parasitic, Viral, and Fungal Infections

arasitic infections, such as *Babesia* (malaria-like organisms), are frequently found in patients with persistent Lyme disease. Along with viral and fungal infections, they can both intensify and cause chronic symptoms for those with Lyme disease and MSIDS. This is especially true when they occur with other bacterial infections and other chronic conditions. How do we know that someone has been infected with *Babesia*? The day sweats, night sweats, chills, fevers, cough, and air hunger that occur for many Lyme disease patients are actually classic symptoms for babesiosis, a parasitic infection that can be carried by the same tick that carries Lyme disease. These symptoms will not respond to classical antibiotic therapy for Lyme disease alone. This means that if you are diagnosed with Lyme but not tested and treated for other co-infections, such as babesiosis, many of your most aggravating symptoms may not go away, even with long courses of proper Lyme treatment.

This chapter explores these types of infections. Understanding them may provide the next clue to helping you or your chronically ill patient improve their overall health.

BABESIA

Ticks carrying Lyme disease and other bacterial co-infections are also frequently carrying several species of protozoa (single-cell organisms), some of which are parasites. The most common of these tick-borne protozoal parasites is *Babesia*, and there are more than one hundred species, which are known collectively as piroplasms. However, most *Babesia* infections that are transmitted to humans are due to a handful of species: *Babesia microti*, *Babesia* WA-1 (*Babesia duncani*), and *Babesia divergens*. Other *Babesia* species are found in animals, such as *Babesia bovis* (the parasite that causes Texas cattle fever, which can occasionally infect humans), *Theileria parva* (a parasite related to *Babesia* that causes East Coast fever in cattle), *Babesia caballi*, *Babesia equi* (found in horses), and *Babesia canis* (found in dogs).

Because ticks can carry one or more of these parasitic infections, as well as other bacterial and viral co-infections, it is possible to get infected with multiple organisms with one tick bite. For example, a recent study performed in New York State showed that 71 percent of the ticks tested harbored one organism, 30 percent had a polymicrobial infection, with two organisms, and 5 percent were carrying three or more microbes. These included *Borrelia burgdorferi*, *Borrelia miyamotoi* (a *Borrelia* species discovered in Japan in 1995 that causes relapsing fever and Lyme-like symptoms), *Anaplasma phagocytophilum*, *Powassan virus*, and *Babesia microti*.

Other studies are now showing evidence of a worldwide epidemic of babesiosis: It is now spreading to parts of the United States, Europe, and Asia, where it had previously been unreported. For example, although Lyme disease has been rampant in parts of the lower Hudson Valley, New York, where I practice, we have only been able to identify babesiosis there since 1998. In the past ten years, however, the scientific literature has shown that the number of positively diagnosed cases of babesiosis in New York State alone has increased twenty times.

Babesiosis is spreading just like Lyme disease because it is transmitted by the same zoonotic cycle, involving ticks, deer, and mice. *Babesia* can also be transmitted from person to person through an infected blood supply, and from mother to unborn fetus. This is a potentially dangerous situation for pregnant mothers, as well as a serious problem for our nation's blood supply. Untreated, *Babesia* can cause significant disability, especially in the very young or elderly with impaired immune systems; in some cases, the disease has been fatal.

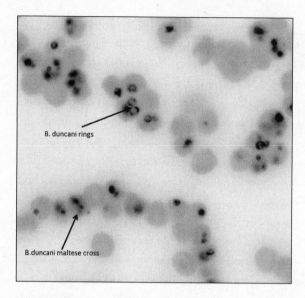

Hamster blood infected with Babesia duncani *(*B. duncani *parasites detected by fluorescent in situ hybridization using a* Babesia-*specific fluorescent labeled probe).*

USED WITH PERMISSION
FROM DR. JYOTSNA SHAH
AND IGENEX INC.

The Symptoms of Babesiosis

Different strains of *Babesia* may cause different sets of symptoms, yet all seem to significantly exacerbate a Lyme disease infection. For example, *Babesia microti* and *Babesia duncani* (WA-1) are both found in the United States, and both vary in their presentations from European strains of babesiosis, such as *Babesia divergens*. Most doctors are taught in medical school that *Babesia* can cause a hemolytic anemia (due to red blood cells breaking down), jaundice, thrombocytopenia (low platelet count), congestive heart failure, and renal failure. Yet this is not the clinical presentation for all patients who have babesiosis with or without Lyme disease in the United States. These patients may initially present with nonspecific symptoms such as fatigue, malaise, and weakness, with an associated fever, shaking chills, and excessive sweating. For many doctors these symptoms might be mistaken for the signs of a seasonal flu or, in certain regions of the world, another insect-borne parasite: malaria. Malaria and *Babesia* share the same set of symptoms, and the infections may look the same to a laboratory technician even under the microscope. *Babesia* and malaria can both produce ring forms (circular structures) under the microscope, although only *Babesia* will produce Maltese Cross forms, and these may not always be present on the blood smear for malarial parasites (Giemsa stain) that the laboratory technician is looking at. Doctors therefore may not consider babesiosis as a cause for this set of symptoms, especially if the patient does not have an associated hemolytic anemia and thrombocytopenia (low platelet counts). It is often only the sickest patients, after admission to the hospital, who will have both the classic textbook presentations combined with the more common malarial symptoms, such as fatigue, malaise, and weakness (91 percent), fever (91 percent), shaking chills (77 percent), and diaphoresis (sweating) (69 percent).

Worse, even if the proper diagnosis is made, some infectious disease doctors are still under the impression that seven to ten days of antimalarial and antibiotic medications, such as Mepron and Zithromax, will "cure" most babesiosis. In my experience, nothing could be further from the truth. Babesiosis occurring in an MSIDS/Lyme patient is one of the most tenacious and dangerous co-infections that I deal with regularly. This parasite exacerbates all of the typical Lyme symptoms, such as an increase in fatigue, joint pain, paresthesias, headaches, and cognitive dysfunction, often with the malaria-type symptoms listed above. Psychological problems, such as depression, anxiety, and mood swings, are also typically worsened with *Babesia*, which is why it should always be considered in patients presenting with multiple systemic symptoms and severe emotional issues that do not seem proportionate to their present situation or history of trauma.

Other classic symptoms of babesiosis that may suggest its presence in sick Lyme disease patients are an unexplained cough and/or a shortness of breath with air hunger, without another, more common, diagnosis to explain these symptoms (i.e., asthma, allergic rhinitis with a postnasal drip, COPD/emphysema, interstitial lung disease, or pneumonia). These can occur with or without the malaria-like signs or symptoms. The most severe form of shortness of breath is acute respiratory distress syndrome (ARDS), which can occasionally be seen in patients with babesiosis and can be fatal to those with compromised immune systems. Other atypical presentations can include severe hemolytic anemia in patients with healthy immune systems and intact spleens, which can be fatal if not properly treated. This is why we need to be vigilant in trying to avoid prescribing drugs that can suppress the immune system (such as high-dose steroids and other immunosuppressant drugs) for patients with Lyme disease, babesiosis, and associated co-infections. An intact immune system and spleen are needed to properly fight these infections.

The Challenge of Identifying Babesiosis

Diagnosing *Babesia* is particularly difficult, because the available testing is not precise. In the summer of 2011 I was invited by the Chinese government to participate in a think tank with their top scientific experts in order to better understand *Babesia* infections occurring in their country. Just as in the United States, these infections were not easily discovered by their standard testing and did not fit the textbook definitions; they were requesting my opinion to explain the discrepancies. I explained that different strains of *Babesia* can cause different clinical presentations in certain patients and are not always easily diagnosed using standard procedures, such as the Giemsa stain, a laboratory test for the *Babesia* parasite on a blood smear. It is taught in medical school as one of the primary diagnostic tests for *Babesia*, but in my experience this test is often insensitive and will miss many patients with babesiosis, especially if the amount of parasites in the blood is not elevated above a certain level (5 percent). I shared the concept of using a *Babesia* panel approach with the Chinese government and Chinese Center for Disease Control (CDC) during our trip to China. This involved using titers (IFA) as well as DNA (PCR) and RNA testing to better diagnose patients with babesiosis. Dr. Harris and Dr. Shah from IGeneX also attended this meeting. It was particularly gratifying to share this information in a way that could significantly benefit a large number of people, and I am grateful I had the opportunity to do so.

My journey in discovering babesiosis in the Hudson Valley started years before, back in the fall of 1995. That year a ray of light finally shone through the clouds and provided one of the answers I was searching for in treating my chronically ill MSIDS patients. I was attending a Lyme Disease Foundation conference, and one of the researchers discussed a co-infection that was being found in ticks in the coastal areas of Cape Cod and Long Island called babesiosis. *Babesia microti* was not supposed to exist in Dutchess County, New York: I went looking for it anyway, since some of my patients did complain of fevers and sweats and malarial symptoms that could not be explained or adequately treated with antibiotics.

I did a review of the medical literature and found that Dr. Peter Krause from the University of Connecticut, in the *Journal of the American Medical Association*, had confirmed that concurrence of Lyme disease and *Babesia* increases the severity and duration of symptoms. There it was. His patients coinfected with Lyme and *Babesia* were much sicker than with *Borrelia burgdorferi* alone. He even reported finding the DNA of *Borrelia burgdorferi* in those patients' blood three times more often than in the blood of patients not concurrently infected with both organisms. *Babesia* was suppressing these patients' immune systems as the *Borrelia* DNA could be found more often in the bloodstream. One piece of the puzzle that I had been searching for had been uncovered: Patients with chronic symptoms didn't always respond because they were coinfected.

I started to order Giemsa stains—the classically accepted method for diagnosing *Babesia*—on my patients through local laboratories. To my dismay, not one Giemsa stain returned positive. Yet something did not fit: The patients all had the nonspecific *Babesia* symptoms the doctor at the conference had described. I decided to call my colleague Dr. Joseph Burrascano and ask him if he had run into a similar problem. He had, and advised me to try IGeneX laboratory in California, which specializes in other types of testing for tick-borne disorders.

I promptly spoke with the director, Dr. Nick Harris, and started to send off *Babesia* titers (IFA) to his lab to look for the elusive organism. Lo and behold, some of the titers started to return positive! IGeneX already had developed a *Babesia* panel, which consisted of a *Babesia* titer (IFA), *Babesia* FISH test (fluorescent in situ hybridization, an RNA probe that binds to *Babesia* and causes it to fluoresce green under the microscope if present), and a *Babesia* PCR test. This last test looks for the DNA of the organism, because occasionally, these elusive parasites can evade the immune system, so finding the RNA or DNA of the organism is another way to prove its presence in the body.

In the several months to follow, I started testing more and more of my Lyme patients, and to my amazement, a large percentage of those resistant to standard treatment tested positive for this malarial-type parasite. Not only were their tests positive, but interestingly enough, many times their Lyme titers were negative and their FISH tests and/or PCR were positive. They also denied traveling to Long Island or Cape Cod, or anywhere else *Babesia* was known to be endemic.

One of my patients put me in touch with Dr. Rick Ostfeld, PhD, a disease ecologist and senior scientist at the Cary Institute of Ecosystem Studies in Millbrook, New York. This particular patient had tested positive for Lyme disease as well as *Babesia*, lived in Dutchess County, and had one of the highest titers for *Babesia* I had ever seen through Quest laboratories.

In 1999 Dr. Ostfeld had already been studying ticks at the Cary Institute for several years. The only co-infection with *Borrelia* that he knew to be present in Dutchess County was ehrlichiosis, the bacterial tick-borne co-infection that can cause high fevers, headaches, fatigue, and severe flu-like symptoms. *Ehrlichia* was, however, easy to diagnose with a standard blood test, and often patients with ehrlichiosis and anaplasmosis would also have low white blood cell counts, low platelet counts, and elevated liver functions on standard blood tests (CBC and biochemistry profiles). So this tick-borne disease seemed easy to diagnose, and seven to ten days of doxycycline was curative.

I called up Dr. Ostfeld. "Have you ever seen *Babesia* in this area?" I asked. Dr. Ostfeld said he had not, although no one had ever tested the ticks for it. "Do you think we could get a sample of your ticks and send them off to IGeneX laboratory in California to see if it is present? I have patients in Dutchess County testing positive for the disease, and I have no way of explaining it."

Dr. Ostfeld kindly agreed, and thanks to his generosity and the generosity of IGeneX, which ran the tests for free, approximately thirty ticks were tested for babesiosis. I got a call one week later: "A significant percentage of Dr. Ostfeld's ticks are positive for *Babesia*." Dr. Ostfeld retested the ticks to confirm IGeneX's results and found a lower percentage, which still confirmed the presence of the parasitic organism. *Babesia* had reached Dutchess County, New York. By 2001 the prevalence of *Babesia* was 5 percent; today, it is up to 41 percent in some areas, with an average of 17 percent. It is also now being discovered that mice, raccoons, and birds, among other animals, are competent hosts.

We then performed a clinical study in conjunction with IGeneX, looking at the frequency of positive or negative testing for babesiosis. The results of that study showed that a whopping 39 percent of patients were PCR positive and/or *Babesia microti* FISH positive while they were IFA antibody negative.

In my practice we now use *Babesia* IFA, PCR, and FISH tests in a panel approach to increase the sensitivity for *Babesia microti* in select patients who present with malarial-type symptoms, especially if they have negative Giemsa stains. The IFA is the standard immunofluorescent antibody test for *Babesia microti*, and a *Babesia* WA-1 (*duncani*) titer should also be included in a *Babesia* panel approach, as standard antibody testing for one species may appear falsely negative due to the diversity of *Babesia* parasites. The combination of these tests may reveal the presence of babesiosis when standard testing with Giemsa stains and IFAs are negative.

I then presented my findings in 2010 at the International Lyme and Associated Diseases conference: The entire eastern United States, from Florida to Maine, had patients testing positive for *Babesia* WA-1/*duncani*. This parasitic disease had spread farther than previously recognized, even by the CDC. This was an important breakthrough, because most doctors, if testing for *Babesia*, typically only test for one species, such as *B. microti*, and do not think of testing for other species, such as *Babesia* WA-1/*duncani*. When the *B. microti* test is negative, doctors may rule out the possibility of the disease being present, so they underestimate the true prevalence of the illness in their communities. For example, antibody tests—performed at LabCorp and Quest—for *Babesia* WA-1/*duncani* are confirming many more cases along the eastern seaboard of the United States.

Initial Ideas for Treating Babesiosis

The standard treatment for babesiosis was the antibiotic clindamycin, along with an antiparasitic drug, quinine, for seven days, the same treatment that is commonly used for malaria. I decided to try this on my Lyme patients with positive *Babesia* titers. It worked! Some of these patients, who had not responded to a classical antibiotic regimen for Lyme disease, improved after seven days of this treatment. Their chills and day and night sweats lessened or went away. Their fatigue, headaches, joint and muscle pain, cognitive difficulties, and even mood swings diminished.

However, the treatment is almost as bad as the disease. The side effects of clindamycin and quinine include nausea, vomiting, skin rashes, and severe ringing in the ears. So although the patients were happy to have some relief from their resistant symptoms, these would recur in a large percentage of them once the seven days of treatment were over, and the side effects were too uncomfortable for most to tolerate.

So I went back to the drawing board. Were there any other drugs that might fight *Babesia*? A review of the malarial literature and discussions with Dr. Burrascano led me to try Mepron (generic: atovaquone). This is another antiparasitic drug that I had prescribed for PcP (*Pneumocystis carinii*) pneumonia in HIV patients at Elmhurst Hospital during my residency. But I had never used this drug in great quantity: Mepron is most commonly used in combination with Zithromax, and it is very expensive. Its nickname is "liquid gold," as it can cost approximately seven hundred dollars a bottle: A prescription of Mepron and Zithromax could cost one thousand dollars per patient per month. By the time I had treated seventy of my patients with unresolved Lyme disease with one month of Mepron and Zithromax, at the tune of seventy thousand dollars in medication costs, I had clearly gotten the attention of my HMO director. Then I met Katherine, and everything changed.

Katherine's Journey with Babesiosis

Katherine came to my office one hot summer day. My nurse called her from the waiting room, and Katherine wheeled herself into my exam room. There was a determination that was evident as she slowly maneuvered her wheelchair next to the exam table. She was thin and lanky, with curly auburn hair, and she had muscular upper arms. Her arms told the story of a fight for independence, as life had not been kind to her. Yet it seemed that she had not been scarred by her battles. Her face was clear and kind, and there was still a slight upturned smile as she spoke, despite her obvious suffering.

"Hi Katherine, I'm Dr. Horowitz. It's nice to meet you. What brings you into the office today?"

Katherine replied: "I'm here to see what else can be done for me. I've been diagnosed with Lyme disease, and despite several years of treatment, I still can't walk. I have no strength in my legs, and every time I try to stand up I feel like I'm going to fall over, because the room spins. I have constant headaches, and I can't get any relief despite all sorts of pain medications. I'm very sensitive to light, so I have to wear sunglasses most of the time, and I'm also sensitive to sound. I need earplugs when I'm outdoors in large gatherings. I also have periods of fatigue that come and go, and generally I'm so tired I need to sleep fourteen to fifteen hours per day. The joint and muscle pain is pretty much all over but does tend to move around from time to time. Occasionally I get such severe chest pain that it feels like I've got a fifty-pound weight sitting on my chest, and I can't get enough air into my lungs, so I feel that I can't breathe. I also can't focus my thoughts. I feel scattered, and often can't remember what I did the day before."

Katherine then handed me a large binder of her medical records. It must have weighed at least five pounds. She had been seeing a Lyme-literate physician for the previous two years who had been extremely meticulous in his record keeping, and she had consulted with ten other doctors as well. Most of her tests were negative, including a cardiac nuclear stress test, an echocardiogram, and a Holter monitor (a test for cardiac arrhythmias). These had been ordered by her cardiologist for her ongoing chest pain and palpitations. Other testing included pulmonary function tests for her shortness of breath from her pulmonologist, which were negative, a CAT scan of the head for her headaches from her neurologist that was also negative, and negative results on tests for rheumatoid factor, anti-nuclear antibodies (ANA, autoimmune disorders), creatine phosphokinase (CPK, an enzyme found mainly in the heart, brain, and skeletal muscle), and sedimentation rate (a common hematology test that is a nonspecific measure of inflammation) for her joint and muscle pain from her rheumatologist. She had a normal complete blood count, a comprehensive metabolic panel (CMP) with normal electrolytes, kidney and liver functions, normal thyroid function, and normal vitamin levels. These tests were done to try and explain her resistant fatigue and memory and concentration problems.

The only positive tests were a CDC-positive Western blot for Lyme disease from Stony Brook laboratory and an MRI of her head that showed some scattered white spots (possible signs of demyelination, which are often seen in patients with persistent Lyme disease), as well as a positive electronystagmogram (ENG, a measure of normal eye movement and involuntary rapid eye movements), confirming a neurological cause for her dizziness. She also had a positive single-photon emission computed tomography (SPECT), which showed a lack of adequate blood flow in certain areas of her brain. Neuropsychological testing confirmed her memory and concentration problems but did not show any obvious depression or anxiety to account for her symptoms.

I then turned to Katherine and asked her: "Did you get any relief from your prior Lyme treatments? Any drugs make you better or worse?"

Katherine had a slightly dejected look. "No, Dr. Horowitz. I've been on antibiotics continuously for the last two years, and although I might feel a little better for a slight period of time, it never lasts."

A review of the antibiotics that Katherine had been taking included long-term use of tetracyclines. She also had been on high-dose amoxicillin, up to 9,000 mg per day. At that point I turned to the questionnaire that Katherine had filled out when she was sitting in the waiting room. Almost every symptom was circled on the list. This is fairly typical for the sickest Lyme patients. I turned to her as I pointed to the first symptom. "How long have you had fevers, sweats, and chills?" I asked.

Katherine replied: "For the past seven years. I often have had low-grade temps in the middle of the day, and sweat, but the sweats are much worse at night. I can be drenched, and need to change my nightshirt several times per night."

Now this was puzzling. Katherine was only thirty-two years old. She was still having regular menstrual cycles, and her labs showed normal estradiol and progesterone levels, as well as normal FSH and LH levels, which would have been elevated if she were in early menopause. She had no complaints of a cough, and her physical examination revealed no enlarged lymph nodes. There were also no enlarged lymph nodes on her chest X-ray, which would have been suggestive of non-Hodgkin's lymphoma, and her chest X-ray showed no prior signs of tuberculosis to explain her fatigue, drenching night sweats, and failure to thrive. She also had never traveled outside the United States, so malaria would be unlikely, although clearly her symptoms had a malarial-type presentation. There was also no evidence of a hemolytic anemia (destruction of red blood cells) on her complete blood count.

"Have you ever heard of *Babesia*?" I said. "I learned about it at a Lyme conference, where they mentioned this parasite can occur in the same ticks that carry Lyme. It causes the same type of drenching sweats you are complaining of, so let's send off some *Babesia* testing and see what we find."

Two weeks later I received a phone call from IGeneX. They let me know that the *Babesia* FISH test had returned positive and that they were definitely identifying *Babesia* under the microscope. "Has the patient traveled to Long Island or Cape Cod?" she asked. "No," I replied. Katherine had told me that she hadn't traveled to any of the most endemic areas for *Babesia*.

I immediately called her. "I think we may have a clue to some of your resistant symptoms. The *Babesia* test returned positive. I would like to give you a drug regimen called Mepron and Zithromax. I'll call in a ten-day supply. Avoid any over-the-counter vitamins with CoQ_{10}, as it can interfere with the effectiveness of the Mepron, and make sure that you stay on a low-carb diet, to avoid yeast, with lots of acidophilus twice a day several hours after you take the antibiotics, to prevent diarrhea." I told Katherine to call me if she had any questions or problems and to come in a few weeks so that we could evaluate her response.

Ten days later Katherine came back into my medical office with tears in her eyes. "I can stand! I can walk!" she exclaimed, as she slowly lifted herself out of her wheelchair and proceeded to take three steps. "I haven't had enough strength to stand in the last seven years. This is the first time I've been able to walk even a few steps!" She hugged me and thanked me. I was speechless. I had never seen anything like this before: Just ten days of treatment reversing a course of symptoms that had lasted for years?

As I treated more and more patients with Mepron and Zithromax, we saw more patients with resistant symptoms ultimately improve, at least temporarily. Just as with persistent Lyme, it became apparent early on that once the treatment was stopped, the fevers, chills, and day and night sweats would return, as well as a relapse of some of the overlapping Lyme symptoms. The improvement was dramatic, however, in some patients, and they were still better than before our treatment.

More Hurdles to Overcome

As the months progressed, Katherine was walking and no longer using her wheelchair after extensive treatment for babesiosis. She even went skiing once. She had been disabled for the previous seven years and had received disability payments from New York State. Now she was finally getting her life back.

At the same time, although I was getting very excited about my discoveries, I was finding that the medical directors of the insurance companies and local HMOs were not so enthused. In fact, after spending approximately seventy thousand dollars on Mepron and Zithromax prescriptions, they terminated me from their HMO and insurance programs. I lost thirteen hundred patients in one month's time, and I lost another six hundred patients after being dropped from a different insurance company several months later. I wasn't sure I could keep my doors open, since I had I lost the majority of my patients in one fell swoop. I had walked out onto a battlefield and had been unaware that a war was even taking place. Chronic Lyme disease and babesiosis didn't exist in our area, according to the medical authorities and insurance companies. But my patients didn't know that, and most of them kept improving with my treatment protocols.

So I did what any extremely naïve, well-meaning physician would do. I called up my local health department and I informed them of my findings. To my amazement, they didn't seem to share the enthusiasm that I had! I received a letter from them several weeks later informing me that *Babesia* definitely did not exist in upstate New York, and thank you for your interest. Not to be deterred, I decided to invite a member of the local health department to my medical office to review charts and discuss in detail my findings. He was cordial but suspicious and let me know that there must be a problem with the laboratory. I explained that the positive results had come not just from the laboratory, but also among treatment-resistant patients. He clearly was not going to be dissuaded from his opinion.

I then received a call from IGeneX letting me know that they were being investigated by New York State. Investigators went all the way to California to check their laboratory procedures, and sent them samples, which were blinded, to be checked for *Babesia*. Thankfully, IGeneX passed the New York State inspection and the California Department of Health investigation that ensued. IGeneX also passed inspections by CMS, which are the U.S. federal regulatory standards that apply to clinical laboratory testing to ensure proper quality. A certificate was issued that they had passed their inspections, yet no mention was made in Dutchess County that *Babesia* had been positively identified there.

This clearly disturbed me. I had hundreds of sick patients who were finding relief from their symptoms with the help of an antiparasitic treatment regimen. Other doctors in my area were probably seeing the same clinical manifestations but did not know what I knew. I decided that I needed to communicate my message more clearly, as no one seemed to believe me—because they couldn't hear me. If I found a treatment that worked, wasn't it my responsibility to spread the word to my colleagues so that they could help their sick and suffering patients?

I presented my data at the 11th International Conference on the Diagnosis and Treatment of Tick-Borne Diseases. I presented a paper on the use of Mepron and Zithromax. This was in a poster presentation format six months before Dr. Krause published his own findings on Mepron and Zithromax in the *New England Journal of Medicine*.

Afterward, I was invited by our local TV station to debate another infectious disease specialist in our area on Lyme disease and what I had just discovered: the existence of *Babesia* in Dutchess County. I had previously cross-covered with this same infectious disease doctor on weekends at our local hospital, or when he was on vacation. Let's simply say that our relationship became strained at that point in time. He never spoke to me again after the television debate.

A year later, after accumulating data on hundreds of patients with Lyme and babesiosis, I was accepted as a presenter at the 12th International Scientific Conference on Lyme Disease and Other Spirochetal and Tick-Borne Disorders in New York City. This was not an ILADS conference but a major international conference attended by researchers and physicians from all over the world who represented emerging, alternative points of view on tick-borne disease. I presented five abstracts, three of which were on *Babesia*. The first was on *Babesia* in upstate New York, with evidence of this co-infection among ticks in Dutchess County. The second was on the failure of Cleocin and quinine and Mepron and Zithromax in Lyme disease patients who were co-infected with babesiosis. The third abstract discussed new treatment regimens for babesiosis, including Lariam, a drug commonly used to prevent and treat malaria. I had found it to be useful in some of my patients who were failing traditional *Babesia* regimens. At the conference, I was onstage with my three heroes: Dr. Sam Donta, Dr. Kenneth Leigner, and Dr. Joseph Burrascano. I spoke for fifteen minutes with a slide presentation summarizing my research on Lyme and *Babesia*. It was a strange twist of fate. I didn't go looking for these diseases, but the raft of life had taken me down a river with unusual twists and turns. I was now onstage discussing diseases I had barely learned about in medical school. The best part was that I could see that the audience response was overwhelmingly positive: I had given them a novel and effective way of identifying and treating some of their chronically ill patients.

The Latest Treatments for Babesiosis

Babesiosis is much easier to treat successfully if it is found in the early stages of illness. If a patient presents with an EM rash and has associated significant day sweats, night sweats, high fevers, and/or shaking chills, then we would clinically suspect an associated co-infection with a malaria-like organism such as *Babesia*. A clinician should therefore consider using Mepron or Malarone early in the illness, while testing for *Babesia* at the initial visit.

Cleocin with quinine remains one of the classical regimens prescribed for babesiosis, but as I stated earlier, it frequently causes severe ringing in the ears, nausea, vomiting, and rashes. I have threatened some patients with this regimen if they are noncompliant with other treatment protocols, and it seems to work quite nicely in getting them to follow my instructions. Due to these severe side effects, I will more commonly use rotations for babesiosis, such as Cleocin and a macrolide antibiotic (Zithromax or Biaxin) with or without Malarone or Mepron. Mepron can also be used with a macrolide, and adding double-strength Bactrim (a sulfa drug) will often significantly increase its efficacy, especially in patients with overlapping *Bartonella* infections (bartonellosis). Other combination regimens that can be tried for resistant babesiosis include:

- Doxycycline: Tetracyclines have been used in the past for malarial prophylaxis, and doxycycline covers the majority of intracellular co-infections seen with persistent Lyme disease. We have found that combining doxycycline and Plaquenil with other antimalarial drugs, such as Malarone, can be an effective combination in some patients.
- Lariam: It can be used alone or with doxycycline and/or Plaquenil/and antimalarial herbs such as artemisia.
- Coartem (lumefantrine/artemether): This may be effective in patients with babesiosis whose previous regimens have failed. This is a classical drug regimen that is used for malaria and is felt to be at least 95 percent effective in eliminating *Plasmodium falciparum* malaria. This is certainly not the case in patients with chronic babesiosis, although it does help to decrease resistant symptomatology in a large group of MSIDS patients. It can be used alone or in combi-

nation with another antiparasitic drug, Daraprim, but Coartem must be taken away from certain drugs (macrolides, quinolones) that can affect the electrocardiogram.

Each of these therapies can be combined with antimalarial herbs, such as artemisia, neem, and/or cryptolepis, to help increase their efficacy, except Coartem. Conventional wisdom is that *Babesia* typically resolves spontaneously or after administration of a seven- to ten-day course of treatment. Unfortunately, it can persist despite months of varied antimalarial therapies: Many highly immunocompromised patients with Lyme and MSIDS who have had the disease for years do not feel significantly better after short-term therapy. *Babesia* can also develop resistance to classical antiparasitic drugs, just as malaria has developed multiple-drug resistant strains. This is particularly important for those who have ongoing chronic symptomatology, especially with malarial-type symptoms, such as ongoing day sweats, night sweats, fevers, and chills. The sickest patients with babesiosis, having high levels of parasites in the blood resulting in the failure of the above regimens, are sometimes given exchange transfusions, in which their blood (which contains the malarial parasite inside its red cells) is taken out of the body and exchanged for healthy, uninfected blood. This can be lifesaving in certain circumstances but carries certain risks.

I reported frequent clinical failures with standard treatment protocols for babesiosis at the International Scientific Conference on Lyme Disease and Other Spirochetal and Tick-Borne Disorders in 1999, and the writer of a recent article published in *Chronic Infectious Diseases* similarly reported drug resistance using standard treatments for babesiosis. Based on these scientific studies, it is clear that not all standard *Babesia* treatments are effective cures. In addition, *Babesia* can persist because it can hide from the immune system, just like Lyme disease.

There are at least four mechanisms that could explain its ability to evade the host immune response:

- Antigenic variation: changing its outer surface proteins to evade the immune system, like Lyme disease
- Different gene expressions: how DNA is produced in the organism

- Cytoadhesion with sequestration: how it binds to cells and hides
- Binding of host proteins to the inner red blood cell surface: binding to cells in ways that allow it to hide and avoid immune recognition

Babesia has been shown to persist in the animal population for long periods of time: It can exist in a chronic asymptomatic carrier state in domestic and wild animals for many years without causing active symptoms. *Babesia* can also suppress the immune system, just like Lyme disease, to a point where it cannot effectively attack certain infections and protect the body. The immunosuppressive effects of *B. microti* infections may contribute to maintaining Lyme disease and other co-infections in the body. *Babesia* does this by affecting our immunological response. There are immune cells in the body called "T helper cells," which are subgroups of lymphocytes (a type of white blood cell) that have an important role in our adaptive immunity. When we are exposed to an infection, proliferating helper T cells differentiate into two major subtypes, called Th1 and Th2 cells. Th1 cells activate our cellular immune system, producing cytokines that help kill bacteria via specialized cells called macrophages. Th2 cells activate B cells (a group of white blood cells known as lymphocytes) and our humoral immune system, increasing antibody production to help kill bacteria. Effective control of *B. burgdorferi* infection depends on a Th2 response within regional lymph nodes. When patients are co-infected with *B. microti*, it may shift the immune response toward a Th1 response, and the body may not be able to effectively combat either Lyme disease or *Babesia*, or any other parasitic co-infections. We also know that *Babesia* impairs the elimination of other parasites from the body, such as nematodes (roundworms), Trichuris (whipworms), and trypanosomes, and it may be the case with another parasite, toxoplasmosis, which is genetically similar to *Babesia*. Toxoplasmosis is often acquired by human contact with cat feces containing it, and it is estimated that between one third and one half of the world's population carries a toxoplasmosis infection. We frequently find that patients in our medical practice have been infected with toxoplasmosis, and that some do not adequately respond to standard toxoplasmosis therapies. Thus, clearing other parasites from the body may be more difficult when *Babesia* is present, leading to increased symptoms.

New Discoveries on the Horizon

Since standard treatment regimens do not always work in babesiosis, we are forced to look for new and more effective drug regimens. But there has not been much in the way of new major research done on *Babesia* over the last few years. We do know that babesiosis responds to classical antimalarial drugs, so we need to look at the antimalarial drug literature to see if there is anything new on the horizon that may be applicable for patients suffering with babesiosis. For example, one novel approach was published in 2011, where scientists invented a new way to disarm the malaria parasite. Researchers from Stanford School of Medicine found the chemical compound isopentenyl pyrophosphate (IPP), which is pivotal to the malarial parasite's survival and is manufactured in a unique structure in the parasite, called the apicoplast. If scientists could create drugs targeting apicoplasts, then perhaps the parasite could be killed more easily.

Drug resistance is commonly seen with malaria, and the World Health Organization (WHO) currently recommends using an herb, artemisinin, in combination with older antimalarial medications to try and prevent resistance. We do this frequently with our *Babesia* patients and often find it to be helpful, although not curative. Reports of resistance are emerging despite this commonly used herb for both malaria and *Babesia*.

Other research options for the treatment of resistant babesiosis include liposomal formulations of artemisinin, for enhancing greater absorption of the herb, beta-blockers (antihypertensive drugs), curcumin, heparin, Stephania root, and cryptolepis, an antimalarial herb from Africa, with or without sida acuta (as per herbalist, Stephen Buhner). The following are some of the most relevant and up-to-date information on these treatments and their possible uses for *Babesia*.

Beta-blockers: Hormones and drugs that control blood pressure (i.e., beta-blockers) can also control malaria infection.

There are specialized proteins in the red blood cells called "G proteins" that receive messages from local hormones and neurotransmitters, which then affect the genetic machinery of the cell. When the malarial parasite is in the red blood cells, the G proteins concentrate around it and, when stimulated, can cause the parasite to reproduce, increasing its infectivity. Beta-blockers, however, can block the effects of the G proteins and prevent the parasite from entering the red blood cell, decreasing its infectivity. We once performed clinical trials in my office, looking at the effects of beta-blockers on the outcomes of patients with babesiosis, but they showed mixed results and were only done in a small clinical cohort. Larger controlled studies are needed.

Heparin: Heparin is a blood thinner commonly used to treat clotting disorders, but it may play other physiological roles in the body. Treatment with various concentrations of heparin has been shown to inhibit the multiplication of *Babesia* parasites and help clear them from the body. These findings indicate that the right levels of heparin can effectively cover the surface of *Babesia* parasites and inhibit subsequent invasion of red blood cells. Further scientific studies need to be done on the use of heparin in the sickest patients with high levels of parasitemia (parasites in the bloodstream) who fail classical treatment regimens.

Curcumin: The herb curcumin contains antimalarial compounds that have been demonstrated to have effects against both malaria and *Babesia*. Curcumin also has powerful anti-inflammatory effects, and helps block some of the same inflammatory molecules found in Lyme disease and babesiosis: It does this by negatively affecting certain inflammatory biochemical pathways by decreasing an inflammatory enzyme called COX-2 or by blocking a switch inside the nucleus called NF-KappaB that turns on the production of inflammatory cytokines. Curcumin shows great promise in the natural treatment of Lyme disease and babesiosis, because of these anti-inflammatory and antimalarial properties, and it should be studied further for these illnesses.

Cepharanthine: This herb goes by many names, including Stephania root and S. cepharantha. *Stephania tetrandra* and *S. cepharantha* are the main species used medicinally. The Japanese have used root extracts, called cepharanthin, to treat chronic inflammatory diseases. It decreases the production of proinflammatory cytokines (matrix metalloproteinase or MMP-9, NF-KappaB, IL-1b, Interleukin 6, and tumor necrosis factor alpha), which are responsible in large part for the symptoms seen in Lyme disease and in patients with Herxheimer reactions. It also has other beneficial effects. Malaria has become resistant to standard drug regimens, like chloroquine (an old antimalarial drug), and when cepharanthine was added to chloroquine, it increased its antimalarial activity by fifteen-fold. It is unclear at this point whether Stephania may be useful and safe in resistant *Babesia* and associated inflammation with chronic Lyme disease (CLD).

When I was in France in 2011, presenting research at a medical conference at the United Nations branch in Paris (UNESCO), I met with Dr. Luc Montagnier, one of the respected winners of the Nobel Prize in Physiology or Medicine. I gave a two-hour presentation on Lyme disease and chronic tick-borne diseases to him and a group of French doctors who had a strong interest in treating Lyme disease and associated co-infections. I did the entire presentation in French, which in itself was nothing short of a miracle, considering I hadn't spoken the language regularly for over twenty years. The other physicians at this conference discussed reports of places in France where certain forms of the herb Stephania had caused renal failure in a small group of patients. This was due to a problem among the herbalists using it, who had not appropriately translated the correct type of Stephania from the Chinese literature into the French literature. No such reports had surfaced in the United States, and there is abundant scientific literature on the benefits of Stephania, but its use must be carefully considered for select patients, using the correct forms of cepharanthine. We need to do further research on this herb, since it is promising with resistant malaria, and we have so many treatment failures of babesiosis in patients using the above classical and herbal regimens.

Cryptolepis: Other options for treating babesiosis may include the use of the herb cryptolepis, a root used for many generations in Ghanaian traditional medicine for the treatment of malaria. The active antimalarial compounds found in it are called indo quinoline alkaloids, and they have been independently shown to have activity against the malarial parasite, including in drug-resistant strains.

A 2010 study from Africa showed the efficacy of cryptolepis in malaria. Forty-four patients were given cryptolepis tea bags three times per day, for five days. The results showed that 50 percent of patients were cleared of *P. falciparum* parasitemia seventy-two hours later, and all were clear by day seven and symptoms of fevers, chills, nausea, and vomiting were clearing rapidly by day three. The overall cure rate was 93.5 percent.

The study concluded that cryptolepis had been shown to be nontoxic and highly effective in the treatment of acute, uncomplicated malaria.

We have now used cryptolepis with hundreds of patients at our medical center for treatment-resistant babesiosis. According to my medical staff, the herb tastes like old lettuce found in the back of the refrigerator for seven days, but it is particularly effective in helping patients with malaria-like symptoms of babesiosis, especially in patients for whom other regimens have failed. Patients can obtain the herb online, and from specialty pharmacies, which also make better-tasting preparations.

Cryptolepis, however, has not been proven to be curative in my MSIDS patients, as I still find that symptoms recur several months after the herb is stopped. We therefore are forced to rotate anti-*Babesia* regimens among patients with positive testing and positive symptomatology.

VIRAL INFECTIONS

There are many vector-borne viral infections that can affect the patient with Lyme disease and MSIDS. Some of these are transmitted by mosquitos, such as dengue fever, Japanese encephalitis, Eastern and Western equine encephalitis, and West Nile virus. Others are transmitted by ticks, such as the tick-borne encephalitis virus (TBEV), Omsk hemorrhagic fever, Kyasanur forest disease (KFD), Congo-Crimean hemorrhagic fever (CCHF), Powassan encephalitis, and the recently discovered Heartland virus. The Heartland virus was first identified in 2012 in two patients in Missouri who were exposed to lone star tick bites. Within five to seven days both patients developed fatigue, fever, loss of appetite, and non-bloody diarrhea, with laboratory values looking like ehrlichiosis. They had marked leukopenia (low white cell counts), thrombocytopenia (low platelet counts), and elevated liver enzymes, yet doxycycline, the treatment for ehrlichiosis, was given and did not improve their symptoms. Researchers then discovered a new pathogen, known as a *Phlebovirus*, as the cause for their symptoms.

Chronic viral infections, like parasitic infections, may also explain some of the resistant symptomatology that we see among the MSIDS population with Lyme disease for whom antibiotic therapy fails. Viruses do not respond to antibiotics, and some of these viruses have already been shown to cause illness in patients with chronic fatigue syndrome and fibromyalgia. Further scientific studies need to be done to clarify the role of viruses in driving chronic illness in patients with Lyme disease and MSIDS, especially in patients for whom traditional therapies fail.

I often screen chronic MSIDS patients for associated viral infections, especially if he or she is presenting with significant fatigue, fibromyalgia, and neurological symptoms. These patients may be carrying viral infections without knowing it, and once they become infected with Lyme disease and other co-infections, it may cause a reactivation of prior viral infections and an exacerbation of their condition.

The most common viral infections that we screen for include:

- Epstein-Barr
- Human herpesvirus 6 (HHV-6)
- Cytomegalovirus (CMV)
- West Nile

Apart from finding previous exposure and occasional reactivation of Epstein-Barr and CMV, we often find elevated levels of HHV-6 in our MSIDS patients. This is important, because there are links to chronic fatigue syndrome and fibromyalgia in patients with HHV-6, and these are the same overlapping symptoms that we see in the Lyme disease population. HHV-6 causes roseola (Sixth disease) in children and nearly 100 percent of adults today have been exposed. It can reactivate later in life secondary to immunological and environmental factors and can lead to hepatitis and meningoencephalitis. It has been linked in the scientific literature as a possible cofactor in ADD, autism spectrum disorder, and multiple sclerosis, apart from its links to CFS and fibromyalgia.

Studies have been done at Stanford University by Dr. Jose Montoya on patients with chronic fatigue syndrome with elevated levels of HHV-6. He found that elevated titers of HHV-6 and a sudden onset of flulike symptoms would herald improvement with antiviral drugs such as Cytovene. Unfortunately, in our patient population, most of the standard antiviral drugs, such as Famvir, Valtrex, and Zovirax do not seem to have a significant effect on reducing chronic fatigue or fibromyalgia symptoms, and IV Cytovene is not a viable option for most patients. Our patients do not always have high HHV-6 titers and flulike symptoms at the onset of the illness, like those helped in the Montoya study. Due to the cost and side effects of the drug, both of which can be significant, Cytovene is not a drug that is easily used in clinical practice. Therefore, since standard antiviral drugs are either expensive, have potentially serious side effects, or are ineffective, we look to integrative therapies for viable treatment options.

We also will occasionally screen for HHV-8, Coxsackie virus, and parvovirus. On rare occasions we may look for Powassan encephalitis or other types of viral encephalitis if the patient is coming in with a particularly severe neurological presentation. The Powassan virus is now found in ticks in different areas of the United States (including in our area in the Lower Hudson Valley of New York) and can be transmitted in as little as fifteen minutes of a tick attachment. It can cause fevers, seizures, focal neurological findings, global neurological deficits, including loss of consciousness, hemiplegia (paralysis of half of the body), and neurological consequences, including mental status changes, visual deficits, hearing impairments, and chronic motor difficulties causing those affected to be unable to ambulate. Other viral encephalopathies are present across the United States and Europe, especially in the regions of the former USSR.

Nutritional Supplements Help with Viral Infections

Lyme disease patients often report that they feel worse and that their symptoms flare up when they come down with other viral infections. It is as if their immune system can only effectively fight so many infections at the same time. Nutritional supplements may help these patients, although most do not see a strong clinical shift in their symptoms.

These products are probably useful in certain groups of patients by helping to prevent reactivation of old viral infections and/or protecting against new ones. Since viral infections are quite common in the MSIDS population, and we have not seen significant clinical results with most of the available antiviral formulas in the sickest of our patients (including both drugs and nutritional supplements), we are presently doing a study on the use of Byron White Formulas. To date we are finding that some patients with elevated titers of HHV-6 and Epstein-Barr virus who complain of chronic fatigue are having a positive response to the Byron White

A-EB/H6 formula, thanks to the specific combination of antiviral herbs. This is encouraging, since antibiotics do not work for a small percentage of patients with Lyme disease.

The following supplements have known scientific efficacy against viruses, usually working through a common mechanism in which they help increase the natural killer cells and/or T cells in the body, the ones that go after viruses and cancer cells.

- Colostrum derivatives, such as transfer factors: antibodies that protect against disease and are produced by mammals during lactation.
- Olive leaf extract: Olive leaves and their active component, oleuropein, was studied by Upjohn Laboratories and found to be virucidal against herpes, influenza A, Coxsackie, and others.
- Mushroom derivatives, including 3-6 beta-glucan: The immune-enhancing properties of the yeast beta-glucan have been the subject of more than sixty years of research and more than eight hundred scientific studies. Preclinical research has shown 3-6 beta-glucan to be efficacious against a range of infectious diseases. Beta-glucan's primary effect is to increase NK cells and the phagocytic capacity of immune cells, and to enhance the movement of these cells to the site of a foreign challenge throughout the body via the mononuclear phagocyte system (the immune system comprising the liver, spleen, and lymph nodes). Clinical research has shown it to have synergistic effects with antibiotics, and 3-6 beta-glucan has been shown to be superior to most other immune supplements. It is therefore useful in patients with Lyme-MSIDS in fighting bacterial and viral infections when patients do not have an overstimulated immune system.

CANDIDA AND OTHER FUNGAL INFECTIONS

Candida syndrome with intestinal dysbiosis (a microbial imbalance in the gut) is not an uncommon health problem among Americans. It should be suspected in any patient with MSIDS who has unexplained fatigue, joint and muscle pain, and neurological symptoms such as brain fog and headaches that are unresponsive to standard treatment regimens. It joins parasitic and viral infections as another infectious cause leading to chronic persistent symptoms, in addition to Lyme disease and the other bacterial co-infections discussed in the prior chapters.

I first learned about *Candida* many years ago after one of my patients had developed a strange set of skin rashes that worsened every time she took antibiotics. She also complained of chronic fatigue, headaches, blood sugar swings, trouble concentrating, and digestive problems. In searching for answers I came across William Crook's book, *The Yeast Connection*. In it he described her set of symptoms perfectly. By placing her on a yeast-free diet and treating the *Candida* with antifungal agents, we were able to reverse all of her symptoms, which had baffled dermatologists and other subspecialists who had been unable to find a cause.

Although we all normally have *Candida* organisms present in our gastrointestinal tract in limited amounts, taking antibiotics for bacterial infections will encourage an overgrowth of *Candida*. Antibiotics kill off those good bacteria that keep our normal level of yeast in check. Furthermore, many Americans have diets high in sugar and refined carbohydrates, which help promote an overgrowth of yeast. Other factors that may contribute to the *Candida* syndrome are: the use of oral contraceptives; immune suppression due to stress; severe illness or chemotherapy; and any drugs that decrease the acidity of the gastrointestinal tract, such as antacids, H2 blockers (such as Zantac), and proton pump inhibitors (such as Prilosec).

When a combination of these factors is present, some patients get a fungal overgrowth in their GI tract and subsequently may manifest a myriad of symptoms. The most common signs and symptoms of candidiasis include:

- Blood sugar swings with overlapping reactive hypoglycemia and a craving for sweets
- Depression
- Dizziness with poor motor coordination
- Fatigue
- Fungal infections of the nails
- Gas and bloating

- Headaches
- Itching and other skin problems
- Mood swings
- Muscle and joint pain that does not migrate throughout the body
- Poor digestion with nausea
- Poor memory and concentration
- Rashes
- Thrush in the mouth (yeast on the tongue and buccal mucosa, which appears as a white, patchy coating)
- Vaginitis (recurrent vaginal yeast infections)

Patients can also present with associated "leaky gut syndrome," which is caused by long branches of the yeast burrowing into the intestinal mucosa and damaging the intestines. When the intestinal cell wall is damaged, it can lead to spreading food intolerances and allergies, as macromolecules of food are able to pass across a damaged intestinal barrier. So if a patient is tested with both an IgE and IgG food allergy panel and is found to be allergic to a multiplicity of foods, one should suspect overlapping *Candida* and leaky gut. These patients need to pay particular attention to their diet and the acid/alkaline balance of their foods, avoiding allergic foods by following a rotation diet. A stool CDSA (comprehensive digestive stool analysis) can also be performed through various labs such as Genova Diagnostics and Metametrix to check for bacterial and yeast overgrowth in the stool, combined with checking for sensitivities to various antifungal agents.

The most important dietary modifications for dealing with yeast are to eliminate malt, vinegar, simple sugars, and carbohydrates (including fruits early on in the treatment), as well as all yeast-containing foods (most breads and cheeses) and fermented foods (e.g., soy sauce, tempeh, and alcohol). Mushrooms should also be avoided (they are a form of yeast), as well as any foods to which a patient is sensitive or allergic.

We prescribe nystatin for both men and women prophylactically if patients need to be on long-term antibiotics, to avoid issues with yeast overgrowth, but often the tablet form of nystatin is insufficient in dealing with severe yeast problems once they have arisen. Powdered nystatin is more effective than tablet and should be used in cases of severe candidiasis.

Despite explaining the necessity of a strict, sugar-free, yeast-free diet to our patients on antibiotics, they often have a difficult time adhering to this regimen. Therefore, we occasionally need to use rotations of antifungal medications such as Diflucan and, rarely, Sporanox. These medications can be very effective, but potential side effects include inflammation of the liver and cardiac symptoms (EKG abnormalities), requiring proper monitoring. If these medications are ineffective or are contraindicated, natural antifungal agents, such as caprylic acid, grapefruit seed extract, garlic, berberine, and oregano oil can be helpful. When combined with good-quality, high-dose probiotics (lactobacillus, bifidobacterium) they can be extremely beneficial in restoring the proper balance of intestinal bacteria and yeast in the colon. We use several strains of high-potency acidophilus and choose brands that are acid resistant and/or coated with sodium alginate to increase the amount of acidophilus that colonizes the small and large intestines.

Not all forms of yeast are detrimental to humans' health. When treating patients with Lyme-MSIDS, apart from giving them high doses of good quality probiotics, and occasionally prebiotics containing fructooligosaccharides (FOS) to prevent antibiotic-associated diarrhea, we also give patients *Saccharomyces boulardii*, a type of beneficial yeast that has been shown to decrease the incidence of *Clostridium difficile* diarrhea. *Clostridium difficile* is a bacteria responsible for 95 percent of pseudomembranous colitis and 30 percent of all antibiotic-associated diarrheas. Saccharomyces is a healthy yeast that acts as a temporary barrier protecting the intestinal mucosa. A 2009 study published in *Infection and Immunity* showed that saccharomyces has a protease that inhibits the effects of *Clostridium difficile* toxins A and B. *Clostridium difficile* has the potential to be life threatening. It is therefore very important to protect against this possibility by using high-dose probiotics and *Saccharomyces boulardii* in patients during antibiotic therapy.

Yeast disorders and *Candida* are among the multiple infections that can cause chronic symptoms in MSIDS. *Candida* can cause fatigue; joint and muscle pain; neurological symptoms, such as brain fog, headaches, and gastrointestinal complaints; and can be confused with antibiotic-resistant Lyme disease. Many patients with adrenal dysfunction and associated hypoglycemia also suffer from candidiasis. These symptoms overlap with those of persistent Lyme disease (except for the latter's migratory nature, where symptoms come and go). Therefore, it is incumbent among health practitioners to include candidiasis in the differential diagnosis of infections in patients who have failed classical Lyme treatment.

MORGELLONS DISEASE

This unusual skin syndrome is occasionally seen in Lyme-MSIDS patients presenting in our office. Although the cause of Morgellons is unknown, it is thought to be due in part to several of the same types of infections we have been discussing in this chapter, including bacterial infections (*Myco-plasma, Borrelia*, etc.), parasitic infections, and fungal infections. There is even a hypothesis that insects may be involved, since the skin lesions appear to extrude a material that is similar to the chitin found in the hard body of insects.

Morgellons disease, or "fiber," disease is characterized by unusual skin wounds that appear to have fibers and specks coming out from the lesions; itching or crawling feelings under the skin (peripheral neuropathy) are also associated with it. According to the Morgellons Research Foundation, it can be characterized by six major signs and symptoms:

1. Skin lesions: both spontaneously appearing and self-generated, with intense itching. The former may initially appear as hives (urticarial-like) or as "pimplelike" lesions, with or without a white center. The latter appear as linear scratches. Even when not self-generated, the lesions often progress to open wounds that heal slowly and incompletely. Often patients with Morgellons syndrome are accused of self-inflicted skin lesions, because no obvious cause is found.

2. Crawling sensations, both within and on the skin surface: may also be described as bugs moving, stinging, or biting intermittently. This can also involve the scalp, nostrils, ear canal, and body hair or hair follicles.

3. Fatigue: may interfere with the activities of daily living.

4. Cognitive difficulties: measurable short-term memory and attention deficits, as well as difficulty processing information.

5. Behavioral problems: common in many patients. Many are diagnosed with psychiatric disorders (obsessive compulsive disorder, attention deficit disorder, attention deficit hyperactivity disorder, bipolar disorder)

and are often labeled as having delusional parasitosis, since well-meaning physicians cannot find an obvious cause for their symptoms.

6. Presence of fibers in and on skin lesions: They are generally described by patients as white or black, but clinicians and patients also report seeing fibers in blue, green, red, and other colors that fluoresce when viewed under ultraviolet light (Wood's lamp). Patients also report seeing black "specks" or "dots" on or in their skin, and objects described as "granules," similar in size and shape to sand grains, can occasionally be removed from either broken or intact skin.

In addition, many patients have been diagnosed with associated conditions, such as chronic fatigue syndrome and fibromyalgia. Other signs and symptoms include many of the ones we have been discussing with Lyme-MSIDS: changes in visual acuity; balance problems; ringing in the ears (tinnitus); and neurological symptoms, including changes in mood and personality, and painful extremities with arthralgias or arthritis-like symptoms. Obtaining appropriate medical assistance for these patients is challenging, since there are no available tests to make the diagnosis.

Although we still do not completely understand this syndrome, I have treated Morgellons patients successfully, starting with using the sixteen-point MSIDS diagnostic map to ferret out any underlying health problems and treating with the same antibiotics used to treat Lyme and associated co-infections. The most effective antibiotics have included tetracyclines (doxycycline, minocycline), macrolides (Zithromax, Biaxin), Septra DS, and quinolone drugs (Cipro, Levaquin, Avelox, and Factive). Often the skin lesions and associated symptoms resolve once the above antibiotics are used in a comprehensive treatment plan.

While the last two chapters have explored co-infections with varying manifestations, the next chapters explore other chronic conditions that are frequently found at the same time in patients suffering with MSIDS. Once these overlapping conditions are discovered and properly treated, most patients find themselves on the road to recovery.

SIX

Lyme and Immune Dysfunction

A utoimmune diseases are caused by an inappropriate immune response in the body; e.g., the immune system mistakes some part of the body as a pathogen, or a foreign invader, and attacks itself. This may be restricted to certain organs or involve a particular tissue, or it may be systemic. More than one hundred diseases are considered autoimmune ones, including: type 1 diabetes, multiple sclerosis, rheumatoid arthritis, Crohn's disease and ulcerative colitis, lupus, psoriasis, and scleroderma. More than fifty million Americans are living and coping with autoimmune diseases, and more than 75 percent are women, making them some of the top ten leading causes of death of women under the age of sixty-five.

It is not uncommon for patients presenting with Lyme-MSIDS to test positively for multiple autoimmune markers in their laboratory blood work. These same patients frequently present with fatigue, joint and musculoskeletal pain with a positive ANA or rheumatoid factor, and sometimes the lab tests show an elevated CRP or sedimentation rate, which are markers of inflammation. Occasionally the patient will also test positive for other autoimmune markers, such as antibodies against double-stranded DNA (which is very specific and sensitive for lupus), have positive Sjögren's antibodies (anti-Ro, SS-A; Anti-La, SS-B), positive anti-ribonuclear proteins (Anti-RNP, which is seen in several autoimmune syndromes), and be HLA DR 4 positive, which can be associated with autoimmune phenomena.

Patients will often come to my medical practice after having seen one or even several rheumatologists, having been given the diagnosis of lupus, rheumatoid arthritis, or a nonspecific autoimmune disease. Frequently their physicians will have tested them for Lyme disease with a basic ELISA test, and when it comes back negative (as it often does, due to the poor sensitivity of this test), they are told that they do not have Lyme disease, but instead have an autoimmune disorder. Then they may be placed on a number of medications for their joint pain, including biologic agents such as methotrexate, Enbrel, Arava, and Cimzia, or on immunosuppressive drugs, such as Imuran or prednisone. Unfortunately, these drugs do not always help patients with MSIDS, and their symptoms will not be relieved. Worse, these medications can have untoward side effects, including the development of certain cancers, reactivation of underlying infections, such as tuberculosis, and exacerbation of active infections, such as Lyme disease and associated co-infections. This is because some of these drugs suppress the immune system and allow latent cancers or other underlying infections to emerge and become much more powerful.

The situation becomes even more complicated if there is a true, previously diagnosed autoimmune disease, like rheumatoid arthritis, as well as an exposure to Lyme disease and multiple co-infections. For example, the patient may have a positive rheumatoid factor as well as a positive anti-CCP (anticyclic citrullinated peptide) antibody, which is a more specific marker for rheumatoid arthritis. He may also have had a negative ELISA test for Lyme and been told that he has rheumatoid arthritis and no other associated diseases. However, a more sensitive test for Lyme disease, such as the Western blot, may yield different results. What's more, the patient may not have been tested for associated bacterial or parasitic co-infections that can also increase joint pain, such as *Babesia, Bartonella, Mycoplasma spc.*, and chlamydia, among others, or for heavy metals, the agents which have been associated with autoimmune phenomenon and can also increase joint and muscle pain through a variety of biochemical mechanisms. Therefore, even the most well-intentioned doctor may have only identified one cause among many that may be contributing to the patient's musculoskeletal symptoms.

However, the MSIDS model requires the medical detective to discover the multiple causes that may be contributing to the varied manifestations of an illness. You can then use the Horowitz sixteen-point differential diagnostic map and the tests listed in Chapter 2 to determine each of the causes that are contributing to an autoimmune response. The fact is, there are four possibilities that may be occurring:

- You may have an autoimmune disease and not know it.
- You or your patient may have an autoimmune disease and know it.
- You may not have an autoimmune disease, but Lyme disease and/or co-infections are mimicking it.
- You have both an autoimmune disease and Lyme disease that, in combination with multiple factors on the MSIDS model, are contributing to making the autoimmune disease symptoms worse.

LYME DISEASE
CAN CAUSE AUTOIMMUNE SYMPTOMS

In the medical literature we find that both children and adults referred to rheumatologists with presumptive diagnoses of diseases such as juvenile idiopathic arthritis (JIA, previously known as juvenile rheumatoid arthritis), or adult-onset Still's disease, (AOSD, a severe form of JIA in adults) were often found to have Lyme disease.

It is interesting that blood levels that indicate rheumatoid arthritis (RA) correlate positively with antibody titers against certain species of Borrelia, especially a commonly found Borrelia species in Europe, Borrelia garinii. In one 1995 study published in Lupus, 57 percent of patients with rheumatoid arthritis also demonstrated previous exposure to Borrelia. Unfortunately, the study's authors dismissed their own findings and assumed these patients had false positive blood tests. As we have seen, many labs are using insensitive testing for the multiple strains of Borrelia, and use CDC criteria to make the diagnosis, which will miss many patients with Lyme disease. This suggests that the authors might have dismissed their own evidence implying a causal link between the two diseases, or at least shows that they may occur together frequently, contributing to the patients' illnesses.

This link has been postulated in the scientific literature, and referred to as "Lyme arthritis," a disease caused by a bacterium that can mimic RA. This finding has begged the question of whether infectious agents could be a contributing factor to autoimmune diseases. In animal models, a causal link has been found between *Borrelia* infection and subsequent developments of rheumatoid arthritis. Some of my patients had been diagnosed with "seronegative rheumatoid arthritis" and not achieved clinical improvement until a diagnosis of Lyme disease was made. But apart from Lyme disease, are there other infectious diseases that may also be driving autoimmune phenomena and joint pain in patients?

Let us look at the situation with two commonly found co-infections we discussed earlier, *Mycoplasma* and *Chlamydia*. *Mycoplasmas* have been shown to affect parts of the immune system (B-lymphocytes, the cells that produce antibodies), which can result in promoting autoimmune reactions and rheumatoid diseases. *Mycoplasmas* have also been found in the joint tissues of patients with rheumatological diseases, suggesting their involvement in the disease process. *Chlamydia pneumonia* also causes arthritis and joint pain, and often more than one bacterial organism can be found in the joint fluid of patients with arthritis. All of these infections are present in MSIDS patients, and all of them may cause joint pain. These infections are also caused by intracellular organisms and are sensitive to the antibiotic minocycline, which goes inside the cell to inhibit bacterial growth. This means that when a rheumatologist prescribes Plaquenil and minocycline and believes that their effects on the body for autoimmune diseases are primarily anti-inflammatory as a disease-modifying agent (DMARD, disease-modifying antirheumatic drug), it may just be that the same drugs are also simultaneously treating Lyme disease, *Mycoplasma*, and *Chlamydia* infections, all of which were not diagnosed.

To complicate matters even further, environmental factors, such as heavy metals may also affect whether bacterial organisms cause joint pain. Mercury has been linked in the scientific literature to many autoimmune conditions, and heavy metal exposure reverses genetic resistance to *Chlamydia*-induced arthritis. Environmental toxins and heavy metals also drive oxidative stress and inflammation and increase the production of inflammatory cytokines such as TNF alpha, IL-1 and IL-6, the specific molecules causing pain, inflammation, and "sickness syndrome" in autoimmune diseases. This may explain the improvement in joint pain in certain patients following chelation therapy when heavy metal burdens have been removed from the body.

Other factors in Lyme-MSIDS that may be responsible for autoimmune symptoms are the shed DNA particles from the surface of *Borrelia burgdorferi* known as blebs. These particles are frequently plasmids, fragments of DNA containing large amounts of chromosomal material. Blebs are highly stimulatory to the immune system, and intracellular blebs convert host cells into targets for the immune system. Therefore, instead of the immune system targeting and killing *Borrelia burgdorferi*, the organism releases pieces of its DNA and diverts the infected host's immunological defenses to go after a decoy. This also allows the *Borrelia* to decrease the effectiveness of the complement pathway, which is another mechanism the immune system uses to clear pathogens from the body. Simultaneously, these blebs can cause an overstimulated immune system to produce the antibodies that mimic lupus or rheumatoid arthritis. The antibodies can kill off the host cells as the immune system goes after cells infected with these blebs.

Garth Nicolson, PhD, and his colleagues found that patients with chronic bacterial and viral infections have other mechanisms responsible for autoimmune responses, which include: molecular mimicry (the immune system cannot differentiate between the patient's antigens and foreign antigens); the release of cell membrane vesicles containing bacterial surface antigens; and intracellular bacteria that cause cell death when bacteria and cell fragments are released into the surrounding environment, increasing inflammation. Furthermore, *Borrelia* can affect the immune system by killing lymphocytes called B cells (which are essential for our proper immune functioning), and when *Borrelia* exits the lymphocyte it surrounds itself with lymphocytic proteins, cloaking itself from the immune system, another mechanism which allows it to persist in the host.

Borrelia burgdorferi has a highly evolved set of defense mechanisms that help explain why many patients who have been diagnosed with rheumatoid arthritis, lupus, and multiple sclerosis may not, in fact, have a "true" autoimmune disorder. Instead, they may have an immune system overstimulated by Lyme disease and *Mycoplasma* and other intracellular co-infections, and exacerbated by exposure to heavy metals and environmental toxins, which further drive inflammation and cytokine production.

Even a well-trained physician may not be able to differentiate between these autoimmune diseases and Lyme disease, especially if they are using inadequate testing. In one study, published in the *Annals of the New York Academy of Sciences,* highly trained pathologists were unable to see any differences under the microscope between Lyme disease and autoimmune conditions. So it should not be surprising that I commonly see many patients in my medical practice who have been misdiagnosed with pure autoimmune disorders. Let's discuss three that are commonly misdiagnosed and their relationship with Lyme disease: lupus, rheumatoid arthritis, and multiple sclerosis. Two others, Crohn's disease and ulcerative colitis and the effects of tick-borne disorders and cytokines on the gastrointestinal tract, will be discussed in a later chapter.

Lupus, Rheumatoid Arthritis, and Lyme Disease

Lupus is one of the most common autoimmune diseases in the United States, affecting women three times more frequently than men. It is characterized by inflammation in many different organs of the body, including the skin, joints, central nervous system, heart, lungs, and kidneys. Individuals with lupus often present with a constellation of many of the following symptoms: fevers, fatigue, skin rashes with sun sensitivity, hair loss, anemia, arthritis, and inflammation in the heart (pericarditis), lungs (pleurisy), arteries (vasculitis), kidneys (nephritis), and brain (cerebritis).

These symptoms can look remarkably similar to many of those seen in unresolved Lyme disease. Often patients come in with these symptoms and have blood tests that show the presence of a number of antibodies: antigens in the nucleus of the cell; against the cytoplasm of the cell (the gel-like substance inside the cell membrane containing all of its metabolic structures); and against the cell membranes. These all may help to characterize the disease. One way to differentiate between Lyme and lupus, however, is to use the double-stranded DNA test (dsDNA), which is 98 percent specific and sensitive for systemic lupus erythematosus. This is part of the new criteria that have been established by the American Rheumatological Society to help establish the diagnosis.

If we look at the biochemistry of lupus and Lyme disease, we see that they have similar immunology and pathology. For example, we can see complement pathway deficiencies in both Lyme disease and lupus. We can also find specific antibodies in both diseases, including antiphospholipid and anticardiolipin antibodies, which are normally thought of as associated only with autoimmune diseases. This is confusing for any clinician who might only think of these as signs of Lupus. What's more, in two studies, positive blood tests for Lyme disease by the ELISA system have been detected in 40 percent of patients with SLE (systemic lupus erythematosus), but since Western blots were not CDC positive, both sets of authors assumed the test results were false positive for Lyme. Worse, these diseases can look so remarkably similar that although we usually think of the butterfly rash on the face as being a clear indication for lupus, facial/butterfly rashes can be seen with Lyme disease as well.

Rheumatoid arthritis can also look like Lyme disease. Like lupus, it is a chronic systemic inflammatory disease that primarily affects the joints, but it also may involve inflammation in tendons, ligaments, muscle, bone, and many organs in the body. To establish a diagnosis of rheumatoid arthritis, the joint score (counting and mapping the joints involved at each visit), the presence of synovitis (inflammation in the synovial membrane surrounding the joints), and the physical exam (range of motion, presence of increased fluid in the joints, nodules, and deviations in the joints) are the focus of the criteria. We can get signs of inflammation in both diseases (including positive ANAs and rheumatoid factors), but the presence of positive anti-CCP antibodies differentiates it from Lyme disease and is a more specific marker for true rheumatoid arthritis.

Rheumatoid arthritis, lupus, and Lyme disease may all respond to similar treatment regimens. The antirheumatic drug Plaquenil is effective not only in lupus and rheumatoid arthritis, but also in Lyme disease. In autoimmune diseases and in Lyme disease, Plaquenil helps modulate an overstimulated immune system to decrease pain and inflammation. Plaquenil has also been shown to be effective in hitting the cystic forms of *Borrelia burgdorferi* and alkalizing the intracellular compartment, making antibiotics more effective and inhibiting DNA gyrase, an enzyme responsible for bacterial replication.

The diagnosis and treatment regimens for autoimmune diseases have drastically changed over the past ten years. For example, for rheumatoid arthritis, doctors used to wait for erosions to be seen on X-rays (implying destruction of the joints) before starting disease-modifying antirheumatic drugs, but now it is the exact opposite, due to the ability of newer drugs called biologics to induce remission. It is therefore essential that we establish a proper diagnosis, to be sure we are instituting the correct treatment.

Judy's Lyme Disease Was Mistaken for Arthritis

Judy traveled all the way from New Hampshire to see me after being referred by her nutritionist. She was forty years old and had a past medical history of rheumatoid arthritis. She had been complaining of chronic fatigue and bilateral joint pain in her hands, knees, ankles, and toes for the past two years, and she finally sought the advice of a rheumatologist. The rheumatologist found that she had an elevated rheumatoid factor (56; normal values are less than 15) and a low positive antinuclear antibody (1:80 positive). Her other autoimmune markers were negative, and she had mild signs of inflammation, with a slightly elevated C-reactive protein and an elevated erythrocyte sedimentation rate (the ESR was 32; normal values are less than 20). He tested her for Lyme disease using the ELISA test, and since this returned negative, she was told that she did not have Lyme disease. Her anti-CCP was negative, which is a specific marker for rheumatoid arthritis, and because of her symptoms and elevated rheumatoid factor, she was told that she was in fact suffering from rheumatoid arthritis. Judy was coming to me for a second opinion, because she did not want to take the biologics and immunosuppressive drugs being recommended by the rheumatologist (particularly steroids and methotrexate).

Judy's physical exam was essentially within normal limits, and she had no redness, swelling, or signs of inflammation in her joints. I sent her for an X-ray of her hands, which did not show any evidence of erosions. My blood testing did confirm the presence of an elevated rheumatoid factor and low positive ANA, but it also came back with a CDC positive Western blot for Lyme disease, evidence of co-infections with *Mycoplasma,* and significant elevations in heavy metals on a six-hour urine DMSA challenge (mercury 22: normal values are less than 3; and lead 18:

normal values are less than 4). All of these factors have the potential for driving autoimmune reactions, and each would have to be addressed to achieve the best results.

Judy was placed on a regimen of Plaquenil with minocycline and nystatin tablets. This is a disease-modifying antirheumatic drug regimen frequently used by rheumatologists, which also happens to address Lyme disease and *Mycoplasma* infections simultaneously. She followed this regimen for one year, showing frequent yet gradual improvements in all of her symptoms, month after month with no side effects, and all of her inflammatory markers eventually decreased into the normal range. We also started a weekly chelation treatment to detoxify her heavy metals until they returned to a normal range, and she no longer complained of fatigue or joint pain. We then stopped the minocycline, continued her on the Plaquenil, and rotated her to an herbal treatment protocol for Lyme disease.

Judy has remained completely well with this treatment protocol for the past two years: Her autoimmune markers decreased over time; her inflammation resolved without joint involvement; and we avoided having to use immunosuppressive drugs for her "rheumatoid arthritis." It was the Lyme disease, possible co-infection with *Mycoplasma*, and heavy metals that were all mimicking an autoimmune presentation. Judy's story illustrates how a patient may not have a true autoimmune disease, and how Lyme disease and various factors on the MSIDS map may stimulate autoimmune phenomena.

Martha's Lyme Overlapped with Her Autoimmune Disease

Now let's look at a patient who had a true autoimmune disease as well as Lyme disease and other co-infections that were exacerbating her symptoms. Martha was a sixty-four-year-old white female with a past medical history of rheumatoid arthritis. She not only had a positive rheumatoid factor but, in this case, also had evidence of a positive anti-CCP, the specific marker for rheumatoid arthritis. When she first started seeing me she was already taking Enbrel and Arava, biologic disease-modifying antirheumatic drugs. She was also on prednisone and methotrexate, with Pred Forte eye drops for the inflammation in the interior part of her eye, known as uveitis. She was taking Synthroid for hypothyroidism and Fosamax with Celebrex for her osteoporosis and joint pain. She had been diagnosed with Lyme disease five years earlier, by a physician-identified EM rash. She was treated by that physician with one month of antibiotics, at which time she reported that all of her symptoms resolved. She had a second EM rash a year later. Her primary physician placed her on amoxicillin, but treated her with it for only six days because she complained of nausea, vomiting, and diarrhea each time she took the antibiotic.

When she came to see me, Martha filled out the symptom questionnaire, and had circled fatigue, right elbow pain, paresthesias (tingling and numbness of the right hand), generalized muscle weakness, decreased balance, memory and concentration problems, and uveitis. Her social and family history was unremarkable, and her physical examination was within normal limits, except that her left eye was slow to react to light.

Laboratory testing revealed a CDC positive IgM Western blot as well as a positive IgG Western blot. IgM Western blots may be positive in early Lyme disease, but also are positive in late Lyme, and is one of the exceptions to the rule to always keep in mind. Co-infection testing was negative for *Babesia* and *Ehrlichia*, but she had a positive *Mycoplasma* IgG and a positive *Bartonella henselae* IgM at 1:16. Her rheumatoid factor and anti-CCP antibody was positive, she was ANA negative, and she was HLA DR 4 positive, which is an immune marker often associated with autoimmune disease and severe joint involvement in Lyme patients. Celiac disease was ruled out with a negative antigliadin antibody and negative TTG blood test.

I started her on doxycycline. She returned one month later after the initial blood tests had returned, and although her fatigue had improved, she had a flare-up of her right elbow pain with no changes in her memory and concentration problems. We therefore added Plaquenil and Cipro to the doxycycline, so that she was now on a double intracellular regimen to extend her coverage against the Lyme and *Bartonella*.

Her follow-up one month later showed that her fatigue, joint pain, paresthesias, and headaches had all resolved. Her resistant uveitis was also now calm for the first time in a year, according to her ophthalmologist. The take-home message was that Lyme disease and co-infections such as *Bartonella* were mimicking and exacerbating Martha's autoimmune disorder and were responsible for some of her resistant symptoms. She had both an autoimmune disorder and tick-borne co-infections. Once we treated her underlying infections, she felt much better, and her resistant eye symptoms improved. This was previously believed to be solely an autoimmune manifestation of her rheumatoid arthritis, but uveitis can be seen in Lyme disease and in *Bartonella* infections. Giving her a double-intracellular drug regimen with a quinolone and tetracycline helped alleviate symptoms that no prior regimen had been able to accomplish. In conjunction with her rheumatologist, we were able to decrease the immune-suppressing drug that she was on (prednisone) that was not completely controlling her symptoms. Treating Lyme disease and co-infections can be an important part of improving clinical symptoms in patients diagnosed with autoimmune disorders.

Is It MS or Lyme?

After rheumatoid arthritis, the most frequent autoimmune disease that may be confused with Lyme is multiple sclerosis. This is a disorder defined by a constellation of symptoms and associated demyelination of nerves—the loss of the myelin sheath surrounding nerves that is essential for proper conduction of electrical impulses—especially of the central nervous system and spinal cord. It can affect the brain, causing white matter lesions to be visible on an MRI, as well as the optic nerve (leading to varying degrees of visual loss), and it can affect the spinal cord, causing numbness, weakness, and tingling of the extremities, as well as urinary difficulties. Other clinical symptoms include difficulty walking, with incoordination, dizziness, hearing loss, difficulties with speech, and pain in varied nerves of the body. It often presents with symptoms that tend to come and go (the remitting/relapsing form of the disease), especially early in its course, and clinically it can be indistinguishable in certain cases from Lyme-MSIDS. In fact, some epidemiological studies suggest an infection may be behind MS, as new outbreaks have occurred in parts of the world only after Westerners arrived. This was the case when the British troops arrived in the Faroe Islands during World War II, where it was not until years after their arrival that the first cases of MS appeared. Genetic and environmental factors have also been suggested to play a role, as MS is more common farther from the equator: some have hypothesized that it may be related to a vitamin D deficiency.

MS is a clinical diagnosis, as is Lyme disease, and there is no available blood test for it. It can be suggested on an MRI of the brain and spinal cord with multiple demyelinating lesions, changes in nerve conduction of the eye (as tested by a VEP, or visual evoked potential), and ear (AEP, auditory evoked potential), with an associated increase in certain markers of the spinal fluid (MBP, myelin basic protein, and oligoclonal bands). Some of these changes, however, can also be seen in persistent Lyme disease, so it is often a diagnosis of exclusion, when other diseases have been ruled out.

The lack of a reliable blood test, and the overlapping of symptoms between the two diseases, would explain the frequent number of patients who I see in my medical office who have been diagnosed with MS when, in fact, they had Lyme disease and MSIDS. For example, I have seen many patients with a previous diagnosis of MS who have failed to improve on commonly prescribed MS drugs, such as Avonex, Betaseron, Copaxone (the ABC prescription regimen), and Rebif; it was then determined that Lyme-MSIDS was responsible for their demyelination and subsequent fatigue, optic neuritis, tingling, numbness, and difficulty walking.

Multiple authors in the medical literature propose that MS is most likely caused by an infection with *Borrelia burgdorferi*, the agent of Lyme disease. There are at least five reasons for the hypothesis that Lyme is the basis for some cases of MS:

1. Spirochetes have been documented in MS pathology specimens.
2. Spirochetal flagellin (the tail of *Borrelia burgdorferi* that allow it to move through the body) is immunologically very similar to human myelin.
3. The demyelination process in MS and Lyme is also similar; they both can cause inflammation in the eye and in the spinal cord, leading to a loss of vision and difficulty walking, making it difficult to differentiate between the two diseases clinically.
4. If a physician were to do a spinal tap trying to differentiate multiple sclerosis from neurological Lyme disease, they would find extremely similar results. As with multiple sclerosis, central nervous system infection with *B. burgdorferi* can cause an increased protein synthesis with IgG antibodies, lymphocytic pleocytosis (increased lymphocytes in the spinal fluid), increased protein, increased plasma cells, and oligoclonal bands. Lyme

that affects the central nervous system can produce both oligoclonal bands that react with *Borrelia burgdorferi* and ones that
do not.

5. We find some of the cystic structures of Lyme disease in the
central nervous system of patients with MS. The cyst forms are
one of the means by which *Borrelia burgdorferi* can persist in
the body for extended periods of time, under extremely adverse
conditions, and reactivate into normal mobile spirochetes when
the conditions are right. Perhaps certain environmental factors
(e.g., low vitamin D) or co-infections with other organisms, such
as *Chlamydia*, are responsible for *Borrelia* coming out of hiding
and reactivating the cysts, driving demyelination and MS-type
symptoms in certain patients.

One of the mysteries that has challenged my medical practice is that as
more and more patients come for help, a large number present with
symptoms of multiple sclerosis. Those coming for help said that the traditional medical establishment had failed to provide them with answers
for their illnesses. Why is this the case?

Patients with multiple sclerosis often complain of intermittent tingling and numbness in different parts of their bodies, and MRIs of their
brains can show varying amounts of white spots. Both of these symptoms and findings are seen in both Lyme disease and MS, and since some
patients have negative serum Lyme ELISAs, they are often told by neurologists that they have MS and are given the ABC regimen, or Rebif. If
these drugs don't help, patients are told that they must have a "relapsing
remitting" form of the disease, in which the symptoms come and go, or a
chronic, progressive form, and are told to remain on these drugs to stabilize their symptoms. However, just as with the patients diagnosed with
lupus or with rheumatoid arthritis, the drugs may not help relieve their
symptoms, or even if they do, we may be treating symptoms and not getting to the true, underlying cause of the disease process.

What is the link between Lyme disease and MS? Do Lyme disease
and/or co-infections somehow provoke the MS autoimmune reaction, just
as it can do with lupus, rheumatoid arthritis, and other inflammatory disorders? Dr. Stephen Phillips, past president of ILADS, has presented evidence at scientific conferences that there is an association between MS

and Lyme disease. He also reported treating an abnormally high number of MS patients in his Lyme practice. Years earlier, Dr. Patricia Coyle of SUNY—Stony Brook presented research on how to differentiate between MS and Lyme at a Lyme Disease Foundation conference. Her work focused on the following:

- Both cause optic neuritis, inflammation of the optic nerve, and blindness.
- Both cause white spots or demyelinating lesions visible on an MRI scan of the brain.
- Both could cause paresthesias—tingling and numbness of the extremities.
- Both can cause bladder dysfunction.
- Both have a relapsing, remitting nature.
- Both diseases can cause elevations of myelin basic protein (MBP) and oligoclonal bands (immunoglobulins) to appear in the spinal fluid.

The primary difference between the two diseases seemed to be that with MS there were more white matter lesions on an MRI and higher amounts of myelin basic protein and oligoclonal bands present on the spinal tap. Moreover, Lyme disease did not usually cause demyelinating lesions in the cervical or thoracic spine. So there were some differences, but the boundaries between the two diseases are easily blurred, and one disease could certainly be mistaken for the other.

One of the early scientific explanations as to why Lyme disease can mimic autoimmune disorders such as multiple sclerosis came out of research by Dr. Norman Latov at New York University. As we have seen, *Borrelia burgdorferi* is a helical-shaped organism, with a head and tails. These tails, or flagella, are how the organism propels itself through bodily fluids and tissues. It is represented by the 41 kDa band (kilodaltons, i.e., molecular weight protein) on the Western blot and is a common band seen in Lyme patients. Although it is nonspecific in nature (it is found with other spirochetal infections as well), the 41 band is part of the CDC criteria for a positive IgM Western blot. If the 23 and/or 39 bands are present with the 41 kDa bands on an IgM Western blot, this is considered diagnostic proof of exposure to Lyme disease.

Some patients also have genetic predispositions for autoimmune diseases. For example, the genes expressed as HLA DR 2 and 4, as well as the HLA B 27 chromosomal markers can predispose certain patients to develope an autoimmune disorder. Dr. Alan Steere has demonstrated that Lyme disease patients who are HLA DR 4 positive have more severe autoimmune rheumatological manifestations. As I said earlier, the immune systems of some patients who are genetically predisposed to autoimmune diseases try to kill off the *Borrelia* causing the Lyme disease by targeting the flagellar (tail) proteins that are biochemically similar to myelin sheaths. This causes their immune system to attack the myelin sheaths surrounding their nerves as well, leading to demyelination, the process that is the hallmark of MS. The immune system in these patients is unable to differentiate between the flagellar protein of *Borrelia* and their myelin sheaths. Since demyelination is part of the disease process underlying MS, and since up to 70 percent of Lyme patients with unresolved symptoms can have demyelination with associated peripheral neuropathy, it would appear that this process is another common denominator in the two diseases.

Yet not all Lyme disease patients have demyelination and neuropathy. Could other bacterial organisms be present, causing these autoimmune reactions and explaining why some patients get these symptoms and others do not? Lyme patients are desperate and searching for answers, so often they do their own extensive scientific literature search when doctors seem unable to help them. I have often learned as much from my patients' research as I have from scientific conferences. For example, one of my patients with MS let me know of a link that had been reported between *Chlamydia pneumonia* and MS. "Just go onto the CPN.org Web site," she said. "You'll get a lot of information there." I went on the Internet and looked up the Web site, and what I found was fascinating.

Chlamydia pneumonia had already been reported in the medical literature as having a possible link to MS. It is an intracellular bacterium, and most physicians are familiar with *Chlamydia* as either causing a pneumonia or sinusitis with *Chlamydia*, Taiwan acute respiratory agent (TWAR), or as being one of the organisms responsible for pelvic inflammatory disease (PID) and other sexually transmitted diseases. In my first several years of practice, positive *Mycoplasma* and *Chlamydia* titers didn't worry me very much, since most of us are exposed to these bacteria, with resulting upper respiratory infections. Most physicians expect that high titers indicate an old exposure and that they probably don't have much clinical significance. Or did they?

In reviewing the literature on chlamydia and MS, I found it interesting that the authors of a protocol to treat *Chlamydia pneumonia* and MS used three drugs I was very familiar with from treating Lyme patients, especially those with intracellular infections such as *Bartonella*: a combination of a tetracycline, such as doxycycline or minocycline, a macrolide, such as Zithromax or Biaxin, and pulsed Flagyl. We had already had a positive experience using this same protocol in our Lyme disease patients, since researchers had demonstrated that Lyme disease can go into the intracellular compartment like many other intracellular infections, including *Mycoplasma* and *Chlamydia,* and would therefore respond to intracellular drugs. So another clue appeared. If the tests for these multiple co-infections were not always reliable, and the patient improved on a combination of intracellular medications, was it possible that other intracellular co-infections were present and causing some of the clinical and autoimmune manifestations that I was seeing in my resistant patients?

Barbara's MS Was Misdiagnosed

Barbara was forty-three years old when she first came to see me in 2006. Her past medical history was significant for multiple sclerosis. Her symptoms began in August 2005, when she complained of numbness in the right upper leg and in the right lower abdomen, which had then moved to the left side and left lower extremity. She was hospitalized at a major New York medical center, and immediately upon admission had a lumbar puncture (LP) to remove spinal fluid for testing. The neurologist on call determined from the results that she had MS. Barbara did not have the results of her LP with her at our initial visit, but my review of her medical records showed that the primary differential diagnosis considered at the time of admission was MS, and Lyme disease had been ruled out.

How did they arrive at the diagnosis? A brain MRI showed several hyperintense lesions around the corpus callosum (which connects the right and left cerebral hemispheres) and an MRI of the thoracic spine showed a T2 hyperintense lesion (bright signal) in the spinal cord at T2–T3. These results were suggestive of demyelination. The cervical MRI

was within normal limits. A CT scan of the spine showed that she had
had a laminectomy (an orthopedic spinal procedure that removes part of
the bone) with a spinal fixation (fusion of the bones) at L4–L5. There was
no associated spinal stenosis (a narrowing of the spinal canal, which
could explain neurological problems, such as tingling, numbness, pain,
and loss of motor control). She had had multiple lumbar spinal surgeries
in 1991 and 2005 for back pain, as well as a history of herniated discs, but
the results of the CT scans could not account for her neurological symptoms, including her difficulty walking.

Barbara was prescribed steroids as an anti-inflammatory treatment
(Solu-Medrol) for her presumed MS while awaiting new lumbar puncture results, which came back with seven white blood cells, all lymphocytes. Elevated levels of lymphocytes in the spinal fluid are sometimes
seen in neurological Lyme disease, whereas in MS, there is usually an
increase in the number of mononuclear white cells. Based on these results, the neurologist called an infectious disease consult to rule out
Lyme disease. A Lyme antibody test was performed, and was negative,
but Barbara informed her physician that she had a history of several tick
bites in 1999, 2004, 2005, and 2006, and the last tick bite was from an
engorged tick on her head. What was interesting to me in reading the
infectious disease fellow's hospital notes is that he stated that the patient
was very convinced that she had Lyme disease: "She knows it mimics
everything, including MS, and says she knows friends who were in wheelchairs and were then diagnosed with Lyme disease and got better with
treatment. The patient seems very invested in being treated for Lyme
disease."

In reviewing the hospital records, I also noted that the physician had
written that the patient had complained of "shifting numbness," a classic
symptom for Lyme disease. However, he did not get a history of all of the
patient's multiple systemic complaints, and once the ELISA test returned
negative, he automatically ruled out Lyme disease.

Barbara had filled out my questionnaire on her initial visit to our
medical office and had twenty out of the thirty-eight questions circled as
positive. She complained of flushing, chills, subjective fevers, and mild
sweats. Her weight fluctuated, and she tired easily. She had irregular
menses and mood swings, with decreased libido and decreased sensation
in the genital area. She had a chronic dry cough without wheezing and

some heart palpitations. She had gas, bloating, and constipation. There were migratory joint pains in her shoulders, knees, and neck, her legs twitched and were numb, and her lower extremities were weak. She often complained of headaches, blurry vision and floaters, poor balance with difficulty walking (she needed a cane to walk), and had difficulty concentrating and reading. She also had difficulties with insomnia, including staying asleep. She denied drinking any caffeine, and there was no prior history of mood swings or depression. Her only other notable past medical history were thyroid nodules seen on the MRI, which were biopsied and found to be negative, as well as a history of reflux disease (GERD), irritable bowel syndrome (IBS), and her L4-5 discectomy and fusion for her long history of back problems. There was also one episode of elevated liver functions in 2004 that had not been explained, with associated fevers, chills, and a headache.

The fevers, sweats, and chills were suggestive of multiple differential diagnoses. Malaria was considered, but she had not traveled abroad. Her night sweats were associated with a cough, but her chest X-ray ruled out tuberculosis or a lymphoma. Her thyroid nodules had been biopsied and found to be benign, and there was no evidence of hyperthyroidism on her laboratory testing. The sweats and chills were therefore most suggestive of babesiosis. The other important clues were her migratory joint pain and paresthesias. Migratory joint pain and tingling constitute two of the most classic symptoms we see in Lyme disease. I have never seen migratory joint pain associated with any other medical illness. It is not seen with rheumatoid arthritis, lupus, fibromyalgia, or osteoarthritis.

This doctor had ruled out Lyme disease based on a negative antibody test result. Barbara had discussed with her physician the possibility that the ELISA had been negative due to the poor sensitivity of the test, but he didn't listen. She knew about the insensitivity of the test based on the experiences of friends who had been misdiagnosed with other diseases because of a negative ELISA.

But what about the elevated lymphocytes on her spinal tap? Lyme disease is known to cause lymphocytic meningitis (inflammation in the meningeal sac surrounding the brain and spinal cord). Although the white cell count of seven was not elevated enough to generate high suspicions of a viral, fungal, or spirochetal infection (the normal range for lymphocytes in the cerebrospinal fluid is between 0 and 5 cells per mcL), that number of lymphocytes still should not be found on a normal spinal tap.

The confounding variable was that when the patient's CSF did eventually come back it was positive for oligoclonal bands that were not present in a corresponding serum sample from the blood. This verified an abnormal synthesis of IgG in the cerebral spinal fluid and was interpreted to be supportive evidence for MS versus a central nervous system infection. But neither a normal spinal tap nor that of someone with MS should contain any significant number of white cells. Lymphocytes are a type of white cell, and they can be found in certain patients with Lyme meningitis. Was it possible that she had both diseases, or was Lyme mimicking MS?

There are certain proteins that are typically elevated in the spinal fluid of patients with MS. These include gamma globulins, especially IgG, but also IgM and IgA, as well as the proteins called oligoclonal bands. They are not specific for MS, as they can also be found in Lyme disease patients, but significantly elevated levels of oligoclonal bands and myelin basic proteins would be more suggestive of an autoimmune phenomenon such as MS.

So with a negative Lyme ELISA, and a negative IgM, IgA, or IgG antibody test for *Borrelia burgdorferi* in her cerebral spinal fluid, she was given a diagnosis of MS, rather than Lyme disease. An abnormal VEP (visual evoked potential) also helped to confirm demyelination of her optic nerve; this again was interpreted to be consistent with MS.

I sent off for a broad range of tests to try and explain her resistant symptoms. Barbara's tick-borne titers came back positive for human granulocytic ehrlichiosis, with an IgG antibody titer positive at 1:80, and her *Babesia microti* IgG titer was 1:80 positive, with a negative *Babesia* PCR and negative *Babesia* FISH test. Her Lyme IgG Western blot was CDC positive, with 5 bands out of 10 being positive (including the 31, or outer surface, protein A and 39 kDa bands, which are highly Lyme specific). Diana's multiple tick bites and positive tests definitely gave her at least three documented potential tick-borne infections, including Lyme, *Ehrlichia*, and *Babesia*.

Her vitamin B_{12} level was in the low normal range at 289 (the normal range being 200 to 914); even though low normal, I suspected a B_{12} deficiency. It is known that patients can have neuropsychiatric abnormalities with B_{12} levels less than 400, and her level of 289 was low enough to warrant a treatment trial of B_{12}, since she had tingling and numbness of her lower extremities with associated memory and concentration problems, which can all be signs of B_{12} deficiency.

Other abnormalities that we found in her blood work included positive tests for food allergies and sensitivity to grains and gluten. We regularly screen patients for celiac disease and gluten sensitivity, using two blood tests: antigliadin antibodies (IgG) and tissue transglutaminase (TTG). Celiac disease, which is a more severe form of gluten sensitivity, can cause fatigue, as well as tingling and numbness of the extremities, which Diana complained of. Her tests returned highly positive for antigliadin IgG antibodies with a negative TTG. These results were suggestive of gluten sensitivity, which can cause neurological symptoms, so a trial of a gluten-free diet was instituted, and it seemed we should consider an upper endoscopy and a small intestinal biopsy if there was inadequate improvement with antibiotics. A food allergy panel was also positive for allergies to wheat, soy, corn, eggs, and milk. Her CBC, comprehensive metabolic profile, thyroid functions, CPK, and complement studies were all within normal limits. The only other abnormalities were a slightly elevated TIBC (total iron binding capacity) with normal iron levels, and a slightly elevated IgM antibody level, consistent with infection.

We started Barbara on doxycycline for the first month to cover her Lyme disease and ehrlichiosis. We also added Mepron and Zithromax for the babesiosis. After the first month of treatment her walking had started to improve, and her right-leg numbness had decreased. Her energy was better, although she still complained of fatigue. Her cognitive symptoms also improved. CBCs and liver functions were routinely tested every four to six weeks while she was on the antibiotic regimens, and these were within normal limits.

Due to her significant ongoing GI intolerance of the medications and the severity of her neurological symptoms, a PICC line was inserted and she was started on IV Rocephin for the second month. Her functioning improved from 60 percent to 85 percent of normal by the end of the second month. The numbness in her right leg was now almost completely gone, and her walking and balance was so much better that she no longer needed a cane. To evaluate a recurring cough, we ordered a CT scan of her chest, which returned negative for cancer or lung disease. Barbara told us that she had stopped taking her Mepron while on the IV therapy. Once the Mepron was restarted with the Zithromax, resuming treatment of her babesiosis, her cough disappeared.

I gave Barbara vitamin B_{12} injections every day with the above antibiotics, and in six months she was back to 90 percent of her normal functioning. We referred her to a Lyme-literate neurologist in New Jersey to help follow her while she was on the antibiotics. He eventually felt as we did: She probably did not have true MS, as she had worsened while in the hospital on steroids. (Prednisone and steroids suppress the immune system and can cause severe flares in Lyme patients and worsen their symptoms.)

Her clinical course was significant for the fact that she felt better and better on antibiotics over time, but every time she tried to come off the antibiotics, she felt worse. This is a classic clinical course often seen with patients with persistent Lyme-MSIDS. Why did she feel worse each time she came off the antibiotics? We decided to recheck her tick-borne tests. Her *Bartonella* titer now returned with a low positive result, and a repeat Western blot showed a significant expansion of her bands. Her 31 band, outer surface protein A (Osp A), was now 4 plus positive on an IgM Western blot, strongly suggesting an active Lyme infection. The Osp A is a very significant band for *Borrelia burgdorferi*, especially in patients who never received the LYMErix vaccine (the LYMErix vaccine was taken off the market years ago, and was the first large-scale attempt to immunize and protect against getting Lyme disease after an infected tick bite. Osp A is its active ingredient and can cause a false positive 31 kDa on a Western blot). She also now had a new positive 93 kDa band, also specific for Lyme disease. The banding on her IgG Western blot had decreased, however, and her *Babesia* titers had turned negative due to the treatment. But the most significant test was the PCR of her serum, which had returned positive for *Borrelia burgdorferi* after two years of antibiotic treatment. In other words, we were able to find evidence of an ongoing infection with *Borrelia burgdorferi* despite more than six months of IV Rocephin and multiple courses of oral antibiotics. This would explain why she complained of clinical relapses of her Lyme disease and MS picture each time she was taken off antibiotics.

Despite these frequent relapses, Barbara responded to retreatment with minocycline plus Biaxin with Plaquenil. This is the classic double intracellular antibiotic regimen we discussed earlier, which is not only commonly used to treat patients with Lyme disease but also patients with MS and Lyme with associated *Chlamydia pneumonia*.

So is MS an autoimmune demyelinating disease without other treatable causes, and does it simply require immune-modulating drugs, such as Avelox, Betaseron, Copaxone, Rebif, and steroids? Not necessarily. Is there an association with Lyme disease and other intracellular bacteria, such as *Chlamydia pneumonia*? The scientific literature says that there is an association. Lyme disease can provoke autoimmune phenomena, making true autoimmune diseases worse, and conversely, autoimmune diseases may be caused by Lyme disease. Do heavy metals like mercury play a role in MS and demyelinating diseases? We know that Lyme disease can cause demyelination, but so does mercury. Mercury can travel up the nerves into the central nervous system and also cause demyelinating lesions. Is there also a role for oxidative stress and environmental toxins damaging neurons, and further increasing demyelination, and do nutritional deficiencies, such as vitamin D deficiency, play a role in driving MS?

The scientific literature suggests that all of these factors may be at work, and we need to look at the MSIDS map to discover if there are multiple overlapping etiologies affecting the patient with an autoimmune disease, from lupus to rheumatoid arthritis to MS. Based on my clinical experience, this approach works in many chronically ill patients for whom standard therapies have failed and offers new hope for those suffering from MS and other autoimmune diseases.

SEVEN

Lyme and Inflammation

The MSIDS map for chronic diseases helps to explain why certain patients with resistant Lyme disease symptoms may not improve with standard treatment regimens: There may be multiple underlying factors driving symptoms that have not been adequately diagnosed and/or treated. At the same time, there is another common denominator that can be found underlying many of the points on the MSIDS model that can help explain various clinical symptoms.

Medicine has been searching for decades to find the magic bullet that would help prevent chronic illness and degenerative diseases. It turns out that there are several biochemical mechanisms that can explain the causes of many common ailments of the twenty-first century, including ones that lead to premature aging. These mechanisms can be summed up in three phrases: free radicals, oxidative stress, and inflammation. Free radicals are atoms and molecules with unpaired electrons. They play an important role in many biochemical reactions in the body, and although they are essential to life, too many can be damaging. We naturally produce free radicals during the oxidative reactions that take place inside every cell, where oxygen is used to create energy. Oxidative stress refers to the production of these free radicals, which are also known as "reactive oxygen species." What's more, oxidative stress has been shown to be an important factor in many diseases. In fact, the number one biological mechanism that seems to underlie most chronic disease states is oxidative stress: When there are too many free radicals, oxidative stress occurs, and it leads to inflammation.

Inflammation is a type of "fire" in the body, and it is defined by five cardinal signs: heat, redness, pain, swelling, and loss of function. It can occur anywhere in the body. You may have recognized inflammation that surrounds a cut or a bruise. Inflammation is also internal and can take many forms, from a headache to nasal congestion to arthritis to heart disease. Any of the disease states that you may have heard of that end in "itis" are forms of inflammation.

Inflammation can be classified as either acute or chronic; with MSIDS we are generally dealing more with the chronic type, except in the case of early Lyme disease and acute exposure to other co-infections. The patients I usually see, most of whom have been sick for years, are suffering from chronic inflammation, which is characterized by the simultaneous destruction and healing of various tissues in their bodies. The major cells involved in this process are immune cells called "mononuclear cells," and they include monocytes, macrophages, lymphocytes, plasma cells, and fibroblasts. These cells produce inflammatory chemicals at the site of the injury known as cytokines, such as interferon gamma (IFN-γ), TNF-alpha, interleukin-1 (IL-1), and interleukin-6 (IL-6), as well as various growth factors and enzymes. Without the proper treatment these cells and their inflammatory products can cause inflammation that lasts for months or years.

When we look at the impacts of free radicals and oxidative stress on multiple organs of the body, we find a broad range of deleterious effects. When free radicals and subsequent inflammation attack the arteries, this can damage the blood vessels and increase atherosclerosis, with oxidized LDL cholesterol eventually leading to heart attacks. Free radicals and the subsequent inflammation can affect the brain and lead to strokes, epilepsy, Parkinson's, or Alzheimer's disease. Inflammation may cause cataracts or macular degeneration of the eye, or dermatitis, psoriasis, or scleroderma of the skin. When it affects the lungs it can worsen asthma or cystic fibrosis. Free radicals and oxidative stress have also been linked to diabetes, aging, and cancer, and to a variety of inflammatory joint diseases, including rheumatoid arthritis.

But are there other ways that free radicals cause inflammation in the body and lead to these varied disease states? Persistent inflammation can be due to multiple etiologies on the MSIDS map, especially chronic bacterial, viral, parasitic, and fungal infections, as well as the type of autoimmune reactions we discussed in the previous chapter. In these circumstances, there is a switch inside the nucleus of cells called NF-KappaB. When free radicals and inflammatory molecules are present in the cell, they turn on the switch of NFKappaB, leading to the production of more of these inflammatory cytokines—IFN-γ (interferon gamma), TNF-alpha, interleukin-1 (IL-1), and interleukin-6 (IL-6)—causing a phenomenon known as sickness syndrome.

What is the sickness syndrome? A good example is seen in the patient who comes down with the flu. They may complain of fever, fatigue, joint and muscle aches, nausea, mood changes, feeling foggy, and wanting to stay in bed and sleep for long periods of time. It is a protective mechanism that is the result of the production of these inflammatory molecules that we have been discussing, TNF-alpha, IL-1, and IL-6. The same cytokines that are produced during the flu also occur in rheumatoid arthritis, causing joint pain, and are the causes of muscle aches and pains in fibromyalgia and chronic fatigue syndrome, the brain fog associated with Alzheimer's disease, and the majority of the chronic symptoms we see in Lyme disease. Ordinarily, sickness syndrome forces the individual to stay out of harm's way at a time when the body's resources are needed to fight off the infection. The medical literature contains extensive evidence on the occurrence of sickness syndrome and how it is linked to a variety of disease processes, including major depression, congestive heart failure, anxiety, pain syndromes, and sleep disorders.

When a Lyme patient with MSIDS complains of fatigue, muscle and joint pain, an increase in neuropathic pain, headaches, flulike symptoms, difficulty sleeping, mood swings, and cognitive difficulties such as brain fog, they are describing manifestations of a dramatic increase in cytokine production and inflammatory molecules in the body: a kind of inflammation gone wild. The most dramatic example of a severe case of sickness syndrome is when a patient with Lyme disease has a Jarisch-Herxheimer reaction. The killing off of *Borrelia* causes a sudden release of these cytokines, leading to a dramatic increase in symptoms.

Medicine has long searched for a common etiologic mechanism to explain diseases that share many symptoms in common, such as chronic fatigue syndrome (CFS), multiple chemical sensitivity (MCS), fibromyalgia syndrome (FM), post-traumatic stress disorder (PTSD), and persistent Lyme disease. Dr. Martin Pall, a professor of biochemistry and basic medical sciences at Washington State University, noticed that the above disease states share many symptoms in common. They include: chronic fatigue; ongoing muscle and joint pains; memory and concentration problems; mood disorders, including depression and anxiety; and an inability to sleep. Back in 2001 he postulated that these illnesses, having similar symptoms, can all be initiated by a variety of factors, such as viral infections, bacterial infections, physical or emotional trauma, or exposure to environmental toxins, such as volatile organic solvents (VOS), pesticides, etc. These diverse stressors can all increase nitric oxide and its oxidant product, peroxynitrite. Nitric oxide was named "the scientific molecule of the year" over ten years ago. Why? It has been shown to have extremely beneficial effects in the body, such as lowering blood pressure, lowering cholesterol, and vasodilating (increasing blood flow) in various arteries in the body, including the coronary arteries. However, nitric oxide can also have deleterious effects under certain conditions. This molecule acts as a free radical and increases oxidative stress, which can damage DNA and proteins inside the cell. It also can stimulate the production of NF-KappaB, which can increase the production of IL-1, IL-6, IL-8, TNF-α, and IFN-γ (interferon gamma). It is therefore logical that apart from needing to address the underlying factors driving the sickness syndrome (i.e., treating the viral, bacterial, parasitic, and fungal infections as well as the physical and emotional traumas and eliminating environmental toxins), our therapy should focus on decreasing the free radicals and oxidant by-products of the nitric oxide biochemical cycle. This would include a regimen of antioxidants, CoQ10, B vitamins, alpha-lipoic acid (ALA), magnesium (Mag++), zinc (Zn++), omega 3 fatty acids, and glutathione precursors such as N-Acetylcysteine (NAC), and glycine.

Fully mitigating the harmful effects of these free radicals and oxidant by-products requires simultaneously treating the three Is—infection, immune issues, and inflammation—and supporting the detoxification pathways, balancing hormones, and addressing nutritional deficiencies, food allergies, and sleep disorders—while eliminating environmental triggers (such as heavy metals) that may also increase inflammation. This is where the Horowitz sixteen-point differential diagnostic map comes into play. Inflammation often underlies many chronic diseases, but the inflammation may not be controlled until all of the points on the MSIDS map have been properly addressed.

INFLAMMATION AND THE BRAIN

Inflammation is an extremely important factor that underlies the symptoms in neurological diseases. In a study published in 2007 in *Lancet Neurology*, researchers reported finding that the neurological syndromes associated with *Borrelia burgdorferi* are also associated with inflammation in the central nervous system, in particular, amyloid metabolism. Amyloids are proteins that aggregate and change the structure of cells, damaging them. They are found in many diseases, including: type II diabetes; autoimmune phenomenon, such as rheumatoid arthritis; and neurodegenerative diseases, such as Alzheimer's, Huntington's, and Parkinson's disease.

Amyloid is just one of several internal neurotoxins (substances that can damage or kill off the brain's neurons) that are produced by inflammation and can alter the normal activity of the cells of the central nervous system. Also, there are external neurotoxins, the most common ones being heavy metals and environmental toxins. In fact, inflammatory processes are involved in the neurotoxicity of many chronic neurologic diseases in addition to Lyme disease: One of them is of the most prevalent and feared neurodegenerative diseases of our time, Alzheimer's disease. Neurotoxins and inflammation both can alter the normal activity of the nervous system in such a way as to cause damage to nervous tissue. Neurotoxicity can result from exposure to substances used in chemotherapy, radiation treatment, drug therapies, certain drug abuse, organ transplants; heavy metals, certain foods and food additives, pesticides, industrial and/or cleaning solvents, and cosmetics; and to some naturally occurring substances. Symptoms may appear immediately after exposure or be delayed. They may include limb weakness or numbness, loss of memory, vision, and/or intellect, uncontrollable obsessive and/or compulsive behaviors, delusions, headache, cognitive and behavioral problems, and sexual dysfunction. Individuals with certain disorders may be especially vulnerable to neurotoxins.

Microglia in the brain (specialized cells that are the first line of immune defense in the central nervous system) are activated by beta amyloid (the primary component of the plaques found in Alzheimer's disease) and proinflammatory cytokines. Activated microglia in turn release more proinflammatory cytokines (IL-1-β, IL-6, TNF-α) that may lead to neuronal death and dysfunction by a variety of mechanisms, including:

1. Enhancement of glutamate-induced excitotoxicity: Excitotoxicity is the pathological process by which nerve cells are damaged and killed by excessive stimulation by neurotransmitters in the brain, such as glutamate.
2. Inhibition of brain neuroplasticity. Neuroplasticity refers to the ability of the brain to recover from injury and is necessary in proper development, learning, and memory.
3. Inhibition of the creation of new neurons in the brain: especially in the hippocampus, the part of the brain essential to memory.

Lyme disease patients, like Alzheimer's patients, often complain of neurocognitive deficits in memory and concentration and difficulties with executive functioning (decision making, for example). Recent studies have reported increased TNF-α levels in the cerebral spinal fluid of AD patients, just as in Lyme disease, and a single genetic change in the TNF-α gene is associated with earlier onset AD. A fascinating study was done on Alzheimer's patients in which the investigators attempted to inhibit cytokine production to see the effect on memory. The study consisted of a trial of the TNF-α inhibitor Enbrel for the treatment of AD. The results were significant improvements in several cognitive and functional assessments (mini-mental state examination, or MMSE, Alzheimers Disease Assessment Scale—Cognitive Subscale, or ADAS-Cog, Severe Impairment Battery). The improvements began at one month and were sustained for the six-month duration of the trial. In other words, inhibiting cytokines significantly helped memory.

This study would not be possible with Lyme disease patients for several reasons. First of all, it is contraindicated to use TNF-α inhibitors in Lyme disease, since it is an immune modulator that could reactivate the infection (this is published in animal studies using the mouse model, and I have seen this effect in patients being treated for rheumatoid arthritis who also had Lyme disease). Second, although Lyme disease patients are often willing to participate in scientific trials, their suffering is such that very few are going to consent to injecting drugs into their cervical spine on a regular basis, especially ones that have been linked to cancer. (They do allow me to use to large needles to administer the bicillin shots on a regular basis, and are happy to receive these injections!) However, since

Lyme disease patients are also known to have increased levels of TNF-alpha in their central nervous systems, as is found in AD, it would explain why my patients improve clinically as we block the production of cytokines and open up their detoxification pathways to remove cytokines and neurotoxins from the body.

This would also explain why certain patients, who had been previously diagnosed with chronic fatigue syndrome, fibromyalgia, autoimmune diseases, neurological diseases such as Alzheimer's, and psychiatric diseases, find that they feel remarkably better once we have treated their Lyme disease and MSIDS. By lowering their inflammatory cytokines, we are treating one of the underlying biochemical mechanisms responsible for their clinical symptoms.

LYME DISEASE AND INFLAMMATION

Lyme disease can cause significant inflammation in the peripheral and central nervous systems, depending on the specific species of *Borrelia*. The manifestations of *Borrelia burgdorferi sensu stricto* (the most common *Borrelia* species in the United States) differ from *Borrelia garinii* (which is found in Europe and is responsible for inflammation in the central nervous system, i.e., neuroborreliosis) and are also different from *Borrelia afzelii* (which is found in Europe and causes skin lesions). *Borrelia burgdorferi* spirochetes express specific lipoproteins on the outer surface membrane of the *Borrelia* cell wall that are known to be proinflammatory. Lipoproteins are structural complexes of both proteins and fats on the outside of the organism, that can stimulate the immune system and increase inflammation. More than 8 percent of the coding sequence of a common strain of *Borrelia*, strain B31, is devoted to lipoprotein sequences, which attract neutrophils, one of the first immune cells to migrate toward the site of the inflammation. These lipoproteins then stimulate these neutrophils and macrophages (other cells of the immune system that also engulf and digest pathogens and produce inflammatory cytokines). A 1994 study published in the journal *Infection and Immunity*, reported that *Borrelia* are so powerful that they can cause a much stronger inflammatory response than common bacteria that produce cytokines (like *E. coli*), one that is fifty to five hundred times stronger. This explains in part the extremely strong inflammatory response that some patients can have when exposed to the bacteria that causes Lyme disease.

The effects of proinflammatory cytokines and the symptoms that they cause depend on whether they act in the central nervous system or peripheral nervous system, as well as on the patient's current health status and their genetic predisposition. If cytokines act in the peripheral nervous system, they can cause pain and inflammation in the peripheral nerves. A study published in 2005 showed that molecular mimicry can also occur in the peripheral nervous system, with *Borrelia*-specific IgM antibodies reacting against the flagellar tail of the organism and cross-reacting with neuronal antigens, causing neuropathy. This explains the overlap in neurological symptoms caused by demyelination in both MS and persistent Lyme disease.

Cytokine activity can also take place in the central nervous system, accompanying demyelination (which is seen as "white spots" or "unidentified bright objects" on a brain MRI). It accounts for many of the neurological symptoms we see in Lyme disease, including headaches, sleep disorders, mood swings, memory and concentration problems, and neuralgia/nerve pain.

One type of cytokine, known as TNF-alpha, has a principal role in initiating a cascade of activations of other cytokines and growth factors in the inflammatory response, causing pain. A 2004 study of the peripheral nervous system found that cytokines induced by TNF-alpha such as interleukin 1-β, can cause the secondary production of other inflammatory molecules, such as nitric oxide, bradykinin, and/or prostaglandins (chemical messengers that regulate pain, inflammation, and smooth muscle contraction). When combined together, these inflammatory cytokines can have a direct effect on the sensory nerves that allow people to feel pain, pressure, vibration, heat, and cold. Lyme disease patients often complain of symptoms relating to these sensory nerves: They feel that they are either too hot or too cold, or experience numbness, tingling, or a significant increase in pain usually described as pinpricks or burning sensations.

Apart from *Borrelia* being able to stimulate proinflammatory cytokines, we must also remember that the MSIDS patient has multiple overlapping factors contributing to the varied symptoms of chronic illness, and that each of these factors must be addressed for the patient to attain well-being. For example, co-infections will significantly increase symptoms.

Mycoplasmal infections increase proinflammatory cytokines, including IL-1, IL-2, and IL-6. *Bartonella* can cause a host of inflammatory reactions, including an encephalopathy and chronic demyelinating peripheral neuropathy (PNP), radiculitis, myelitis, vasculitis, and inflammatory ophthalmologic manifestations. *Chlamydia* causes reactive inflammatory arthritis, and frequent viruses found in MSIDS, such as Epstein-Barr, cytomegalovirus, and human herpesvirus-6, can cause inflammation. We know that with HHV-6 there is a link to chronic fatigue syndrome and fibromyalgia, which are syndromes that overlap with MSIDS. HHV-6 can reactivate later in life secondary to immunological and environmental factors, leading to inflammation in the liver (hepatitis) and the brain (meningoencephalitis). It is also considered by some authors to be a cofactor in autism, ADD, and MS. So the patient needs to be adequately diagnosed and treated for all of these co-infections, since treating only one of them will leave the patient vulnerable to ongoing inflammation and symptoms of the sickness syndrome.

Similarly, we find other common factors on the MSIDS map that can increase inflammation. For example, I frequently find that my patients suffer from food allergies and food and chemical sensitivities. Food sensitivities can cause a complex immune reaction, involving cellular activation of sensitized T cells and natural killer cells, as well as recruiting different types of white blood cells (eosinophils, basophils, monocytes, and neutrophils) that release different inflammatory mediators, such as cytokines, leukotrienes, histamine, and prostaglandins. These inflammatory molecules play an important role in the pathogenesis of pain, as well as asthma and allergic reactions.

Mineral deficiencies can also have a profound effect on inflammation. Patients may have copper deficiency, and copper is necessary in superoxide dismutase (SOD), an enzyme essential for controlling free radicals and oxidative stress. We also frequently find zinc deficiency in my MSIDS patients, and this can lead to increased levels of inflammatory cytokines and IL-10. In a National Institutes of Health–funded study, elderly patients with zinc deficiencies who were given zinc supplements had decreased incidences of infections, decreased levels of TNF-alpha, and decreased plasma oxidative stress markers. These are not tests commonly performed in a physician's office, but addressing any deficiencies in essential minerals can profoundly help the patient with MSIDS control inflammation.

SLEEP AND INFLAMMATION

The MSIDS population generally does not sleep well. In fact, they have some of the most resistant and profound insomnia that I have ever witnessed. That is why many patients with Lyme disease and MSIDS are misdiagnosed with CFS and fibromyalgia, which are also syndromes associated with fatigue, aches and pains, mood disorders, and poor sleep. Sleep deprivation is one primary cause of the production of inflammatory cytokines. How does impaired sleep cause these same symptoms? It is because sleep deprivation increases inflammation and the production of inflammatory cytokines, causing similar symptoms in these patient populations. Impaired sleep correlates directly with impaired immune functioning, and sleep disorders are commonly associated with chronic inflammatory diseases, such as rheumatoid arthritis, fibromyalgia (FM), and CFS. Chronic sleep restriction also leads to elevations in IL-6 and pain. Since we already see elevated levels of IL-6 in Lyme disease, sleep deprivation compounds the effects of the elevated level of this inflammatory cytokine.

In 2010, the American College of Rheumatology updated the diagnostic criteria for fibromyalgia. They concluded that 20 percent of patients with rheumatoid arthritis, lupus, osteoarthritis, and other diseases had overlapping FM. It may be secondary to the underlying disease or a completely separate condition. Therefore, widespread pain in a number of areas of the body along with gradations in the severity of fatigue, sleep disturbance, cognitive dysfunction, and other somatic symptoms are the clinical signs for fibromyalgia. These are the same symptoms found in Lyme-MSIDS. You see how easy it would be to mistake MSIDS and Lyme disease for much simpler diagnoses of sleep deprivation and fibromyalgia.

INFLAMMATION WAS AFFECTING VICKI'S RECOVERY

Vicki was fifty-eight years old when she first came to see me. She had a past medical history significant for hypertension, hyperlipidemia, metabolic syndrome, obesity, hypothyroidism, anxiety and depression, and severe osteoarthritis of the knees. Her arthritis and weight problem was so severe that she needed a wheelchair to get around because walking was simply too painful for her. She had been diagnosed with Lyme disease and babesiosis several years earlier, with evidence of exposure to *Barton-ella*, *Mycoplasma*, *Chlamydia*, and several viruses, including Epstein-Barr virus (EBV) and HHV-6. She also tested positive for elevated levels of mercury and lead with a six-hour urine DMSA challenge, and her dehy-droepiandrosterone (DHEA)/cortisol levels showed evidence of mild ad-renal dysfunction.

Vicki was taking multiple medications, including Altace for her blood pressure, Zocor for her hyperlipidemia, Glucophage for her metabolic syndrome, Levothroid for her hypothyroidism, Paxil and Wellbutrin with intermittent benzodiazepines for her depression and anxiety, and Ambien with trazodone for sleep. She also required the regular use of non-steroided anti-inflammatory drugs (NSAIDs) (including high doses of Motrin), and Percocet four to five times per day for the extreme pain that she lived with day after day.

When Vicki first came to us, her chief complaints were extreme fatigue, severe pain in her joints—especially her hands and knees—a stiff neck, headaches, intermittent tingling and numbness of her extremities, chest pain, palpitations, shortness of breath, intermittent night sweats, severe memory and concentration problems, and overlapping depression, anxiety, and insomnia. She had been an extremely active woman with her family and her church and was mourning the loss of her prior state of health. Yet despite all of these challenges with her health, Vicki main-tained an exceptional sense of humor, and she showed great warmth in her relationships with others. She had a wonderful spirit and was not one to give up.

I treated Vicki with some of my standard protocols during the first several months that we were together. This would include rotations of cell wall, cystic, and intracellular drugs, while giving her adrenal support and removing her heavy metals. We treated her *Babesia* intermittently, whenever the night sweats would return and increase (she had a positive *Babesia* FISH test after one year of *Babesia* therapy), and although this would help temporarily, the sweats would often return several months later. She was well into her menopause, and her thyroid functions were within normal limits, so there were no other obvious reasons for the in-termittent night sweats.

The primary problem that we faced with Vicki was that every time we would give her antibiotics to treat her Lyme and co-infections, she would have extremely severe Jarisch-Herxheimer flares. She would feel worse on the regimens, and feel better temporarily whenever they were stopped. We therefore tried her on multiple herbal protocols, including traditional Chinese herbs, Samento, Banderol, Cumunda, and several Byron White remedies, but even herbal protocols would cause severe flares. What was there left to do?

When I reviewed Vicki's laboratory work, I noticed that all of her autoimmune markers were negative. Her 1-25 to 25 hydroxy-vitamin D ratios were within normal limits. An elevated 1-25/25 hydroxy-vitamin D ratio (greater than 2:1) has occasionally been seen in patients with inflammation. The X-rays of her knees did show severe osteoarthritis, but her joint pain would flare up independently of her using her knees, and her joints would occasionally be hot, red, swollen, and painful. Her sedimentation rate, a sign of inflammation, was within normal limits, but she did have a slightly elevated C-reactive protein, at 4.5 (normal is less than 3) in her past blood work. She was taking an 81 mg baby aspirin per day for her history of an elevated CRP. CRP is an indirect marker of elevated levels of interleukin-6, one of the inflammatory molecules that increases the symptoms of Lyme disease patients.

At that point I went back to my sixteen-point differential diagnostic list to see what other options we had not yet considered for Vicki. Her inflammation was a red flag, so I decided to send a cytokine panel to Lab-Corp to evaluate her for other markers of inflammation. Her TNF-alpha level came back within normal limits, but her IL-6 returned extremely elevated. Yet we had already tried multiple anti-inflammatories and pain medicines to treat her resistant symptoms, and these had been ineffective. She had also been to a rheumatologist in the past, and she had avoided using stronger disease-modifying drugs for her pain, such as TNF-alpha blockers and prednisone, because these drugs are known to exacerbate the symptoms of Lyme disease by suppressing the immune system. What else was left to do?

I reviewed Vicki's history and realized that she had not yet been given a dose of IV glutathione for her resistant symptoms or certain detoxification supplements or anti-inflammatory herbs for her severe Jarisch-Herxheimer reactions. She signed a consent form, and we gave her IV glutathione while she was in my medical office. I went out to see another patient and came back twenty minutes later. Already Vicki was brighter, calmer, and in less pain. She also noticed that she could think more clearly, and she was having an easier time with word retrieval and forming sentences. I brought her husband, Brian, into the room to discuss her case, and so that he could also witness the change in Vicki's health. Brian was amazed at the improvements. I then asked Brian whether anything had changed recently with Vicki, i.e., new medications, supplements that I was not aware of, new changes in sleep patterns, chemical exposures, etc. Brian thought carefully and then said, "No, Doc. Nothing has changed. We did, however, recently have the exterminator come into the house to spray and get rid of the fleas. He comes four times a year, and I do put pesticides on the lawn in the springtime, but we have been doing this for years."

Was it possible that Vicki had chemical sensitivity and was having difficulty with the extra chemical exposures in her environment? Could that have been playing a role in her resistant symptoms apart from her Lyme disease, co-infections, heavy metals, and adrenal dysfunction? Her response to the glutathione was remarkable in how effective it had been in decreasing her symptoms within minutes. Was the glutathione helping to remove fat-soluble toxins as well as cytokines, such as the elevated levels of IL-6 that Vicki had tested positive for? We reviewed Vicki's list of medications. She was on multiple medications that would require the use of the same liver detoxification pathways, and this could be a problem with the extra chemical exposure from the environment, requiring enhanced detoxification. Also, some of the drugs she had been taking had side effects associated with memory loss and amnesia. This included the Ambien, for sleep, and the statin drug (Zocor) for her elevated levels of cholesterol. There are reports in the medical literature of patients sleepwalking on Ambien, and getting confused, as well as amnesia and memory problems with patients on statin drugs.

We decided to stop her statin and Ambien and to give her a different sleep medication. We also increased her detoxification with oral phosphatidylcholine (an essential fatty acid in cell membranes) and liposomal glutathione (a better absorbed form of oral glutathione), added N-Acetylcysteine (NAC) with alpha-lipoic acid (an important antioxidant) to promote the body's own production of glutathione, and had her stop any further chemical exposure in her immediate environment. We also tried using herbal drainage remedies, to assist in removing toxins from her body; had her try an herbal Herxheimer compound of redroot, boneset, and *Smilax*; and a German product known as Itires, which is an herbal blend that assists lymphatic drainage. We had seen positive clinical results with this protocol in a group of our patients who had problems with detoxification. It is necessary to move the toxins out of the body, and the lymphatic system is one important means to do so. These herbs have been scientifically studied and validated to be effective in helping to decrease inflammation and cytokine levels, and to help with Herxheimer flares.

Vicki returned one month later. She had clinically improved with her new regimen. Her fatigue, joint pain, and cognitive problems had improved, since she was finally able to sleep with a new medication (Remeron), and an aggressive detoxification protocol helped decrease her elevated cytokine levels. She was also off medication that may have been causing overlapping symptoms, which could have been confused with ongoing Lyme disease.

Vicki's symptoms were linked to inflammation, which was making her recovery more difficult. She did not have positive autoimmune markers. Inflammation was there, and the Lyme was exacerbating it. That is part of the reason the rheumatologist was also in agreement that we should avoid using stronger disease-modifying drugs. She did not have a true autoimmune disease. By decreasing the aggressiveness of her antibiotic treatment, to decrease Jarisch-Herxheimer flares, helping her to sleep, opening up her detoxification pathways, and eliminating medication with overlapping side effects, we were able to help Vicki finally achieve significant clinical improvement. Until we made all of the above changes in her regimen, we could not shut off the inflammation that had been reflected in the elevated IL-6 levels in her blood.

HEAVY METALS AND INFLAMMATION

Assessing heavy metals, especially mercury, in chronically ill patients is critical for identifying other potential sources of inflammation. I am finding mercury exposure in the majority of my patients, using a six-hour urine DMSA challenge. Heavy metals such as mercury increase oxidative stress with subsequent changes in cytokines, and it has been suggested that it causes a multiplicity of autoimmune disorders, such as lupus, in which mercury can act as a hapten on the outside of the cell. A hapten is a small molecule that can elicit an immune response only when attached to a large carrier, such as a protein, on the outside of the cell. Some haptens can induce autoimmune disease.

According to a 2006 article published in *Critical Reviews in Toxicology*, mercury can also cause an increased susceptibility to infections, not a desired effect in the MSIDS patient who may already have multiple co-infections. When the patient is already overwhelmed with multiple infections, such as Lyme disease, parasites such as *Babesia*, viruses, and *Candida* simultaneously, we certainly do not want any other factors increasing his or her susceptibility to infections. By detoxifying the patient using chelating agents such as Dimercaptosuccinic acid (DMSA) and Ethylenediaminetetraacetic acid (EDTA), and removing these metals, some of our most difficult to treat patients find that their fatigue, muscle and joint pain, and cognitive difficulties improve as their inflammation decreases.

Heavy Metals and Minerals Were Affecting Steve's Health

Steve is one example of the necessity of checking for mineral deficiencies in patients with severe pain and inflammation. He came to see me from the Midwest approximately two years ago. He was a young man with a history of severe fatigue, joint pain, headaches, memory and concentration problems, drenching night sweats, and a complete loss of libido. He had seen multiple subspecialists without finding a cause for his symptoms, including eight different rheumatologists for the severe, unremitting joint pain he felt throughout his body. His autoimmune markers were all negative, and his Lyme ELISA test was negative, even though he reported that he had been bitten by multiple ticks over the years, some of them engorged and on him for days. Because the rheumatologists couldn't find a cause for his resistant pain, he was diagnosed with seronegative rheumatoid arthritis. He had been placed on rotations of high-dose prednisone, methotrexate, Enbrel, Arava, and other antirheumatic drugs over a three-year period. None of them helped his symptoms, and he continued to get worse over time. Eventually he became disabled at twenty-eight years old, unable to work in his profession. He had also been seen by a pain specialist and was on morphine sulphate with oxycodone several times per day for breakthrough pain, yet he still complained of severe, unremitting pain throughout his body. He also had a history of severe kidney stones, and was treated with a high-dose diuretic, chlorthalidone. This was necessary to stop his production of stones, for every time he stopped the diuretic, the stones reappeared.

My battery of tests painted a different picture. His Lyme Western blot was positive, his *Babesia* test was positive, and his *Bartonella* test was negative. He tested positive for exposure to mercury and lead, was severely deficient in testosterone, and had severe mineral deficiencies of zinc, iodine, and magnesium. I wasn't surprised by this finding: The diuretics he was taking are known to decrease levels of key minerals in the body.

Once we replaced his minerals, lowered his heavy metal burden, treated his hormone deficiency and Lyme and *Babesia*, Steve began to feel significantly better, and he was able to get back to work for the first time in years after being disabled.

HORMONE PRODUCTION AND INFLAMMATION

The last diagnostic category on the MSIDS map that frequently is affected by cytokines are the hormonal abnormalities often seen in persistent Lyme disease. We often see the hypothalamic-pituitary-adrenal axis (HPA), the master control center for all hormonal production throughout the body, affected by inflammation, and it is specifically affected in Lyme disease and FM. Cytokines can affect hormone levels positively and negatively. For example, research has shown that cortisol, an antiinflammatory hormone, is able to shut down the production of cytokines in a healthy individual. However, in someone with Lyme disease and FM, although cortisol production increases, it becomes ineffective due to cortisol resistance, and the result is increased, uncontrolled inflammation. We'll cover hormonal changes in more detail in Chapter 11.

TREATING INFLAMMATION

How do we regulate cytokines and inflammation? We have found, using the Horowitz sixteen-point differential diagnostic map, that a multifaceted approach works best, especially for patients with overlapping chronic fatigue syndrome or fibromyalgia who present with severe fatigue, headaches, cognitive dysfunction, neuralgia, myalgias, and arthritis.

The antibiotics and herbal regimens discussed in Chapter 3 do treat the pain that comes with Lyme disease, and usually the sickest patients will require a combined approach, using pharmaceuticals and nutraceuticals. If we focus on decreasing the production of inflammatory molecules produced along the nitric oxide pathway, and decrease oxidative stress while increasing the functioning of the biochemical pathways in the liver that help with detoxification, many patients will experience a significant benefit. Combining drugs such as low-dose naltrexone (LDN) with nutraceuticals that decrease inflammation (curcumin, broccoli seed extract [sulforpaphane], and glutathione and its precursors [NAC], among others) are generally effective in helping with pain and inflammation. The probable mechanism of action of these antioxidants and phytochemicals is to act on nuclear factor-like 2 receptors (Nrf2) and the antioxidant response element (ARE) genes inside the nucleus of cells. These are DNA-binding sites that primarily activate phase II enzymes in the liver (with a minor effect on phase I) plus numerous other enzymes that protect the cells from oxidative stress. When we activate the ARE genes, this helps enhance detoxification and decrease inflammation. This mechanism may explain many of the observed beneficial effects of phytochemicals, since a variety of substances activate Nrf2, such as sulforaphane (broccoli sprouts), resveratrol (the extract from red wine), curcumin (the spice turmeric), and green tea (EGCG). A diet high in these phytochemicals is known to be protective against many disease processes and is excellent in assisting detoxification and lowering inflammation.

If we hope to conquer the chronic infectious and degenerative diseases associated with MSIDS, we must put out the fire of inflammation that is slowly destroying our health. A comprehensive testing approach using the sixteen-point differential diagnostic map for chronic disease states, to determine which factors may be driving inflammation, is essential to getting to the root cause of these illnesses.

EIGHT

Lyme and Environmental Toxins

A ten-year-old boy once told me, "Doc, I've been to so many doctors. No one can tell me what's wrong. I was told that I probably have chronic fatigue syndrome with fibromyalgia and depression and that it's 'all in my head.'"

In the summer of 2002, Aaron came to see me with his mother. They lived in rural Maryland, and he had a history of multiple tick bites. His symptoms started in the second and third grades with reading problems, difficulty retaining information, and temper tantrums. He had a "real attitude problem" according to his mother, who was growing frustrated with his "acting out" at home and at school.

When I reviewed the physical symptoms that he circled on the questionnaire, I noticed that Aaron complained of fatigue, muscle pain, joint pain, neck stiffness, headaches, chills with hot and cold feelings, tingling of his extremities, palpitations, and insomnia, along with significant memory and concentration problems. To others, his behavior might seem like he had ADD. But I've seen these symptoms all too often: He was doing an excellent job of "acting out" like an inadequately treated Lyme disease patient with multiple co-infections.

I sat across from Aaron and looked him squarely in the eyes. "What bothers you the most?"

"Doc, I keep losing my wrestling matches. They're kicking my butt. You gotta help me." Not exactly what I expected to hear as the worst symptom, but I wasn't living in his ten-year-old world where WWF and Duane "the Rock" Johnson were king.

So we did a physical exam, which was unremarkable, and I sent off his blood to test for Lyme disease and co-infections. His Lyme IFA, his IgG Western blot, and his Lyme dot blot through IGeneX were all positive. He also had a positive *Bartonella* PCR through MDL Laboratories, as well as a positive Lyme antibody test and a positive *Babesia* test. As we have seen, babesiosis and *Bartonella* can both significantly increase the severity of Lyme symptoms, and account for an increase in mood swings, as well as memory and concentration problems, all of which bothered Aaron.

I started Aaron on a rotation of different antibiotics. The first rotation in which he showed significant improvement was high-dose amoxicillin, which covers the cell wall forms of *Borrelia*, with probenecid to improve the levels of amoxicillin in the central nervous system. We added to this regimen Mepron and Biaxin for the *Babesia* and *Bartonella*. Within one month's time the majority of his symptoms had improved, although his energy was inconsistent. His stamina continued to fail him at the gym during wrestling matches. However, he did get up to 98 percent of what he considered to be "normal functioning" during six months of treatment, so we decided to stop the antibiotics and give him Diflucan, an antifungal medication, to clear out any associated yeast.

Before we started the next rotation, Aaron told me that although his energy levels were better, he was still tired in the middle of the day, especially after meals, and around 3:00 P.M. after coming home from school. I suspected reactive hypoglycemia as one of the causes for his fatigue and lack of stamina, but knew that I would have a difficult time convincing him to stay away from pizza, hamburgers, fries, and ice cream, which make up a regular part of the typical ten-year-old's diet. I sent him for a five-hour glucose tolerance test with insulin levels. The test came back positive for significant hypoglycemia, so I thought that I had uncovered the final piece of the puzzle. If he could stay on a reasonably strict hypoglycemic diet his energy levels would be stable, and he would be able to get out of a full nelson in his matches.

Unfortunately, that was not the case. Aaron returned two months later. He had a frustrated look on his face and reported sadly that all of his symptoms were returning now that he was off the antibiotics. Once again he had increasing fatigue, aches and pains, and decreasing memory and concentration, and his grades were worsening in school. His irritability and temper were worse, and neither he nor his mother was happy. I wasn't happy with these results, either. Although in 2002 I was making significant progress for the vast majority of my patients, I was still confounded by the fact that some patients continued to have resistant symptoms. I am not only a medical detective, I also am a perfectionist. I wanted 100 percent of my patients to be back to normal, and so did they. What else was I missing?

Soon after receiving the news that Aaron was relapsing, I got a call from Randy, a dentist friend of mine. He had developed a strong interest in nutritional and functional medicine over the years, and integrated these protocols into his dental practice. We had become friends after we had both been on the medical advisory board of a nutrition company specializing in functional medicine. We would often chat about biochemical issues in chronic-disease states. Randy was often light-years ahead of his colleagues as he pushed the boundaries of nutritional medicine and dentistry with his patients. I was used to hearing his excitement, and he is one of the most passionate health-care providers I have ever met. He would often discover nutritional protocols that he would institute in his patients, and then excitedly call me up about how much help his patients were getting with resistant dental problems. But this time something was clearly different. Randy was even more excited than usual during this phone call in September.

"Richie," he said. "You won't believe what just happened. I decided to test myself for mercury poisoning since I'm around mercury vapor all the time with my patients. I just got back the test. My levels were ten times over the toxic range."

Mercury is a neurotoxin that contaminates fish and poses a health risk to people and to wildlife that eat them. The effects on health will depend on four variables: the patient's total load of toxins, their nutritional status, immune function, and the status of their detoxification pathways. Symptoms after exposure include fatigue, joint pains, muscle pains, tingling and numbness, memory and concentration problems, and emotional problems. These were the same symptoms that Aaron complained of, and are also frequent complaints of other Lyme disease patients in our practice.

"Do you have any symptoms?" I asked.

"Richie, I'm in my sixties," he replied. "I have a few little things here and there, but generally I feel well. The problem is that after I tested myself, I tested some of my patients. They also were coming back high for heavy metals. I think you should check yourself."

I didn't quite know what to make of this, but his call was an interesting synchronicity. I had just gotten back from the dentist for a root canal. In the days following it, I started to develop severe back spasms. I never had muscle spasms before. Nothing had changed at work or in my exercise regimen. However, the dentist had recently drilled out a silver mercury filling, and filled the root canal with a substance called eugenol. I did some research, and discovered that some patients who are chemically sensitive do not react well to certain materials used in root canals, and may have increased exposure to mercury after removal of their amalgam fillings. Is that why I suddenly noticed new physical symptoms I had never had before?

I decided to check myself for heavy metals, and subsequently started testing my patients. Heavy metal burden is a term that refers to exposure to metallic elements whose specific gravity is about 5.0 or greater, especially those that are poisonous. The most common heavy metals include mercury, lead, arsenic, cadmium, nickel, and aluminum. Back in 2002 there were only two laboratories in New York State that were doing the majority of heavy-metal testing among integrative doctors: Metametrix and Doctor's Data. I already had a relationship with Dr. Alexander Bralley, who was the laboratory director of Metametrix, since he was also part of the same scientific advisory board that Randy and I participated in for the nutrition company. So I asked Dr. Bralley for his advice on the best ways to test for heavy metals. He advised me to do a twenty-four-hour urine test using an FDA-approved chelating agent known as DMSA, dimercaptosuccinic acid. He told me to use a 500 mg dose and collect urine for the next twenty-four hours. The DMSA would bind to heavy metals in the tissues, and then it would be excreted in the urine, where it could be collected and tested. He sent me a Metametrix test kit, and one week later I received the results. I had highly elevated levels of mercury, lead, and cadmium. Mercury, lead, and cadmium cannot be metabolized by the body and, if accumulated, can cause toxic effects by interfering with various physiological functions.

I called up Randy and gave him the results. "You were right," I said. "Damn, you're good." We discussed the potential implications of the tests. Elevated levels of mercury have been linked to chronic fatigue syndrome, fibromyalgia, joint and muscle pain, tinnitus, memory and concentration problems, tingling and numbness, a host of autoimmune disorders, and can impair the immune system. I didn't have any of these symptoms except for muscle spasms, but my Lyme disease patients surely did. In fact, every one of the symptoms of an increased heavy metal burden looked remarkably similar to every one of the symptoms exhibited by my patients. So I asked the next logical question. If I have it, and Randy has it, I wonder how many of my Lyme disease patients have been exposed to heavy metals, and if these levels might be the cause for some of their resistant symptoms?

I had occasionally tested patients in the past for mercury and lead poisoning, since I was aware that Lyme symptoms overlapped those of an elevated heavy metal burden. Yet these tests always returned negative. Why? I had been taught to use a blood test to measure the levels, and I discovered that these blood serum levels were not highly reliable unless there had been a recent acute exposure. That would explain why prior blood tests for mercury and lead were negative in my patients, and why I had assumed heavy metals were not present. I also found out that some doctors ran a hair analysis, and others did the same DMSA urine testing on their patients. I sent off a hair analysis on myself while simultaneously doing a urine test provoked by DMSA. The hair analysis did show a certain amount of elevated levels of heavy metals, but were nowhere near the elevated levels that came back on the DMSA urine challenge. I repeated this on several patients. It was always the same outcome. The urine test consistently showed higher levels of mercury, lead, arsenic, and other heavy metals when DMSA was used as a provocation agent.

I then contacted Dr. David Quigg, a PhD researcher at the commercial laboratory, Doctor's Data, and asked him about the discrepancy. Doctor's Data did a lot of the heavy metal testing among integrative practitioners, and although their results are considered by some mainstream physicians as being highly controversial, they are certified by the New York State Department of Health as well as being CLIA certified, CAP certified (College of American Pathologists), and certified by the Centers for Toxicology in Québec. Dr. Quigg's explanation for the discrepancy was that the hair was a dumping ground for excess heavy metals. The provoked urine test would have the DMSA go into the tissues where the metals had been deposited, bind the metals, and, therefore, ultimately lead to higher levels since it was going into the storehouse where the metals were being stored. Dr. Quigg gave me another reason that the urine test was showing higher levels. His lab was using a different protocol than Metametrix, basing the test on the patient's weight. He had recently discovered that a 30 mg/kilogram challenge of DMSA (a weight-dependent dose) with a six-hour urine collection yielded superior results to a twenty-four-hour collection with just 500 mg of DMSA, where the dose was independent of the patient's weight. After all, did it make sense in a three-hundred-pound individual to use the same dose of DMSA as in a one-hundred-twenty-pound person? A study published in the *Journal of Nutrition and Environmental Medicine* in 1998 suggested that better yields could be obtained with DMSA given at 30 mg/kg followed by six-hour urine collection, and that I might find higher levels of heavy metals using this protocol. The reasoning for this is that only 20 percent of DMSA is absorbed from the GI tract, and almost all DMSA is cleared by the kidneys in approximately four hours, so there was no need to collect urine for twenty-four hours.

The first low-dose DMSA challenge I performed in my office was using 500 mg, and was independent of body weight. The second study was using 30 mg per kilogram of DMSA with a six-hour urine DMSA challenge. The differences were striking. The lead level went from 9 to 70, and the mercury level went from 1.4 to 9.3 using the higher dosage of DMSA, in the same patient. The high-dose DMSA challenge yielded evidence of elevated levels of heavy metals in a significantly greater percentage of patients in the second study, and we have now used this protocol in several thousands of patients. High dose DMSA (30 mg/kg) has been safe and well tolerated with only a rare patient reporting nausea, flulike symptoms, and a rash if there is an unknown sulfa sensitivity. High-dose DMSA should, therefore, be considered as a preferred screening technique for testing the heavy metal burden in patients with chronic unexplained symptoms, especially those suffering from chronic fatigue, fibromyalgia symptoms, neuropathy, cognitive difficulties, tinnitus (ringing in the ears), and neuropsychiatric symptoms. All of these symptoms can be caused, and/or increased, by exposure to heavy metals.

I started doing tests through both laboratories using the same protocols to confirm results. I reported the research data at the 16th International Scientific Conference on Lyme Disease in 2003. Out of ninety-three patients initially tested with a twenty-four-hour urine challenge with DMSA, forty-three patients were tested by Metametrix laboratories and fifty patients were tested by Doctor's Data. Among the patients tested by Metametrix, 41 percent showed evidence of elevated heavy metals (mercury 29 percent, lead 21 percent, aluminum 47 percent, arsenic 3 percent, cadmium 9 percent, and boron 18 percent). Among the patients tested by Doctor's Data, 58 percent showed evidence of elevated levels of heavy metals (mercury 52 percent, lead 8 percent, arsenic 8 percent). Combined results from both laboratories showed that 56 percent of my Lyme disease patients tested positive for elevated levels of heavy metals on a twenty-four-hour urine provoked challenge. However, when we changed the protocol to the 30 mg/kilogram DMSA challenge over six hours suggested by Dr. Quigg, the numbers went up even further.

Heavy metals can accumulate for years in the body, leave the bloodstream where they are no longer measurable there, and then start compartmentalizing in body tissues. DMSA diffuses into and effectively competes with the tissue binding sites for the metals, thereby releasing them from sequestered sites in the tissues. They then will redistribute into the blood as a stable complex, and be eliminated in the urine where they can be measured.

Just as I was discovering the role of heavy metals in my chronic resistant Lyme patients, and finding them in myself, a friend invited me to attend a medical conference in Maryland. So I flew to Maryland to attend the course, held in a lovely hotel on the Chesapeake Bay. The restaurant's specialty was Maryland crab cakes. After having just found that I had elevated levels of mercury, lead, and arsenic, and reading about the levels of heavy metals in seafood, it was a bit difficult to find something non-metallic on the menu. All that I saw on the menu was: "Salmon with a delicate cream sauce covered with delicious PCBs," "Swordfish, in a butter and wine sauce with a creamy mercury topping," "Tuna, sushi style, with a mercury and parasite roulade," and "Crab cakes, spiced and lightly

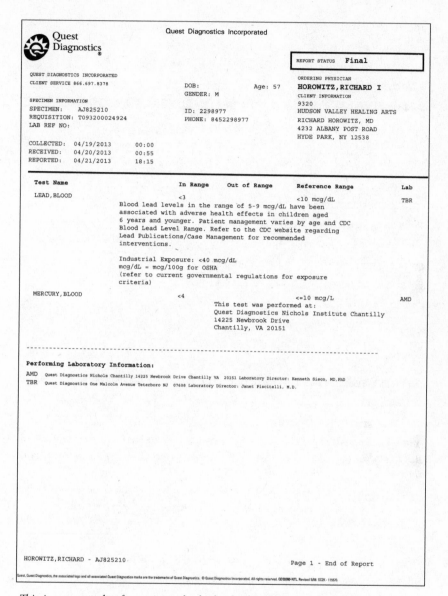

This is an example of a patient who had a lead and mercury level drawn in blood. According to Quest Laboratories, there was no evidence of mercury.

REPRINTED WITH PERMISSION FROM QUEST DIAGNOSTICS. © 2013 QUEST DIAGNOSTICS.

LAB #:	CLIENT #: 26262
PATIENT:	DOCTOR: Richard Horowitz, MD
ID: .	
SEX: Female	4232 Albany Post Rd
AGE: 50	Hyde Park, NY 12538 USA

Toxic Metals; Urine

TOXIC METALS		RESULT μg/g creat	REFERENCE INTERVAL	WITHIN REFERENCE	OUTSIDE REFERENCE
Aluminum	(Al)	11	< 35		
Antimony	(Sb)	0.2	< 0.4		
Arsenic	(As)	9.3	< 117		
Barium	(Ba)	2.4	< 7		
Beryllium	(Be)	< dl	< 1		
Bismuth	(Bi)	< dl	< 15		
Cadmium	(Cd)	1	< 1		
Cesium	(Cs)	5.9	< 10		
Gadolinium	(Gd)	1.5	< 0.4		
Lead	(Pb)	17	< 2		
Mercury	(Hg)	11	< 4		
Nickel	(Ni)	3.4	< 12		
Palladium	(Pd)	< dl	< 0.3		
Platinum	(Pt)	< dl	< 1		
Tellurium	(Te)	< dl	< 0.8		
Thallium	(Tl)	0.2	< 0.5		
Thorium	(Th)	< dl	< 0.03		
Tin	(Sn)	0.8	< 10		
Tungsten	(W)	< dl	< 0.4		
Uranium	(U)	< dl	< 0.04		

URINE CREATININE	RESULT mg/dL	REFERENCE INTERVAL	-2SD	-1SD	MEAN	+1SD	+2SD
Creatinine	42.4	35- 225					

This is the same patient after taking a six-hour urine DMSA challenge to evaluate heavy metal burden. These are similar to many of the test results that I am finding among the thousands of patients that I have seen with Lyme-MSIDS.

REPRINTED WITH PERMISSION FROM DOCTOR'S DATA, INC. (Any opinions expressed by Dr. Horowitz about the test results are those of the author and do not necessarily reflect the positions of Doctor's Data INC.)

fried with just a touch of lead and arsenic." Sometimes medical knowledge is a dangerous thing. It was clear that I would no longer follow the "see-food" diet that I had been on in the past.

THE PREVALENCE AND TOLL OF HEAVY METALS

Most doctors do not do regular testing for heavy metals unless there is a history of some acute poisoning with lead, mercury, or arsenic, for example, in the workplace. But why would I test positively for so many different elevated metals, and why were so many of my patients showing such high levels? When my arsenic levels came back elevated, my first thought was to turn to my wife and ask her if she still loved me (she said she did). The answer was simply that these heavy metals are now ubiquitous in the environment, and they accumulate slowly in our bodies over time. That is why many patients do not get acutely ill from chronic low-level exposures.

But the story is different when we consider those who already have been exposed to other chronic illnesses. When patients complain of fatigue, muscle pain with fibromyalgia symptoms, joint pain, tingling and numbness of the extremities, and neuropsychiatric abnormalities with memory and concentration problems, and standard medical testing fails to reveal a cause for their symptoms, many doctors tell them that they are experiencing the "aches and pains of daily living." These are actually the words that are used by certain infectious disease doctors who have published guidelines on the diagnosis and treatment of Lyme disease. They propose that these are simply classic manifestations of getting old, or so-called "normal aging." Unfortunately, the problem is not that simple. Lyme disease, associated co-infections, and heavy metals all overlap in their clinical presentations, and are off the radar screen for most physicians.

Where do these metals come from? A National Wildlife Federation study from 2003 showed that more than 98 percent of the rain samples in Texas contained levels of mercury far exceeding what the EPA considered safe for people and wildlife. Well fine, that's Texas. We all know what drilling for oil wells and all those barbecues could do to the environment. But what about New York? It turned out that the highest mercury level measured in New York rain (29.9 ng/l) was 8.5 times the EPA human health standard for mercury in lakes. Eight times! Eighty-four percent of the rain samples in New York exceeded the EPA human health standard for mercury in lakes and the average rain sample collected in New York was nearly two times the EPA's human health standard for mercury. The same year, the CDC published a $6.5 million study in which 116 different pollutants including 13 heavy metals, 14 combustion by-products, and 10 pesticides were found in their sample of 2,500 citizens. The Environmental Working Group in Washington, DC, also did a study that found 167 different chemicals in people's bodies, including PBDE (flame retardants) and multiple pesticides, even in human breast milk. I suppose that's fine if you don't want your baby to catch on fire or be eaten by insects, but somehow I didn't think that this was a good thing! Metametrix Laboratories and Doctor's Data are government certified laboratories, and the same governmental and nongovernmental agencies confirmed that multiple toxins including heavy metals were appearing in human tissue and breast milk. But what role were these toxins playing in patients that were chronically ill?

Heavy metals have multiple potential deleterious effects on the body including increasing oxidative stress, which can damage cell membranes. Perhaps damage to the mitochondrial cell membranes, the organelles responsible for the energy production of the cell, could also be the cause of resistant fatigue. This seemed likely, and the scientific literature had postulated that a certain percentage of patients with chronic fatigue syndrome improved once damaged mitochondrial cell membranes were repaired using nutritional supplements like glycosylated phospholipids.

Mercury has also been linked in the scientific literature to autoimmune disorders. The Carolina Lupus study, published in *The Journal of Rheumatology* in 2004, found increased odds for autoimmune diseases in patients with occupational exposures to mercury (especially dental technicians). Many of my Lyme disease patients have autoimmune manifestations. Were my patients who were ANA positive or had positive rheumatoid factors having an overstimulated immune system because of the blebs shed from *Borrelia burgdorferi*'s surface increasing these immune reactions? Or was it the mercury acting as a hapten on the outside of the cell causing these autoimmune reactions? Or perhaps *Mycoplasma fermentans* was causing nonspecific B and T cell stimulation in the body and provoking autoimmune manifestations in my patients. The plot thickened. I was learning that multiple factors and different causes might be driving similar symptoms in these chronically ill patients. Mercury and associated heavy metals might not always be directly responsible for their suffering, but might be a secondary cause.

AS WITHOUT, SO WITHIN

Whatever toxins have found their way into the external environment will invariably find their way into our bodies. We breathe them in, ingest them from the food and water supply, or absorb them through the skin.

There are a variety of toxins to which we are exposed on a regular basis. Many of them, e.g., heavy metals, have long-term profound health effects. Some of the most common heavy metals we are exposed to are mercury, lead, arsenic, cadmium, and aluminum. These are some of the oldest toxins known to man and are ubiquitous. However, they are only one of several categories of toxicants. Others include industrial compounds and chemical by-products, such as volatile organic solvents, plasticizers, pesticides, insecticides and herbicides, combustion and incineration pollutants, and food and cosmetic additives. Scientific studies have demonstrated that we are exposed to many of these environmental toxins on a daily basis. But how significant is our actual exposure? Do these toxins really play a role in affecting our long-term health, contributing to chronic illness?

A 1997 Mercury Study Report to Congress stated that the best estimate of U.S. emissions of mercury from 1994 to 1995 was 158 tons. You read that number correctly. In the mid-1990s we were dumping 158 tons of mercury into the environment every year. In 1999 the EPA's Office of Prevention, Pesticides, and Toxic Substances reported that over four billion pounds of pesticides are used annually in the United States. This amounts to *eight pounds* for every individual in the United States each year. If you want to give a laboratory rat Parkinson's disease, immune dysfunction, or cancer, scientific studies have shown that you can do so just by exposing it to one good dose of pesticides. Another interesting study comes from the Environmental Protection Agency and their 1982 U.S. EPA National Human Adipose Tissue Survey. In this study, fat biopsies were performed on subjects living in different regions of the United States, from New York to California. They found that of those individuals tested, 100 percent were positive for different chemicals, including styrene, dichlorobenzene, xylene, ethyl phenol, and TCDD (Dioxin). Why should we be concerned about finding these chemicals? These and other environmental toxins are primarily acting as xenoestrogens (foreign-based estrogens), and have been linked to a variety of cancers, including cancer of the breast, prostate, lung, colon, cervix, and uterus. These environmental toxins are now showing up in all individuals tested.

In the 2003 CDC study mentioned earlier, 2,500 subjects across the United States were found to be carrying 116 different pollutants. One of those toxins, trichloroethylene (TCE), was responsible for a leukemia outbreak in Woburn, Massachusetts. TCE frequently causes paresthesias (tingling and numbness) and learning disabilities. Based on this 2003

CDC study, could TCE, combined with heavy metals such as mercury, which affects memory and concentration, be one of the many factors responsible for some of the ADD and learning disability epidemics in children in the United States and worldwide? Could these also be affecting the memory and concentration of my Lyme disease patients when these toxins are combined with the effects of *Borrelia burgdorferi* on the brain, and/or perhaps be an overlapping cofactor driving dementia among Alzheimer's disease patients?

The reason that these environmental toxins are so important is because their effects can mimic just about every medical condition found in the doctor's office. Just as Lyme-MSIDS can mimic most disease processes, so can environmental toxins. They can cause exactly the same symptoms we see in persistent Lyme disease, including such varied symptoms as tinnitus, headaches, fibromyalgia symptoms, fatigue with chronic fatigue syndrome, memory loss, psychiatric symptoms with mood swings, panic attacks, and learning disorders.

Because they are silent destroyers of our health, and are not commonly tested for in the medical community, it is impossible for most physicians to differentiate when these environmental toxins are actually the root cause of the patient's illness. However, when we look at the magnitude of exposure to these toxins, we see that they may have far-reaching implications not only for our health, but especially the health of our future generations. Pregnant and nursing women are exposed to these toxins, potentially harming the developing fetus and nursing infant. Remember, the Environmental Working Group found that multiple chemical toxins such as pesticides and flame retardants were present in the breast milk of women living in California. This does not imply any increased risk from living in California, but what is quite striking is that the women participating in the study lived a healthy lifestyle including eating organic foods. Similar results were found in studies of Eskimo women who were breast-feeding, subjects far away from the source of these environmental toxins. These toxins have now spread worldwide, and no one is exempt from their effects. This exposure must be evaluated if a child is in poor health and not developing properly. An infant or young child's immune system is not fully developed, and subsequently is unable to process these environmental toxins properly. This is why integrating a detoxification regimen into normal preventive medical care may be necessary to help prevent certain chronic illnesses of the twenty-first-century.

Apart from heavy metals, other toxins may also be present in the Lyme-MSIDS patient. These include PCBs, dioxins, plastics and plasticizers, pesticides, VOS's (volatile organic solvents), as well as exposure to mold neurotoxins. It is always important to ask the patient about possible mold exposure at home, such as *Stachybotrys*, since this is often a silent factor that can cause a whole host of physical, musculoskeletal, and neurological symptoms.

Some toxins, however, are internally produced in the body, and can cause devastating neurological symptoms. These include quinolinic acid, which is a neurotoxic metabolite of certain biochemical pathways in the body (such as the nitric oxide pathway previously discussed), which when produced in the brain by activated microglia and macrophages is involved in neurodegenerative diseases such as Parkinson's disease, Lou Gehrig's disease (ALS), Huntington's disease, MS, and Alzheimer's disease. Lyme disease patients, however, have also been shown to have increased levels of quinolinic acid. This toxin may be playing a key role in the cognitive processing issues and mood disorders that Lyme patients frequently complain of after having been exposed to *Borrelia* and associated co-infections. It could explain in part why certain patients continue with ongoing symptoms despite seemingly adequate antibiotic therapy. The scientific literature has shown that once you suppress the production of quinolinic acid, using antioxidants such as curcurmin, or the ones found in green tea (epigallocatechin), or protect against the effects of quinolinic acid using COX-2 inhibitors (like the medication Celebrex), patients will clinically improve. Detoxifying patients from chemical compounds like quinolinic acid may also make them better. This gives us new avenues of treatment for patients who fail classical therapies.

CHEMICAL SENSITIVITY AND ENVIRONMENTAL ILLNESS

All of us are continuously exposed to internal and externally produced toxins, but not everyone feels their effects. Some patients, whether due to their genetics, their total load of these toxins, or their inability to properly detoxify, become ill when the load of toxic substances reaches a certain level. How does it manifest clinically? Every symptom that we find in Lyme disease and co-infections can be mimicked by heavy metals, and those that suffer from these symptoms may also be experiencing chemical sensitivity and/or environmental illness (EI). These are patients who are particularly sensitive to the effects of the toxins from the environment. These patients may suffer from:

- fatigue
- fibromyalgia symptoms
- joint pain
- paresthesias
- cognitive dysfunction
- anxiety
- depression
- loss of balance and/or incoordination
- varied abdominal complaints
- urinary symptoms
- visual symptoms
- auditory symptoms
- changes in weight
- increased susceptibility to infection
- cardiac symptoms (palpitations, chest pain)

All of these symptoms can be caused by or exacerbated by environmental toxins and heavy metals, and no level of heavy metals in the body has been shown to be "safe" and without possible long-term side effects. This is because of the general mechanisms of their toxicity: They can increase free radicals and inflammation, cause neurotoxicity, and bind to sulfhydryl groups, which are essential for the biochemical pathways of the body to function properly.

In a 1993 U.S. FDA report on the amount of lead in shellfish, they reported that "Presently, there are no levels of lead exposure for children or adults at which it may be considered that no adverse effects occur." We can assume the same is true for all of the heavy metals. A small increase in exposure to a toxic metal can lead to a disproportionate increase in the number of individuals who will experience symptoms of toxicity, and additive/synergistic effects among toxic metals may occur.

If we then look at the specific symptoms for mercury poisoning, we find that mercury can bind to sulfhydryl groups in the body, increase oxidative stress, which can further drive cytokine production and inflammation, and penetrate into the nerves and bind to acetylcholine receptors in the brain, resulting in neurological dysfunction. Mercury can also affect the central and peripheral nervous systems. It can move upward from the peripheral nervous system by traveling along axons, and penetrate into the central nervous system, causing denervation of nerve fibers similar to the pathology that we can see in multiple sclerosis, and also leading to a peripheral neuropathy. In a recent study published in *Archives of Pediatrics and Adolescent Medicine*, prenatal exposure to mercury was found to be associated with symptoms of attention-deficit/hyperactivity disorder in childhood. Children whose mothers' hair samples tested positive for mercury levels were at increased risk for impulsivity and hyperactivity. This highlights the importance of these environmental toxins on expectant mothers and their developing fetuses. So when a patient presents with an MS-type picture, we need to rule out whether Lyme disease, co-infections, and heavy metals such as mercury are each playing a role in creating the same symptoms.

Similar overlapping symptoms are seen with lead. Lead can cause fatigue, encephalopathy with impaired concentration, short-term memory deficits, GI symptoms, insomnia, anxiety and depression, irritability, and peripheral nerve dysfunction. Once again we see that these are the same symptoms in patients with Lyme-MSIDS. Lead also can cause anemia, and chronic renal failure with elevated blood pressures. Lead is stored in the bones, and may be dumped into the blood as men and women go through hormonal changes and develop osteopenia and osteoporosis. Since lead can raise blood pressure, lead may need to be considered as one of the comorbid conditions causing hypertension, which is now being found in over 50 percent of the aging population. As reported in a 2012 *New York Times* article, preliminary results from a New York State Health Department study show that more than half the eggs tested from chickens kept in community gardens in Brooklyn, the Bronx, and Queens had detectable levels of lead. Lead exposure may therefore be more common than most people think, since exposure may be coming from multiple sources.

Arsenic can cause multiple cardiac, vascular, and neurological symptoms including paresthesias and peripheral neuropathy (apart from other effects such as causing aplastic anemia and cancer). Where would we get arsenic from? Arsenic toxicity is now a growing problem, as arsenic is being found in a wide variety of frequently ingested foods, especially rice, rice products, apple and grape juice, according to a recent FDA report in September 2012. Eating one serving of rice at the highest levels found in these studies could expose a person to more arsenic than the EPA allows in drinking water, putting adults at risk for cancer and heart disease, and children at risk for neurological symptoms and poor brain function. Arsenic exposure has also been linked to type 2 diabetes. So regular exposure to arsenic may underlie some of the most common diseases in the twenty-first century, and physicians generally are not checking for exposure to this toxic metal. What's more, there are no federally approved safe levels for arsenic ingestion.

Cadmium, which is also found in trace amounts in some foods, has been linked to chronic fatigue syndrome and toxic brain syndrome, as well as hypertension and vascular disease, emphysema, osteopenia, prostate cancer, and renal dysfunction with proteinuria and subsequent loss of amino acids. Aluminum is a potent neurotoxin and has been associated with increased neurofibrillary tangles and brain degeneration and is known to accumulate in the neurons of patients with ALS and Parkinson's disease. It can cause an encephalopathy with abnormal speech, similar to the encephalopathic symptoms that we see in severe chronic neurological Lyme disease with associated co-infections like *Bartonella*. These toxic effects will depend on how much of the metal reaches the systemic circulation, as well as its ability to reach essential target sites within the body, including membrane and structural proteins, membrane lipids, enzymes, and DNA molecules. Once at a target site in sufficient concentration, the metal can displace a mineral of physiological importance and alter its function. This is the case with cadmium as it competes for zinc binding sites.

Zinc is known to play a central role in immune function and those suffering from a zinc deficiency experience more susceptibility to a variety of pathogens. Zinc effects multiple aspects of the immune system including B cell and T cell immunity. Macrophages, essential cells of the immune system that help to engulf and then digest cellular debris and pathogens, are also adversely affected by a zinc deficiency. This can lead to poor intracellular killing, and increased inflammation with elevated cytokine production. That is why it is so essential to test patients with chronic infections for mineral deficiencies like zinc.

Treatments for Removing Heavy Metal Toxins

There is no one "right way" to remove heavy metals, known as chelation. It is individualized, and based on the patient's levels of heavy metals, possible drug allergies, preferences, and side effects (although these are few and far between, except in patients with extremely poor detoxification abilities).

In 2003, I attended a three-day seminar given by the American College for Advancement in Medicine (ACAM) to become certified in chelation therapy, which is one of the most effective ways for binding heavy metals and removing them from the body. This way I would be able to offer chelation therapy to my patients to see if this improved patient outcomes. I learned about many different ways to remove heavy metals from the body, using oral medications, such as DMSA and Cuprimine, as well as intravenous (IV) therapies, such as with EDTA. At the conference I spoke to many integrative physicians who had a variety of protocols that they were using for chelation. I didn't want to do IV EDTA chelation if possible, due to the cost and possible side effects, as well as the fact that it required a four-hour infusion in the office: a huge time commitment for my patients. I wanted to find a protocol that was easy to administer, inexpensive, relatively side effect–free, and since many of my patients were coming from long distances, one that could allow them to be treated at home. After much research I decided initially to use Dr. Sherry Rogers's protocol of using DMSA three days on and eleven days off. I was acquainted with Dr. Rogers's work on environmental toxins from having read all of her books. She described links between environmental illness and abnormalities in our nutritional biochemistry, and she had extensive scientific documentation on environmental toxins and their effect on health. So we tried her DMSA protocol, and although it worked, several Lyme disease patients had severe Jarisch-Herxheimer reactions during chelation, as the metals were being pulled out of their bodies. We therefore used N-Acetylcysteine (NAC), alpha-lipoic acid, chlorella (green algae), and a host of other supplements to naturally chelate the heavy metals, while trying to decrease the reactions to the chelation protocol.

Some of our patients still found chelation difficult to tolerate. I experimented with a variety of dosages and found that very low doses of DMSA were well tolerated and could easily be mixed with EDTA suppositories if a high lead level was also present. This became our standard protocol for most chronically ill Lyme patients with evidence of heavy metal burdens who were resistant to standard antibiotic therapies.

The initial results were encouraging. As we continued to chelate more and more Lyme-MSIDS patients, we found that the protocol was effective in a small group of resistant patients. More important, the protocol we used was found to be safe and well tolerated, with no long-term effects on the patients and without any biochemical abnormalities in the kidney or liver functions, or hematological parameters. Our experience is important, because there are many misconceptions about chelation and its safety. We have never seen a life-threatening reaction, nor any long-term problems chelating several thousands of patients using the protocols that I am describing, and many patients have experienced the clinical benefit. Although some scientific studies have not found consistent benefits with using various chelating agents, approximately 20 percent of my resistant Lyme-MSIDS patients had improved fatigue, decreased muscle and joint pain, and improved neurocognitive functioning following chelation therapy. This included a reversal of memory loss and improved concentration, with fewer mood swings. This improvement was independent of any antibiotic protocols used to treat these same patients. So although it was not helping a large percentage of the patients, I clearly had identified one more piece of the puzzle that could be causing some of the suffering in the Lyme patients failing antibiotics.

Chelation first requires performing a six-hour urine DMSA challenge, which evaluates the level of heavy metals in the body, and then uses specific chelating agents to remove these heavy metals. The most common agents include: oral DMSA, which will remove mercury, lead, cadmium, arsenic, and other toxic metals; oral and IV 2,3-Dimercapto-1-propanesulfonic acid (DMPS), which is more specific for the removal of mercury; and rectal and IV EDTA, which is specific for the removal of lead. These all exist in oral forms, although they are not all well absorbed, and many physicians choose to use IV DMPS for significant mercury toxicity, with IV EDTA for elevated lead levels. Cuprimine can also be used as a chelating agent for patients who are allergic to DMSA, but it is more labor-intensive to use and may have more side effects. We also frequently use oral liposomal glutathione in combination with these medicines, to both help chelate heavy metals and protect against any side effects and associated increased oxidative stress.

I do not use IV chelation, and have found that combining oral DMSA with EDTA suppositories (Detoxamine) if high levels of lead are present will work well without significant side effects, for the vast majority of patients. DMSA should initially be started in low doses to test for tolerance (100 mg every third night), as some patients may get Jarisch-Herxheimer reactions with chelation if their detoxification pathways are not functioning properly. Other chelation protocols we have found to be effective include oral DMSA three days on, eleven days off (or two days on, five days off), again using oral liposomal glutathione, NAC, and alpha-lipoic acid with chlorella at bedtime to support the detoxification pathways and protect against increased free radical exposure. Patients should avoid taking mineral supplements on the days of chelation—such as antacids, including Tums, multivitamins with minerals, or calcium supplements with magnesium—since minerals may bind to the chelating agents, making them ineffective. These supplements, especially magnesium, should be taken on the days not chelating, because they are essential in helping to prevent any side effects, such as muscle spasms, because chelation can pull magnesium out of the body. If high levels of aluminum are present, we will also add malic acid (a natural substance found in fruits) to our chelation regimen. This is because aluminum is a heavy metal with three positive charges, and it does not bind well to DMSA, which only binds well to molecules with two positive charges, such as mercury, lead, and arsenic. Malic acid is naturally found in apples and grapes, and also can be taken as a nutritional supplement. By adding DMSA and other natural chelating agents to our treatment regimens, we found that we were able to help certain resistant patients, such as Aaron.

Aaron had come back to my office with his mother after a return of his fatigue and pains, along with relapsing memory and concentration problems when off his antibiotics, despite following a hypoglycemic diet. We performed a six-hour urine DMSA challenge and found that his lead level was five times above the normal range, his mercury almost twice the normal range, and his nickel and aluminum were also high. I asked him if he had been playing with thermometers, eating the paint off the wall, swallowing loose change, or eating the siding on his house. I told him these elevated levels of heavy metals could explain why he's a little denser than some of the other children who came to see me. He did not appreciate my humor, and tried to wrestle me to the ground.

I started Aaron on oral chelation therapy with DMSA. Do not try and convince a ten-year-old budding wrestler to do EDTA suppositories for elevated levels of lead, although the process of describing it to him and convincing him to do it was quite amusing. After doing a course of chelation, he still complained of some resistant symptoms. Yes, his compliance was not ideal, which could explain some of the inadequate results, but overall we saw a significant improvement in his health over time. Each time that we discovered another piece of the medical detective puzzle, whether it was hypoglycemia or heavy metal burdens, Aaron would improve. How was I sure? "I'm kicking their butt in wrestling" was his joyous response when I asked him how he was feeling. He was now Aaron the Invincible. He was King of the Hill.

Some patients doing a chelation regimen will only notice mild improvements, but for others it may be much more dramatic. But even for those patients who do not notice a clinical shift in symptoms, it is still wise to chelate these heavy metals. Heavy metals have been linked to autoimmune diseases and may be responsible, with *Borrelia* infections, for some of the autoimmune manifestations we see contributing to the chronic illness in these patients. This includes mercury's effect on nerves, causing neuropathy, a common symptom seen in this patient population. Second, heavy metals, such as mercury, can increase oxidative stress and increase inflammation, which we have shown to be a common denominator in causing symptoms of Lyme disease and MSIDS, as well as those of many other chronic illnesses. Finally, mercury has been shown to increase susceptibility to chronic infections, which is a problem in patients with MSIDS, who already have an impaired immune system that is overwhelmed by multiple co-infections.

We also need to remove these toxins because a heavy metal burden may lead to mineral deficiencies. As we began testing our new patients for serum mineral levels, we learned that up to 25 percent of our chronic MSIDS patients with heavy metals are deficient in one or more minerals, such as iodine, magnesium, and zinc. We also learned to check red blood cell mineral levels, such as magnesium, since 99 percent of the body's magnesium levels are intracellular and cannot be adequately tested by serum levels alone.

Proper levels of trace minerals (micronutrients) are essential for optimal biochemical functioning at the cellular level. Minerals are also essential components in complex biochemical detoxification reactions. For example, magnesium is necessary in approximately three hundred detoxification enzymes in the body. A magnesium deficiency can result in muscle spasms, tremors, anxiety, Raynaud's phenomenon, and cardiac arrhythmias. Copper is involved in the production of superoxide dismutase (SOD) which is an essential enzyme in dealing with free radicals and oxidative stress. Copper is also found in other enzymes: polyphenol oxidase, which is necessary to detoxify chemicals, tyrosinase and dopamine oxidase (essential for neurotransmitters), and cytochrome c oxidase (essential for energy production).

Zinc is necessary for over ninety enzymes to operate correctly, including alcohol dehydrogenase, which is one part of the liver's detoxification pathways, when it converts alcohols to aldehydes. If zinc levels in the body are low, we develop a biochemical bottleneck: Aldehydes shift to chloral hydrate, causing toxic brain symptoms. We also know that older patients generally have significantly lower levels of zinc, which is associated with increased levels of inflammatory cytokines and plasma oxidative stress. In one NIH-funded study, the zinc-supplemented group had a decreased incidence of infections, lower levels of TNF-alpha, and lower levels of plasma oxidative stress markers compared to a placebo group. Many of our Lyme-MSIDS patients are zinc deficient. When these patients complain of cognitive dysfunction, they may have any one or all of the following: active spirochetes or coinfecting organisms in their brains; neurotoxins, such as quinolinic acid or mercury, in the central nervous system that cannot be detoxified; or a buildup of chloral hydrate, which can cause toxic brain symptoms. If all of these factors are not adequately dealt with, the patient's neurocognitive and neuropsychiatric symptoms may not get better.

For mineral replacement, I generally prescribe calcium, magnesium, and zinc, with other trace minerals, for the days that the patient is not chelating. I will test the patient's mineral levels every several months (serum magnesium, red blood cell magnesium, zinc, and iodine) as well as get a CBC and biochemistry profile to check their liver and kidney functions. I have never seen any long-term adverse effects of using DMSA in this fashion, although an occasional patient may become chemically sensitive to DMSA over time and sulfa sensitive, and develop a rash. However, there are patients who are sensitive to sulfa (i.e., cannot take drugs like Bactrim or Septra double strength) and are able to tolerate DMSA without a problem. If chelation is absolutely necessary, and DMSA must be used, and there is any possibility of an associated sulfa sensitivity (history of a rash), an H1 blocker (i.e., over-the-counter Allegra, Zyrtec, or Claritin) or H2 blocker (over-the-counter Zantac or Pepcid) can be used simultaneously to help prevent allergic reactions, by blocking all of the histamine receptors. This seems to prevent any significant reactions in patients who have questions about sulfa sensitivity, and can be used for the initial DMSA challenge, although it is of course up to the treating physician as to whether this testing and treatment is safe for an individual patient.

Tom Was Carrying a Load of Heavy Metals

Tom was a pleasant thirty-seven-year-old male who lived in New York City. He was in excellent health until five years earlier, when he found an engorged deer tick on his right arm. Three weeks later his arm became very swollen and painful. He saw a physician in Illinois who gave him thirty days of doxycycline, and all of his symptoms went away. Five months later his symptoms returned again, with fevers, fatigue, flulike aches and pains, and headaches. He saw another physician and was given amoxicillin for a relapse of his Lyme disease, and again felt improvement, but he did not ever feel completely well. He moved to Illinois after this episode, and although he did feel better for a period of time in the warmer weather (Lyme disease patients often report this), his symptoms worsened again. He developed a panoply of symptoms, including: chest pains and shortness of breath; migratory joint pain; increased fatigue, sweats, chills, and fevers; muscle pain and twitching; headaches, neck cracking and stiffness; tingling and numbness of the extremities; blurry vision; light-headedness; brain fog; memory and concentration problems; and mood swings. His Illinois doctor told him that he likely had the flu, but his symptoms persisted. He subsequently returned to New York and saw several MDs, but the cause of his multiple symptoms remained elusive.

He finally found a nurse practitioner in New York who evaluated him for Lyme disease. His blood tests were positive for it; he had a positive Lyme ELISA and a positive IgM and IgG Western blot. She treated him with an IV antibiotic (IV Claforan) and he felt tremendous improvement. After his treatment was completed, he felt well for one month, but then symptoms returned. He was then tried on IV Rocephin, but he did not get as much help as with the Claforan, and he then was switched to amoxicillin with Zithromax. This helped the symptoms, but as with most of my patients, all of his symptoms worsened once he was taken off his treatment.

After Tom was seen in our office, we sent off a standard battery of tests and evaluated him for co-infections. We sent out titers and PCR's for *Babesia*, *Bartonella*, *Mycoplasma*, *Chlamydia*, Rocky Mountain spotted fever, Q fever, and viruses. The only laboratory abnormalities that returned were a positive *Mycoplasma* titer, an elevated C-1 Q immune complex, reflecting an overstimulated immune system, a low vitamin D-3, and a six-hour urine DMSA challenge for heavy metals, which showed elevated levels of lead at 16 (normal is less than 5), and mercury at 12 (normal is less than 3).

We clinically diagnosed him with Lyme disease, babesiosis (based on the drenching sweats and chills with normal thyroid functions, and a normal chest X-ray), and a significant heavy metal burden. We started him on Mepron with Zithromax, as well as bicillin LA injections (an extremely effective form of intramuscular penicillin for Lyme disease) since he previously responded to oral amoxicillin. Plaquenil was not started, as he had a history of psoriasis (it can exacerbate the symptoms), and grapefruit seed extract was used instead to address the cystic forms of *Borrelia*. Cymbalta (an antidepressant that increases serotonin and norepinephrine levels) was started for his fibromyalgia and mood disorder, as well as for his neuropathic symptoms.

Tom returned one month later, having improved from 30 percent to 70 percent of normal functioning. He felt remarkably better. All of his sweats and chills had improved from the *Babesia* treatment, although he still complained of some residual fatigue, joint pain, and brain fog. For the elevated heavy metals, he was started on Chemet (DMSA) every third night, with chlorella, Alamax (a long-acting form of alpha-lipoic acid), and NAC. We replaced his minerals for the next two days postchelation with a multivitamin packet containing calcium, magnesium, zinc, and other trace minerals.

When Tom returned for his follow-up visit, he stated: "I am definitely feeling better with the antibiotics, but I really notice a difference the next day after doing the chelation. My fatigue, joint pain, and memory and concentration are definitely better the day after doing the DMSA." Heavy metal burdens, with chronic bacterial and parasitic infections, were all playing an important role in keeping Tom ill. Tom had MSIDS with elevated levels of heavy metals. There were multiple causes for his illness, and we needed to address all of them in order for him to regain his health.

Detoxification and the Role of Glutathione

There are four main ways to remove unwanted chemicals and toxic substances from the body: sweating them out through the skin; clearing them out of the colon; transforming them in the liver to less toxic substances; and eliminating them through our kidneys.

The liver plays a key role in the transformation of these toxins to less toxic substances, and by supporting liver functions, we can enhance the detoxification of chemicals that would otherwise be difficult to remove from the body. The liver helps transform chemicals, drugs, hormones, and toxic compounds into nontoxic substances. This takes place through two essential phases, known as phase I (oxidation) and phase II (conjugation). In phase I, an electron is added to a molecule (oxidizing it) by a series of enzymes in the liver called the cytochrome P 450 system, which prepares it for phase II. Then biotransformation of the chemical compound takes place: It shuttles through one of six different detoxification pathways, where a series of molecules are added (conjugation) to help make it more water soluble, increasing its ability to be excreted out of the body through the kidneys.

A novel approach to removing toxins from the body via the liver in phase II involves glutathione (GSH), a protein with three amino acid side chains: glycine, glutamic acid, and cysteine (with a sulfhydryl group, SH). Glutathione is made by the liver to help the body detoxify foreign chemicals, as well as to help remove hormones and medications that we may be taking. Glutathione takes fat-soluble toxins stored in our tissues that are not easily eliminated and helps make them water soluble, so they can be removed from the body. It also helps with many other important metabolic functions in the body, such as making enzymes, hormones, and new genetic material. We make glutathione all the time, but if you have inadequate stores of it, because of increased exposure to internal and external toxins, the glutathione levels in the body will be depleted. Hence, less glutathione would mean a possible increase in toxic chemicals from the environment, or in the case of a Lyme patient with MSIDS, an inability to properly deal with a sudden release of cytokines during a Jarisch-Herxheimer flare, making the patient sicker.

Prescribing glutathione has been shown to be a safe treatment in clinical trials. We ran a trial of GSH in our medical office to determine its role in patients with Lyme disease with chronic resistant symptoms: 118 patients with Lyme disease were given IV GSH over a five- to ten-minute period; 80 patients were given 1,000 mg of GSH; and 38 patients were given 2,000 mg of GSH. Patients' symptoms scores before and after (0 percent to 100 percent self-reported scale) were recorded after a thirty-minute interval. The results were the following: Among 80 patients given 1,000 mg of GSH, 36 percent had no clinical improvement, 40 percent had a mild clinical improvement, 6 percent had a moderate clinical improvement, and 18 percent had a marked clinical improvement. Among 37 patients given a higher dose of glutathione, i.e., 2,000 mg of GSH, 27 percent had no clinical improvement, 46 percent had a mild clinical improvement, 16 percent had moderate clinical improvement, and 11 percent had a marked clinical improvement. Mean improvement in symptoms after thirty minutes of 2,000 mg of IV GSH was 9.5 percent. What does this mean? Within minutes to hours of giving IV glutathione we saw improvements in patient's symptoms, such as less fatigue, decreased headaches, improvements in memory and concentration problems, fewer word-finding problems, less joint and muscle pain, and improved mood, especially a lessening of anxiety.

Improvements from a single dose of IV GSH lasted from several hours to two to three days before patients experienced a relapse in symptoms. There were no significant adverse effects. An occasional patient complained of temporary nausea, rare, fleeting pressure in the head, and a temporary increase in tingling in the extremities. These symptoms all disappeared within several minutes of the injection. One patient felt faint, nauseous, and dizzy after the needle was inserted but before receiving the glutathione. This was secondary to a vagal reaction, which is a sudden lowering of the blood pressure that can happen with fear or a perceived increase in pain. Also, two patients experienced an increase in their Lyme symptoms after the injection, which also subsequently resolved.

There were eight Lyme disease patients in a second part of the study, who underwent a one- to two-month GSH trial, with doses ranging from 400 mg IV three times a week to 2,000 mg per day. These were patients for whom multiple antibiotic regimens had failed in the past and were considered treatment resistant. Among that group, one patient had no clinical response, but the other seven sustained positive clinical improvements, ranging from 10 percent to 35 percent, with a mean improvement of 20 percent. These patients reported consistent improvements in cognitive functioning, energy, headaches, muscle strength, and muscle and joint pain. There were no adverse side effects from longer-term use of GSH. These were also the patients who experienced the most significant benefits from glutathione.

Why did glutathione help improve symptoms in these chronically resistant patients when other treatment regimens had failed? Glutathione plays many important roles in the body. The metabolic functions of glutathione include DNA synthesis and repair, protein synthesis, and the synthesis of prostaglandins, a type of chemical messenger involved in regulating inflammation, sensitizing neurons to pain, causing constriction or dilation in vascular smooth muscle cells, and controlling hormone regulation and cell growth.

Glutathione is also involved in activating essential enzymes in the body, metabolizing toxins and carcinogens, preventing oxidative cell damage, and helping the immune system to function more efficiently. This is especially important in the MSIDS patient with chronic inflammation and/or autoimmune manifestations: A 2009 study published in *Autoimmunity Reviews* showed that glutathione also may play a key role in modulating autoimmune reactions. Antioxidant defense mechanisms have been demonstrated to be lacking in patients with chronic degenerative diseases, especially inflammatory and immune-mediated ones. In patients with chronic inflammation there is sustained production of reactive oxygen species (ROS, i.e., free radicals), which increases oxidative stress. Glutathione is the principal component of the antioxidant defense system in living cells, and part of its role is to either stimulate or inhibit the immunological response in order to control inflammation. If there are inadequate levels of glutathione present in cells, this may have a detrimental effect on those autoimmune conditions caused by oxidative stress reactions. You may remember that oxidative stress causes Nrf2 to be released from its receptor sites, go to the nucleus of the cell, and switch on NFKappaB, which subsequently causes the production of inflammatory cytokines, like TNF-alpha, IL-1, and IL-6. As discussed previously, these are inflammatory molecules that cause the sickness syndrome. Since many patients reported improvement in fatigue, joint and muscle pain, mood swings, headaches, balance, dizziness, speech problems, and cognitive difficulties within thirty minutes of GSH administration, glutathione may be acting to metabolize toxins and cytokines in the short term, and may have an effect on prostaglandins, interleukins, oxidative stress, and immune modulation in the long term. Alternatively, the rapid initial improvement in symptoms may have been a placebo response due to the novelty of trying a new treatment approach; however, the sustained response among patients given longer-term treatments was less likely to be due to a placebo effect.

Although this clinical report suggests that IV GSH may be useful to patients with symptoms that persist after antibiotic treatment, of course only a placebo-controlled trial can determine its true efficacy. However, we continue to use both a liposomal form of oral glutathione and IV glutathione with thousands of resistant Lyme-MSIDS patients on a regular basis. Overwhelmingly, I have found that for treatment-resistant patients with symptoms unresponsive to antibiotics and other interventions, we clearly see marked clinical improvement when we enhance their detoxification pathways using glutathione. That is why we recommend a three-step process of detoxification, chelation, and nutritional supplementation to all patients who come to our office.

Detoxification can be most efficiently accomplished by accessing all of the detoxification pathways of the body. Far infrared saunas, a specific type of sauna therapy, are extremely effective at helping patients detox multiple chemicals by sweating them out through the skin. The use of nutritional fiber, probiotic supplementation (Acidophilus), and occasional colon cleanses will help move toxins through the intestines and out of the body. Drinking two to three liters of fluid per day will help flush toxins through the kidneys. We also recommend using high-quality protein with essential amino acids, combined with specific vitamins, minerals, herbs, and nutritional supplements, to support phase I and phase II liver pathways and help to convert toxic substances from fat-soluble toxins that are stuck in body fat to water-soluble substances that can be more easily eliminated. Since glutathione is one of the primary molecules produced in the liver phase II detoxification pathways to help eliminate fat-soluble toxins, are there ways to help increase glutathione naturally in the body?

Supplementing with N-Acetylcysteine (NAC) can enhance the body's production of its own glutathione, and alpha-lipoic acid can facilitate the regeneration of glutathione. Alpha-lipoic acid also has other beneficial effects, such as providing antioxidant support against free radicals and lowering inflammation (which causes the sickness syndrome) that we see in Lyme disease and associated inflammatory disorders. Alpha-lipoic acid also helps with insulin resistance, is used at high doses for diabetic neuropathy, and is a mild chelating agent of heavy metals. For these reasons we use NAC and alpha-lipoic acid on a regular basis in our patients with heavy metal burdens, inflammatory disorders, detoxification problems, insulin resistance, and neuropathy, with very good results.

Glutathione Unloaded Trudi's Chemical Burden

It was a beautiful spring day at the Hudson Valley Healing Arts Center. The outside flower beds were starting to bloom, and the world was becoming green again. Patients were arriving in colorful short-sleeved shirts, including Trudi and her husband, Jack, who had just driven for over three hours from New Jersey for their monthly office visit.

Everything initially seemed normal at our medical center, until it became clear that Trudi couldn't walk a straight line into the waiting area. She was off-balance and slurring her speech, and my receptionist probably was thinking that she must have had a six-pack of beer to wash down her Egg McMuffin that morning. My nurse immediately got me out of one of the exam rooms. By the time I got to the waiting area, Trudi had fallen into the wall and was lying on the floor, curled up in a ball. The waiting room was filled with new patients. I bet they wondered what type of medical practice they had walked into.

"What happened?" I asked Jack.

"Oh, Doc, she's been like this for days," he said. "She goes in and out of these spells when she can't walk or talk. She's okay for a couple of hours, and then it happens again."

Trudi was a hardy soul. She exercised every day and was physically quite strong. She smiled when she saw me coming. "Trudi, are you OK?" I asked.

"I'm okay, Doc. But if you could help me up, I'd appreciate it. The view is not great from down here."

Jack and I lifted Trudi and got her into a chair. My nurse ran to get a wheelchair, and we wheeled Trudi down the hall into an exam room. Her vital signs were normal. Temperature was 98.8, pulse 92 and regular, respiratory rate, 16 per minute. She had full motor function in her extremities. She was, however, slurring her speech and had great difficulty getting out more than three or four words in a coherent sentence. When I tried to stand her up and observe her walk, she couldn't coordinate her muscles to take more than one or two steps. She would fall over if we weren't holding her.

"What have you been drinking?" I asked. "Looks like some good stuff."

"Oh, Doc," she said, "You know me, I don't drink. Not that I don't think of it from time to time, being married to Jack." Trudi had a wicked sense of humor.

"Okay, so any new drugs you've been taking?" I asked.

"Nope, nothing, Doc. I've just been on the same antibiotics for the Lyme disease for the last month."

Trudi was taking a new antibiotic. She had been diagnosed with Lyme disease over a year earlier, and despite a variety of oral medications, her memory and concentration were still terrible. She was only forty-two years old, and she couldn't remember her friends' names and phone numbers. She had severe word-finding problems and no ability to multitask. So, recently we had inserted a PICC line in order to start her on IV Rocephin. She was also on Actigall, to try and prevent gallbladder complications, and Plaquenil and Zithromax, to cover the cystic and intracellular forms of *Borrelia*.

"Have you been flaring, Trudi?" I asked. "Have you been having any increase in your symptoms with Jarisch-Herxheimer reactions, such as increased fatigue, joint pain, or more brain fog?"

"Nope. I was starting to feel better on the Rocephin." She slowly and painfully had to enunciate each word and often had to repeat a word several times to get it out in a sentence. I turned to Jack. "Have there been any new chemicals or chemical exposures?" I asked.

Sometimes patients have difficulty tolerating new chemicals when they are on several different medications. Their detoxification pathways can't handle the load of one more chemicals, and the system starts to back up. Trudi looked encephalopathic; she was confused, dizzy, and off-balance. Working long hours in city hospitals during my medical training and residency I saw numerous long-term alcoholics with end-stage cirrhosis; this is how some of them acted. Their mental confusion was from an overload of ammonia in their systems that couldn't be properly detoxified in the liver. But what I couldn't figure out was what Trudi was reacting to, and I didn't think it was a TIA (transient ischemic attack with fleeting neurological symptoms) or a stroke. She didn't report any permanent motor deficits or any unusual tingling or numbness. There was no history of a loss of consciousness, tongue biting, or urination to suggest that she was having a grand mal seizure, but perhaps this was a partial seizure or an absence seizure?

I turned to her and said, "Trudi, can I try something to help you? You look toxic to me, and I'd like to try a new medication. Can I inject this through your PICC line?"

Trudi had gotten to know me well over the previous year. She and Jack drove from their home to my office almost monthly, and we had established a solid friendship. She knew that I had her best interests at heart, and we would often joke together as a way to relieve the stress and difficulties she was experiencing with her illness.

"You can do to me whatever you want, Doc." I turned to Jack. "Does she ever say that to you?" I asked. "Not a chance," he said. "I've been married to Trudi for five years. I couldn't get her to listen to me from the beginning."

So I walked out of the room and went to the refrigerator where we store the medications. As I walked down the hall, I thought of Tom, an ALS patient of mine who had encouraged me to order some glutathione. When he began seeing me he had heard reports about a protocol in which IV glutathione was being used to detoxify neurologically impaired patients with ALS with some positive results. Tom couldn't travel long distances to get this treatment, and he was desperate for help. After doing some research I had called up one of the primary specialized pharmacies making this drug, Wellness Pharmacy in Birmingham, Alabama. I reviewed the scientific literature that they sent me. Glutathione had been used for various applications in medicine for years, and it appeared safe, so I had ordered it. So here I was walking to the fridge to get some of the vials of glutathione that I had recently ordered for Tom. As I picked up the vial, I first saw the word "Wellness" and I thought to myself, "Ah, a magic wellness elixir." If only that could be true.

I followed the instructions from Wellness Pharmacy to prepare the glutathione. It can't be exposed to light and was kept covered in the refrigerator to prevent it from oxidizing, which would render it less effective. One cc was equal to 200 mg of glutathione, and the instructions were to mix 10 ml (2,000 mg) with 10 mL of 0.9 percent normal saline. I pulled out two sterile needles and syringes and first pulled up 10 mL of saline, changed the needle, and then put the needle into the bottle of glutathione, and pulled back immediately with force to prevent the vacuum from pulling the saline into the bottle of glutathione.

Trudi signed a consent form for administering the IV glutathione after I explained the potential side effects, such as nausea, a temporary pressurelike sensation in the head, or possible allergic reaction to the drug. Once she signed, I unclamped the IV line coming out of her left arm, cleaned the head of the IV access (Luer lock) with alcohol, and proceeded to inject the glutathione slowly. Within sixty seconds Trudi sat up on the exam table suddenly, as if a lightning bolt had struck her. In perfectly enunciated English she said, "It couldn't be working this fast, could it?"

Jack and I looked at each other in amazement. His falling down, drunklike wife looked like she had just sobered up. She started speaking quickly and coherently. Words flowed out effortlessly.

"Can I get up, Doc?" she asked. "I feel stronger."

Trudi stood up, got off the exam table without assistance, and walked out of the room. She excitedly walked up and down the corridor connecting the exam rooms, joyfully exclaiming, "I can walk, I can walk, I can talk, I can talk!" She walked past a couple in an exam room next door who had been out in our front waiting area when Trudi arrived. Without missing a beat the woman looked at Trudi and said to me, in *When Harry Met Sally*-style: "Whatever she got, I'd like some of that."

I then looked back over Trudi's chart to find other clues to explain her present illness. She had complained of associated headaches, tingling and numbness in her extremities, and severe aches and pains, with symptoms that would wax and wane, as they frequently do in patients with unresolved Lyme disease. Her brain MRI showed multiple areas of demyelination in the frontal and parietal lobes. The radiologist had read it as "nonspecific," with the differential diagnosis including small vessel ischemic changes, migraines, Lyme disease, or a nonspecific demyelinating process. EEGs were also negative, ruling out a seizure disorder. Since she had intermittent chest tightness and palpitations, she was also sent for a stress echocardiogram and a nuclear stress test, with adenosine and thallium, which were both negative. The only study that returned with a positive result was her sleep study. She complained of fatigue and headaches, and was full-figured, and the sleep study did reveal obstructive sleep apnea. The only problem was that her obstructive sleep apnea would not explain her bizarre intermittent neurological symptoms. Then I noticed one final detail: In Trudi's initial consultation she described how going into some department stores would make her ill (I told my wife she had the same problem, and therefore couldn't go shopping, but it didn't work). Now that she was feeling better she told me that she had been back to one of those stores recently and, shortly after returning home, had such severe fatigue that she was unable to get out of bed. Did Trudi have chemical sensitivity/environmental illness?

Trudi also suffered from a host of all too common medical disorders, such as hypertension, hyperlipidemia, obesity, diabetes, and hypothyroidism. On top of that, our office had received positive test results for Lyme disease, babesiosis, *Mycoplasma*, and Q fever exposure. Now I realized that I could also add chemical sensitivity and environmental illness (EI) syndrome to that list.

I first learned about EI years ago, when another patient complained of similar symptoms. She had no history of Lyme disease or co-infections at the time. Specifically, she reported that her worst symptoms were severe muscle spasms in her extremities, with lower back pain, irritable bowel syndrome (IBS), and asthma. I wondered if there was a common denominator for her symptoms, such as magnesium deficiency, to explain the spasms in the various parts of her body. When I checked her serum magnesium level, it was low. After reading about magnesium deficiency, I was reminded that 99 percent of the body's magnesium was intracellular, so then I checked her red blood cell magnesium level. It was far below the range of normal, implying that her body was severely depleted of magnesium.

I excitedly returned to my patient, believing that I had discovered one of the key problems causing her to feel chronically ill. I gave her oral magnesium, but it had limited results. We then began intramuscular shots of magnesium sulfate, and the results were astounding. The majority of her symptoms cleared up. It wasn't until years later, doing further medical detective work, that we discovered the cause for her severe magnesium deficiency. She had significant pesticide exposure at home. She therefore was using up her body's magnesium in an attempt to detoxify that ongoing chemical exposure.

I sent her to see Dr. Sherry Rogers as well as Dr. William Rea, who are experts in environmental medicine, and she eventually ended up going to Dr. Rea's clinic, the Environmental Health Center in Texas. They discovered not only various mineral deficiencies, but also multiple food allergies and sensitivities, as well as other chemical exposures. When she was detoxified using infrared sauna therapy, "purple ooze" started coming out of her pores. This turned out to be the pesticide sprayed in her home, which had settled in her air-conditioning and heating duct system. Every time the heating/AC system would come on, trace amounts of these chemicals were released into the ducts, and she would become severely ill.

Trudi reminded me of this patient with EI. If she was already taking multiple medications for a host of medical disorders, had a large toxic load of chemicals in her body and compromised detoxification pathways, then it is likely her body was unable to handle any further chemical exposure. Trudi's department store visit likely started her on a declining health spiral, with severe encephalopathic-type symptoms. The most likely chemical exposure was formaldehyde, which can be found in pressed-wood products used in new construction, and this department store was new in her area.

Many toxic chemicals are fat-soluble, so they have a direct pathway to the brain, which is comprised of 60 percent fat. These then disturb the brain chemistry, causing a host of "unexplained" neurological symptoms. When the detoxification pathways are overloaded, or when there are nutritional deficiencies affecting the phase I and phase II liver detoxification pathways, these chemicals will back up and produce aldehydes and chloral hydrate. These chemicals produce neurological symptoms such as dizziness, brain fog, headaches, slurred speech, exhaustion, and mood swings (Trudi also reported experiencing periods of sudden rage that would disappear just as suddenly). Glutathione likely improved her functioning because it unloaded some of those chemical toxins responsible for her neurological symptoms.

Apart from having miraculous results with using glutathione, we also used intramuscular magnesium sulfate whenever Trudi had encephalopathic symptoms with associated joint and muscle pain. Often she would get relief of her symptoms using magnesium, as did my other patient with EI. It wasn't just her Lyme disease and co-infections that were making her sick. Yes, she felt better on antibiotics for her Lyme disease and antimalarial drugs to treat her *Babesia*. However, the key to turning around Trudi's health during these extreme encephalopathic episodes was supporting her detoxification pathways with glutathione and magnesium.

We cannot continue to ignore these factors and their overlapping roles in chronic illnesses. Could it be that so-called normal aging does not have to mean that we will face the challenge of heart attacks, strokes, cancer, Parkinson's disease, Alzheimer's disease, and a host of other illnesses? In some individuals it may be that chronic bacterial, viral, and parasitic infections, mixed with long-standing exposures to environmental toxins, are depressing their immune systems and increasing chronic inflammation, with all of the resulting consequences.

As we explore the universe of possibilities of causative agents in patients who suffer with chronic illness, we are likely to find that what some would label "new age" treatments, such as detoxification, chelation, and nutritional supplementation, lie at the heart of any good prevention and treatment program. We must make sure that the patient with chronic illness has the nutritional, biochemical, and detoxification support necessary to deal with the burden of these environmental toxins. What's more, for those of us who are not sick and wish to maintain our current good health, detoxification, chelation, and nutritional supplementation may be the future of preventive medicine.

We are all living with toxins inside of us. Yearly physicals, when we check our blood pressure, blood sugar, and cholesterol, and go for preventive screening exams, are certainly useful, but in no way will affect these potential silent killers inside of us, nor tell us whether some of the minor symptoms and "aches and pains of daily living" are due to these chemicals. There likely will be few double-blind placebo-controlled trials any time soon to determine the effects of detoxifying these chemicals from our bodies. But sometimes just observing the numerous health epidemics facing our families, friends, and neighbors can make us wonder whether assessing the role of toxins on our health is the next logical step in preventive medicine of the twenty-first century.

NINE

Lyme, Functional Medicine, and Nutritional Therapies

Functional medicine" offers a different perspective from the way medicine is commonly practiced, which is primarily concerned with naming a disease and then finding drugs to treat it. According to the Institute for Functional Medicine, "functional medicine is a science-based healthcare approach that assesses and treats underlying causes of illness through individually tailored therapies to restore health and improve function." One of the ways we do this is by looking at nutritional and metabolic profiles that address the various organ systems of the body. For example, through specialized functional medicine laboratories such as Metametrix and Genova Diagnostics and Doctor's Data we can look at a range of specialized profiles. These include specific tests of our gastrointestinal function, immunity, toxicity, nutrient and toxic elements, amino acids and fatty acids, vitamins, oxidative stress, and endocrine profiles that are not typically performed in standard laboratories. These allow us to look at the body through the eyes of a nutritional biochemist, evaluating illness at the deepest cellular and biological levels.

These profiles are extremely important in patients who may present with a plethora of symptoms, who have seen ten to twenty doctors and been screened for every imaginable disease without finding an adequate cause, like the typical MSIDS patient. They may be suffering from the toxic effects from PCBs, volatile organic solvents, pesticides, and a host of other environmental toxins, and do not detoxify these chemicals well, subsequently becoming and remaining ill without obvious cause. Standard laboratories do not adequately screen for environmental toxins and for specific detoxification problems. These patients often require testing through a functional medicine laboratory such as Metametrix, where the lab's specific metabolic profiles (such as the ION or Organix tests) will measure levels of organic acids, amino acids, fatty acids, nutrient and toxic elements, vitamins, and antioxidants and can give a comprehensive biochemical picture of the patient's health. They are an important option for some patients in discovering the underlying cause of their chronic illness when other testing fails to reveal a cause.

Other examples of how we might use functional medicine testing include evaluating for *Candida* (intestinal fungal overgrowth), leaky gut (increased intestinal permeability), and food allergies and sensitivities in those with resistant fatigue, aches and pains, headaches, and gastrointestinal complaints. Standard allergy testing may only look at IgE antibodies (antibodies involved in immediate reactions to allergens), but functional medicine laboratories also do extensive IgG food antibody panels (antibodies involved in delayed immune reactions against foods) and can therefore pick up food sensitivities and allergies missed by other labs. Similarly, standard stool cultures do not give us the detailed analysis necessary to rebalance the microflora in the intestine and see if digestive enzymes may be necessary. By ordering a comprehensive gastrointestinal stool profile, which looks at digestive and pancreatic functions as well as levels of bacteria, yeast, and parasites in the intestine, we can get a much better look at the gut and determine how best to treat the patient. Why is this important?

Nutrition and enzyme deficiencies that cause digestive disorders are commonly seen with chronic fatigue syndrome (CFS). These enzyme deficiencies lead to poor digestion of proteins, carbohydrates, and fats, thereby causing a deficiency of vital nutrients necessary for proper cellular function. Remember, we are bombarded by toxins every day, and healthy detoxification is a necessity if we wish to maintain our health and live a long and productive life. Detoxification reactions of environmental chemicals require an ongoing supply of essential vitamins, minerals, amino and fatty acids, and phytonutrients to be effective, and the higher the toxic load, the more likely nutritional deficiencies will be present. What's more, the standard American diet (SAD) typically does not include large amounts of fruits, vegetables, and whole grains—the foods that have the highest volume of vitamins and minerals—so we are even more challenged to detoxify all the chemicals entering our bodies every day. We must evaluate the levels of these essential nutrients and help patients increase their intake in order to help their detoxification pathways work correctly.

We are what we eat, drink, breathe, and touch. The growing list of toxins that can affect our health include: industrial chemicals and combustion pollutants (i.e., halogenated hydrocarbons such as PCBs); over eight hundred pesticides, insecticides, and herbicides; multiple endocrine disrupters (PCBs, DDT, bisphenol A(BPA), plastics, and phthalates); heavy metals; as well as food additives, preservatives, and drugs. So the problem is not just one individual toxin, as we discussed in the last chapter, but all of these toxins simultaneously affecting our bodies. They are also fat-soluble, and can accumulate in the body tissues, reaching much higher doses than environmental concentrations would suggest, as well as acting in an additive manner if they exert their toxic effects through the same pathways. Decreasing the total toxic load and supporting our detoxification pathways by providing proper nutrition for the GI tract and the liver are essential components in achieving better health. These areas are the first line of defense, for as toxins enter the body, at least 25 percent of our detoxification initially takes place in the gut, and they are then processed in the liver, the main detoxification powerhouse of the body.

There are six basic functional medicine detoxification principles that need to be a part of every good health plan for the Lyme-MSIDS patient:

- Minimize toxic exposure
- Ensure hydration
- Optimize bowel health
- Increase antioxidant reserves
- Optimize mitochondrial function
- Assist and balance liver biotransformation

MINIMIZE TOXIC EXPOSURE

Do not use pesticides in your home or close to the home, and try to avoid using chemical products indoors. Use natural cleaning products when possible. Use of water and air purifiers may be helpful in decreasing further toxic exposure.

ENSURE HYDRATION

The kidneys are among the main organs of detoxification. Drink at least two to three liters of fluid per day (unless you have a medical condition which requires fluid restriction, such as congestive heart or kidney failure); as Dr. Sherry Rogers says, "Dilution is the solution to pollution." When you drink copious amounts, you are more easily flushing toxins from the bloodstream and out through the kidneys. Fluids also help us maintain proper bowel health, preventing constipation and moving toxins more quickly through the GI tract.

The water should be pH neutral, and preferably alkaline. A neutral pH for water is around 7.0 to 7.4, and acidic water has a pH below 7.0, while alkaline water has a pH of 7.5 or higher. Test strips can be purchased at a local pharmacy or through a company that specializes in water testing (i.e., Culligan or swimming pool and hot tub suppliers), and you can determine the pH of your water at home. Reverse osmosis systems take minerals out of the water, making it more acidic, and alkalizing water purifiers are commercially available to correct this problem. We need a proper acid/alkaline balance for our cells to function, which is a blood pH between 7.34 and 7.45, so drinking the right type of water is important to help maintain that balance.

Drinking regular purified water (not distilled water, which has no minerals, and not club soda or other carbonated beverages, as they contain carbonic acid and are acidic in the body) is the easiest way to achieve your daily intake. Neither caffeinated coffee or tea counts in your total fluid intake, as the caffeine can cause additional excretion of fluids and can lead to a negative fluid balance, with dehydration. Fresh vegetable juices are also an excellent option, as these are high in vitamins and minerals, and are alkaline in pH.

One easy way to tell if you are adequately hydrated is by observing the color and smell of your urine. A dark, strong-smelling urine usually means that you are not drinking enough of the proper fluids.

Chronic health conditions such as MSIDS can create a tremendous buildup of acid by-products in the body that need to be balanced by an alkaline diet, which means eating a diet high in fruits and vegetables.

OPTIMIZE BOWEL HEALTH

Maintaining colon health is an essential part of any detoxification plan. We need good bowel health for several reasons. The GI tract is one of the first lines of defense for protecting us from certain pathogenic bacteria and viruses. We also need a healthy GI tract to properly absorb all of our essential vitamins and nutrients, and the bowels play an important role in detoxifying chemicals and toxins that may enter the body through the foods we eat or the fluids we drink.

We can maintain proper bowel health by drinking adequate amounts of fluids and by taking in high amounts of fiber (which helps prevent constipation and diverticulosis, a potentially painful condition which can lead to inflammation in parts of the colon). Occasionally colon cleansing may also be necessary in certain individuals who are chronically constipated, as toxins that are not properly removed from the colon may find their way back into the body through the enterohepatic (intestinal-liver) circulation. We also can maintain a healthy colon by taking in the right types of nutrition that support the enterocytes (cells that line the intestines), and by using high quality probiotics.

Probiotics are important in maintaining bowel health, even when we are not depleting our beneficial bacteria, i.e., while taking antibiotics. Probiotics produce substances that prevent harmful bacteria and yeast from establishing themselves in the colon. These include lactic acid, bacteriocins, and hydrogen peroxide (H_2O_2). They also inhibit dangerous bacteria, such as *Salmonella*, from attaching to the intestines. Other important functions of probiotics include specific metabolic activities, such as the breakdown of microbial toxins and the modulation of the immune system, the latter by helping to regulate certain proteins and signaling molecules, such as interleukins and cytokines. Remember, these molecules actively participate in inflammatory and autoimmune reactions in the body, and also have regulatory effects on sleep patterns, which we will discuss in Chapter 13. For all of the above reasons, we routinely use a variety of high-potency probiotics with the Lyme patients who are on long-term antibiotics.

The probiotic *Lactobacillus rhamnosus* is a type of acidophilus that has been shown in nearly two hundred clinical studies to help prevent antibiotic-associated diarrhea, as well as preventing *E.coli, Salmonella,* and *Shigella,* which are pathogenic organisms that cause diarrhea, from adhering well to the intestinal lining. *Lactobacillus rhamnosus* accomplishes this by lowering the intestinal pH where the lactic acid produced inhibits the growth of the harmful bacteria responsible for outbreaks of gastroenteritis and diarrhea.

Another organism that is frequently associated with diarrhea is *Clostridium difficile*, which is normally present in the colon, but antibiotic use increases its production, leading to inflammation in the colon. It is the gut bug responsible for 95 percent of pseudomembranous colitis (a serious and potentially life-threatening inflammation of the colon). Based on a 1999 study published in *Infection and Immunity*, we've long since known that by using a different type of probiotic, *Saccharomyces boulardii*, which is a healthy yeast, we can create a temporary barrier in the colon protecting the healthy intestinal bacteria. There are three documented actions of *Saccharomyces boulardii*. First, it stimulates secretory IgA and intestinal IgG production along the mucosal lining of the intestine. IgA and IgG antibodies play a critical role in mucosal immunity, and provide protection against harmful microbes that may multiply in the intestines.

IgA is also important because it participates in "immune exclusion," i.e., it helps to decrease allergic and autoimmune reactions to certain foods. Secondly, it releases polyamines, which are agents that help repair and reestablish intestinal health. Finally, it also secretes an antitoxin against gram negative bacteria, other pathogens, and their toxins. The toxins secreted by these pathogenic bacteria are directly responsible for the inflammation in the colon (colitis) and severe diarrhea we see in outbreaks of gastroenteritis with organisms such as *Clostridium difficile*. Clinical studies have shown the protective effect of *Saccharomyces boulardii* in preventing *Clostridium difficile* diarrhea. Although we can use different drugs to treat *Clostridium difficile* (Flagyl, Vancocin, Dificid), the drugs are not always 100 percent effective. Newer aggressive treatments include fecal transplantation of healthy bacteria into the colon, but using *Saccharomyces boulardii* helps to prevent this serious inflammation in the bowel from occurring.

We can also assist detoxification by adding fiber to the diet, which cleanses the bowel of toxins by increasing bowel movement frequency. Food sources of dietary fiber include the indigestible portion of plants, which contain two main components, soluble and insoluble fiber. Soluble fiber is readily fermented in the colon into gases and active by-products, and insoluble fiber may be metabolically inert, and it facilitates the bulking of the stools. Insoluble fibers can absorb water as they move through the digestive system, making it easier to have a bowel movement.

However, some forms of insoluble fiber, such as wheat bran, may actually decrease bowel frequency in some patients, so choosing the right type of fiber is important. Flaxseeds that can be added to food is a good choice. Current recommendations from the United States National Academy of Sciences' Institute of Medicine suggest that adults consume 20 gms to 35 gms of dietary fiber per day and 1 tbsp to 2 tbsp per day of milled flax. One hundred grams of ground flaxseed supplies 28 gms of fiber and 20 gms of protein. Flaxseeds contain an insoluble fiber that can increase bowel frequency, and also has high amounts of lignans, a type of fiber that modulates hormone levels and may be useful in treating hormonal imbalances that can occur with premenstrual syndrome (PMS), perimenopause, menopause, and postmenopause. Lignans may also have anticancer properties, especially against hormone-sensitive cancers such as estrogen-receptor-positive breast cancer, as they can inhibit aromatase activity, preventing the conversion of testosterone to estrogen. This is equally important for men, as they can convert too much testosterone to estrogen, which can be a risk factor for prostate cancer.

GI Dysfunction Is Linked to Other Medical Conditions

When there are inflammatory conditions in the gut (e.g., inflammatory bowel diseases such as Crohn's disease and ulcerative colitis), which produce symptoms of abdominal pain, cramping, frequent bowel movements, and/or bloody diarrhea, we also may benefit from using other strategies that support colon health. The functional medicine approach suggests that we reduce the burden of toxic substances in the body, especially the GI tract and liver. This approach recommends nutritional support for gastrointestinal and liver functions. For example, glutamine, which can come from either foods or dietary supplements, is a naturally occurring amino acid and essential for recovering from illness or injury. Dietary sources of L-glutamine include beef, fish, chicken, eggs, wheat, dairy products, cabbage, spinach, parsley, beets, and vegetable juices.

Glutamine provides essential fuel for colon cells, enabling them to act as a functional barrier to dangerous microorganisms that can cause inflammation. This same inflammation can cause the conditions for leaky gut syndrome, in which large molecules of food pass across the intestinal barrier, creating increased food sensitivities, food allergies, and further inflammation. Leaky gut syndrome has been identified in the medical literature in such diverse conditions as ankylosing spondylitis (a chronic, inflammatory arthritis in which immune mechanisms affect joints in the spine and the sacroiliac joint, leading to eventual fusion of the spine), rheumatoid arthritis, asthma, eczema, and inflammatory bowel disease (IBD). In 1990, scientists examined the relationship between increased intestinal permeability and inflammatory joint diseases. They found that the gut is the likely source of the antigens causing inflammatory arthritis. Antigens are usually proteins or specific sugar molecules that are found in bacteria, viruses, and other microorganisms. These molecules make their way into the gut, but because the intestinal barrier is damaged, they can pass into the bloodstream, where they cause the production of one or more antibodies that contribute to these inflammatory joint diseases. By supplementing with glutamine and probiotics, we are strengthening the intestinal cells, and a stronger barrier is created, so that these organisms and their antigens cannot pass into the bloodstream.

Another nutritional supplement that may support gastrointestinal function includes larch arabinogalactan, an immune-enhancing polysaccharide. Polysaccharides are components of soluble dietary fiber that can bind to bile acids in the small intestine, making them less likely to enter the body. This helps to lower cholesterol and sugar levels (decreasing the risk of diabetes), while also lowering the levels of toxins, as some are bound to bile acids. Once polysaccharides are fermented in the colon, they can also produce short-chain fatty acids (SCFA), which engage in broad physiological activities. Arabinogalactan has been shown to increase the production of short-chain fatty acids, which can stimulate natural killer cell function and enhance other aspects of the immune system.

There are protein sources that can support the immune system and control inflammation in the gastrointestinal tract, such as immunoglobulins found in some food sources (whey protein) and supplements. Although most proteins we ingest are broken down by our stomach acid and digestive enzymes into smaller amino acids, some immunoglobulins survive the conditions of the digestive tract. Other immunoglobulins are produced by the B-cells of our immune system and help to identify and neutralize harmful bacteria and viruses. For example, immunoglobulins have been looked at as a treatment for inflammatory bowel disease.

Immunoglobulins may also neutralize endotoxins, the molecules found on the outer cell membranes of dangerous bacteria, which are made up of lipids and sugars (lipopolysaccharides). Large amounts of endotoxins can be released when these bacteria are killed or destroyed, and these endotoxins go on to produce fever and lower blood pressure (causing hypotension) and activate inflammatory and coagulation pathways in the body, leading to sickness and even death. Increasing your intake of immunoglobulins can help neutralize endotoxins and prevent and treat infections caused by pathogenic bacteria, viruses, parasites, and yeast, and are an important addition to antimicrobial prescription medications.

In the table that follows you can see the relationship between the gastrointestinal system and the liver and the overlapping syndromes found in Lyme disease and MSIDS. The diseases shown below are ones that we would not normally consider to be related to problems in the gastrointestinal tract, such as fibromyalgia, which produces pain and cognitive impairments as well as neuropsychological symptoms. We have seen that it is in part driven by inflammatory cytokine production, as is the case with chronic fatigue syndrome and Lyme disease. Helping to establish a healthy GI environment and lowering inflammatory cytokines, by decreasing the absorption of endotoxins and preventing leaky gut, can positively influence these varied disease processes. What's more, lowering the toxic burden in both the GI tract and the liver while providing the nutrients essential to their proper functioning also contributes to the treatment of these diseases.

INCREASE ANTIOXIDANT RESERVES

Environmental toxins create large amounts of free radicals and reactive oxygen species (ROS). This results in oxidative stress, causing increased cytokine production and inflammation. It is therefore essential to have adequate amounts of antioxidants to decrease free radical damage to our various organs and to prevent the turning on of NFKappaB (the switch inside the cell's nucleus which increases the production of the cytokines IL-1, IL-6, and TNF-α), which increases inflammation.

Certain nutrients and antioxidants can modify detoxification reactions and promote enzymes that make glutathione. These include glutathione reductase, glutathione S transferase, and glutathione peroxidase.

Table 9.1: GI Dysfunction and Other Medical Conditions

Inflammatory Bowel Disease	• Glutamine is a primary fuel for the formation of healthy intestinal cells. • Fiber/probiotics promote the formation of short-chain fatty acids (SCFA). • Essential oils promote healthy GI function.
Chronic Fatigue Syndrome	• Bowel permeability results in systemic translocation of toxins, which may uncouple adenosine triphosphate (ATP), causing fatigue.
Fibromyalgia	• O_2 deprivation (Krebs cycle) results in cell death and tissue damage, leading to tender muscles.
Chronic Inflammation (Arthritis)	• Bowel permeability results in the uptake of antigenic protein, which may be deposited in joints.
Food Allergies	• The translocation of antigenic proteins results in allergic reactions or sensitivities with subsequent inflammation.
Hormone Imbalance (PMS, Menopause)	• Enterolactone (good estrogen) is formed in the bowel by the bacterial fermentation of fiber (i.e., flaxseed, lignans). • Impaired liver function (phases I and II) results in excessive circulating estrogens.
Cognitive/Neurological Dysfunction	• Impaired liver function facilitates free radicals attacking the CNS (myelin sheath). • Heavy metal deposits in neurons result in neurological disorders (e.g., aluminum and Alzheimer's).

Glutathione is one of the most important antioxidant systems that we have in the body, along with superoxide dismutase (SOD). Whey-based proteins and nutritional supplements such as N-Acetylcysteine and glycine will help in the production of glutathione, because they contain amino acids that are essential parts of the glutathione molecule.

Alpha-lipoic acid is another excellent nutritional supplement. It decreases free radicals and ROS and increases the production of other antioxidants, such as vitamins C and E and glutathione. It can function in both aqueous and lipid environments, as well as in the intracellular and extracellular compartments, making it an extremely effective antioxidant throughout the body.

A 2002 study published in *Alternative Medicine Review* showed that alpha-lipoic acid has the ability to chelate heavy metals, and that it plays an important role in the treatment of toxicity of mercury and other toxic metals, such as arsenic and cadmium. It is also useful for treating metabolic syndrome with insulin resistance, polycystic ovarian syndrome (PCOS), and diabetes, as it helps lower blood sugar and reduces one of the primary neurological conditions in diabetes, diabetic neuropathy. ROS are now thought to be directly involved in many neurological disorders, and an examination of the current research reveals the protective effects of alpha-lipoic acid in: cerebral ischemia/reperfusion (decreased blood flow to the brain, as occurs in strokes); excitotoxic amino acid brain injury (the pathological process by which nerve cells are damaged and killed by excessive stimulation of neurotransmitters, such as glutamate); mitochondrial dysfunction (inefficient energy production by the mitochondria, the powerhouse of the cells), and other causes of acute or chronic damage to brain or neural tissue. Therefore, alpha-lipoic acid is a very versatile and powerful antioxidant, and it should be an integral part of any detoxification program.

A diet high in protein and proper nutrients is also essential for the detoxification systems to work correctly. Dietary protein is essential for the synthesis of glutathione. Amino acids such as glycine, glutamine, cysteine, and taurine (which are found in most proteins, dairy products, grains, and vegetables; each can be also be taken as a nutritional supplement) are also involved in the conjugation of drugs and their metabolites as well as aiding in detoxifying environmental chemicals. Conjugation reactions are one of the six essential phase II detoxification reactions that take place in the liver. These phase II reactions help to make fat-soluble substances (such as toxins) that cannot be excreted from the body into water-soluble molecules, which can then be eliminated through the kidneys.

Many antioxidants and phytochemicals, the active nutrients of fruits and vegetables, are also important in strategies to decrease cancer risk. Cancer and Lyme disease are not known to be related, yet we are seeing both in epidemic numbers. One of the common factors is inflammation and free radical oxidative stress, which are damaging the cells of the body. In MSIDS, those free radicals cause the production of inflammatory cytokines. In cancer, the free radicals have been shown to damage the DNA of the body, causing mutations that can lead to cancer.

Antioxidants and Epigenetics

Scientists previously believed that our genetic code is essentially fixed and unchangeable. Our present understanding, however, is that nutrients in foods can modulate genetic expression: They do not change the DNA sequences, but by modifying the proteins surrounding the DNA (histone proteins), or through adding certain nutrients from foods (such as methyl groups) to the DNA, they can change how the genes express themselves. The study of epigenetics has now demonstrated that nutrients have long-term influences on what genetic characteristics are expressed, and that chronic disease may be related to the interaction between our genetic inheritance and lifestyle. This allows us the possibility to use diet, nutrition, and exercise as a means to influence chronic illness, which is essential for the MSIDS patient, who has multiple overlapping factors simultaneously affecting their health.

The human genome is made up of forty-six chromosomes, which contain approximately thirty-five thousand genes and over three billion nucleotides, the individual structural units that make up our RNA and DNA. The challenge for the human body is how to pack and retrieve all of this genetic information from inside each cell. The way this is accomplished is through DNA compaction. Our DNA is compacted into nucleosomes (the primary unit of DNA packaging), and then into chromatin (the combination of DNA and proteins that make up the contents of the nucleus of a cell), and finally into the genes contained in our chromosomes.

The epigenome is a record of the chemical changes that take place during our lifetime to the DNA and histone proteins, and the latter are responsible for packaging and ordering the DNA in our cells, protecting it, and helping with gene regulation. These changes can be passed down to our offspring, and are determined by our diet, exercise, and environmental exposure to chemicals and infectious agents. Epigenetic modifications primarily take place through two mechanisms: DNA methylation of genes (adding methyl groups without changing the DNA structure) and biochemical modifications of histones (removal of acetyl groups, i.e., histone deacetylation). Representative clinical conditions that have been suggested to have epigenetic origins include allergies, diabetes and metabolic syndrome, coronary heart disease, cancer, and certain neurological diseases, such as Alzheimer's, Parkinson's, ALS, and autism spectrum disorders. Epigenetics therefore needs to be considered as another important factor if we are to control these chronic disease states that are now spreading worldwide.

The question naturally arises: Why are some children and adults susceptible to these epigenetic effects, and why are others not? The answer lies in the fact that certain genes appear to be more epigenetically sensitive than others. These are described in the medical literature as "metastable epialleles." It has now been demonstrated that in the developing fetus these genes are capable of being environmentally marked, and not only are the genes themselves marked, but so are the histone proteins. What's more, the changes can then be passed on from one generation to another. Michael Skinner has defined this phenomenon as "transgenerational epigenomics," in which "the ability of environmental factors to promote a disease state are not only for the individual, but also for subsequent progeny for successive generations." So although environmental toxins and endocrine disruptors may not directly promote genetic mutations in our DNA, they do have the capacity to alter our epigenome, as well as the epigenome of future generations.

Nutrition becomes information for our epigenome: What a mother eats during pregnancy "imprints" the fetus with epigenetic tags. This is the future of medicine and prevention, in which nutritional supplementation can play an important role in affecting how genes and DNA express themselves in an individual. We know that in the animal model, early changes in nutrition affect future disease risk. For example, some mice have a high risk of obesity, diabetes, and cancer, but supplementing the mouse mother with zinc, methionine, choline, folate, and B_{12} lowers the risk of cancer, diabetes, and obesity, and it prolongs life in the off-spring.

There are other instances when diet and nutrition have been shown to impact the epigenetics of the developing human fetus. It is well-known that maternal metabolic conditions during pregnancy, such as diabetes, hypertension, and obesity, are associated with children who have an increased incidence of autism spectrum disorder, developmental delays, or impairments in specific domains of development, but the specific epigenetic effects are not as well-known. Having Lyme disease and MSIDS also can confer an increased risk on the fetus, since *Borrelia burgdorferi*, *Bartonella henselae*, and other associated tick-borne disorders can be transmitted transplacentally. We need to pay closer attention to the effect of chronic infections, nutrition, and metabolic conditions on the fetus if we wish to control preventable illness in our present and future generations.

These dietary effects on epigenetics also apply to the adult population. We have ample evidence that caloric restriction, which refers to consuming at least 25 percent fewer calories than what we are eating right now, can affect gene expression not only in children, but also in adults. In a 2011 article published in the *New England Journal of Medicine*, caloric restriction was found to directly affect the sirtuin genes (SIRT1, for example), the ones responsible for preserving cells and influencing age-related diseases such as cancer, heart disease, osteoporosis, diabetes, and neurodegeneration. The activation of these genes also has an anti-inflammatory effect. As we previously discussed, the biological mechanisms that seem to underlie most chronic disease states are oxidative stress and inflammation. Free radicals create inflammation that drives atherosclerosis and, along with oxidized LDL cholesterol, can eventually cause heart attacks. Free radicals can affect the brain and lead to diseases such as stroke, epilepsy, Parkinson's, and Alzheimer's. Free radicals and oxidative stress have also been linked to downstream effects with diabetes, aging, and cancer. Controlling inflammation at the level of the sirtuin gene would be equivalent to discovering a hidden fountain of youth in the body. These are exactly the types of effects we are looking to induce in MSIDS patients, who suffer from an overabundance of inflammatory molecules, which increase their symptoms.

We know that caloric restriction, combined with exercise, can prolong life, and has an epigenetic effect, yet very few follow these guidelines. Another way to achieve the same effects of caloric restriction is with the supplement resveratrol. Resveratrol is an important antioxidant that is derived from grapes and other dark berries. It also works with the sirtuin genes, and has important anti-inflammatory effects: It increases the production of Nrf2, which prevents us from turning on NFKappaB and producing large amounts of proinflammatory cytokines. In rat and other animal studies another advantage of resveratrol has been shown: It up-regulated (increased) a significant number of genes that are involved in mitochondrial function, which, when disrupted, is known to result in neurodegenerative disorders. This will be further discussed in Chapter 10, when we discuss Lyme disease and mitochondrial dysfunction.

Other nutrients and phytochemicals can either inhibit or activate enzymes that effect DNA methylation or modify histones. These include: zinc; choline; betaine; pyridoxine; B vitamins, such as niacin, niacinamide, and cobalamine; as well as SAMe and 5-methyltetrahydrofolate (5-MTHF). We discussed earlier the important effect that zinc has on immune function, inflammation, and cytokine production, and in supporting phase I detoxification reactions for foreign-based chemicals in the liver. Combining zinc with methylation cofactors, such as methylcobalamin, SAMe, and 5-MTHF, we find that many of our patients improve their overall functioning. These nutrients are not just acting at a cellular level; their effects may also have a regulatory effect on our epigenetics.

Other nutritional substances that have an effect on our epigenetics are compounds found in fruits and vegetables. The American Cancer Society suggests that we consume as many as five to eight cups of fruits and vegetables every day to maintain health. Many of the colorful compounds found in a variety of fruits and vegetables contain important antioxidants and phytochemicals. The phytochemicals that have been found to have an epigenetic effect include: broccoli compounds such as sulforaphane; the red wine/grape extract resveratrol; curcumin (turmeric), epigallocatechin gallate (EGCG) from green tea; hops; and genistein from soy. These nutrients and phytochemicals literally "talk" to our genes and help to affect our epigenetics in a positive way.

OPTIMIZING MITOCHONDRIAL FUNCTION

The mitochondria are the energy powerhouses of the cell. If they are damaged by free radicals and toxic chemicals, they are unable to work correctly. The end-stage result may be fibromyalgia, chronic fatigue syndrome, as well as a host of neurological symptoms, including neuropathy, as shown in a 2012 article published in the *International Journal of Clinical Medicine*. We can optimize mitochondrial function by taking the vitamins, minerals, complex carbohydrates, and phospholipids necessary for proper energy metabolism, such as CoQ10, acetyl L-carnitine, D-ribose, and glycosylated phospholipids. These all help to ensure more efficient ATP and energy production. This will be discussed in more detail in Chapter 10, Lyme and Mitochondrial Dysfunction.

ASSISTING AND BALANCING LIVER BIOTRANSFORMATION

The liver is one of the primary organs that help transform chemicals, drugs, hormones, and toxic compounds into nontoxic substances. This takes place through biotransformation in the phase I and phase II pathways in the liver. Biotransformation refers to the metabolism of a drug or toxin in the body, making it more water-soluble and increasing the body's ability to excrete it through the urine. This takes place through the chemical reactions in the liver of a series of enzymes known as the cytochrome P450 system, such as adding an electron (oxidation) in phase I reactions, which then prepares the substance for phase II, when a molecule is added (conjugation), making the compound more water-soluble. It requires energy and a steady supply of nutrients to be effective.

Good quality protein—such as lean red meats, chicken, turkey, cottage cheese, Greek-style yogurt, and nut butters—is especially important in phase I and phase II reactions. The enzyme systems present in the liver that are involved in phase I detoxification reactions (which are called "the cytochrome P450 system") are dependent upon certain essential amino acids, such as lysine and threonine. If these essential amino acids are not present, these enzyme systems will not work effectively. Similarly, in phase II reactions, dietary protein is essential to promote the synthesis of glutathione, and certain amino acids, such as glycine, glutamate, cysteine, and taurine, are also necessary in conjugation reactions, to eliminate drugs and their metabolites as well as environmental chemicals from the body.

There are other food and dietary compounds that help modulate the phase I and phase II metabolic pathways and make them more efficient. These are known as "bifunctional modulators," meaning that they can affect both the phase I and phase II pathways, by either increasing or decreasing the enzymatic activity of the pathway, depending on what is most beneficial to the body. The foods that have an effect on modulating phase I enzymes include:

- Ellagic acid (found in pomegranates)
- Green tea
- Watercress
- Silymarin (milk thistle)

The compounds that affect the six detoxification pathways in the phase II enzyme systems include:

- Alpha-lipoic acid
- Artichoke leaf
- B_6
- B_{12}
- Ellagic acid
- Folic acid
- Glutathione
- Glycine
- Magnesium
- NAC
- Pantothenic acid
- Silymarin
- Sodium sulfate
- Watercress

Other important nutritional supplementation includes the use of broccoli compounds and cruciferous vegetables. These contain active compounds, such as indol-3-carbinol, di-indol methane (DIM), and sulforaphane, that help modulate the phase I and phase II liver detoxification pathways and convert toxins acting as xenoestrogens (foreign chemicals with estrogenic effects) into healthier compounds.

LYME NUTRITIONAL THERAPIES

Beginning in 2002, I started using herbal protocols for treating Lyme disease. The majority of my patients were relapsing once they were taken off antibiotics, especially the ones that had been ill for many years before receiving a proper diagnosis. However, I knew that I couldn't leave my patients on antibiotics forever. I had heard about a variety of herbal protocols that were being used to treat Lyme disease. Then, in 2002, I was at a Lyme Disease Association meeting where I was introduced to Dr. Qingcai Zhang, a Chinese medical doctor who had moved to the United States and was practicing traditional Chinese medicine (TCM), specifically focusing on herbs and acupuncture. He was living in Westchester County, an area known to be highly endemic for Lyme disease, and over the years had been seeing more and more patients with it. He had therefore developed an effective system of herbal therapies to treat it and associated co-infections, such as *Babesia*. He let me know that these herbal protocols were based on traditional Chinese herbs that had been studied in China for similar bacteria and parasitic infections, such as syphilis and malaria, and that there were published references in the Chinese medical literature on their use and safety. I then accepted his invitation to train with him.

Within three weeks time I found myself at his home with his lovely wife, Lee-Lee, and son, Yale, and he was explaining the protocols to me in between bites of freshly cooked, delicious Chinese food. I left his home with a satisfied stomach and newfound hope that I had discovered another piece of the puzzle that would help my chronically ill, relapsing patients.

For the next three years I tried Dr. Zhang's protocols on patients who were either failing on antibiotic therapies or had frequent relapses. The protocols consisted of using several herbs in varied combinations. One combination was allicin (the active component of garlic) with a mixture of herbs called HH and Circulation P (which helps get the herbs deeper into the tissues). This clearly was helpful in certain patients, especially if they had an overlapping *Candida* problem (garlic compounds can be useful in yeast infections), but the smell of the garlic often was a limiting factor. I could always see how stable a marriage was based on how their spouse reacted to the strong odor that emanated from them day and night. Some patients complained so bitterly that I even took it myself to show them that it wasn't so bad. However, my wife, who is Italian and cooks with garlic, couldn't take the smell after several months either.

So we often ended up rotating to other combinations, which were odorless, such as *Coptis*, HH, and Circulation P, or a third protocol using an herbal combination known as R-5081 with HH and Circulation P. We also added the herbs *Cordyceps* when there was significant fatigue and lack of stamina, Puerarin if there were memory and concentration problems, *Artemisia* if there were ongoing sweats and chills with babesiosis, and, finally, the herbal product AI#3 (autoimmune III), when there was evidence of an overstimulated immune system with inflammation. These protocols were helpful: I was able to keep approximately two thirds of my patients off antibiotics for long periods of time while they remained on these herbs. Ultimately, however, many of them relapsed as they tried to come off the herbs, and some relapsed while staying on a traditional Chinese medicine protocol. The protocols were clearly helpful but not curative.

As I was searching for answers, one more clue appeared in fall 2006. Doctors often train with me as part of a teaching program sponsored by ILADS. Timothy Callaghan, an ILADS member and MD from North Carolina, came to learn about Lyme disease. He had an interest in integrative medicine, and as we discussed cases, he informed me of an herbal regimen that was just starting to be used for Lyme disease, called the Cowden protocol. It came from a company called NutraMedix, and it involved using various herbs, such as Samento, Banderol, Cumunda, *Quina*, parsley, and Burbur. The combinations of herbs were designed by Dr. William Cowden, an internist and cardiologist who specialized in integrative medicine, and who was getting good results helping people with Lyme disease.

Dr. Cowden told me that his protocol was highly effective in helping to relieve the symptoms of Lyme disease, and that his herbs had also been studied in the laboratory for efficacy and safety. I then asked him if anyone had ever done a clinical study to verify the results. He said that they hadn't, but that NutraMedix, the company making the Cowden herbal protocol, would certainly be willing to provide free herbs to my patients to participate in a study to prove their efficacy. It seemed like an overly generous offer, and one I couldn't refuse, so I agreed to do a study in my office.

We designed a six-month study, evaluating the herbs Samento, Cumunda, Banderol, *Quina*, parsley, and Burbur in four different combinations. Samento, Banderol, Cumunda, and *Quina* target *Borrelia burgdorferi* and may affect different co-infections by their antibacterial, antiviral, antiparasitic, and antifungal effects. Burbur and parsley are used to help support detoxification during treatment, especially during Jarisch-Herxheimer reactions. Patients took these herbs both while on and off antibiotics, and used either a limited version of the Cowden protocol or a more extensive full Cowden protocol. The limited Cowden protocol used these herbs but without more extensive supplements for detoxification and removal of heavy metals (trace minerals, magnesium, *Chlorella*, and zeolite), treatments for biofilms (Serrapeptase), or treatment for anxiety and insomnia (Amantilla, valerian root in liquid form).

The study compared four treatment groups against my patients who were taking only antibiotics:

Group 1: Full Cowden herbal protocol; no antibiotics
Group 2: Limited Cowden herbal protocol; no antibiotics
Group 3: Full Cowden herbal protocol; with antibiotics
Group 4: Limited Cowden herbal protocol; with antibiotics

These were the questions that we set out to answer: Is this herbal protocol safe? Is it efficacious? Are there any effects on associated co-infections, like *Babesia* and *Bartonella*? Is there an effect on removing heavy metal toxins? Were there any side effects, such as Jarisch-Herxheimer (JH) flares, and if so, what was the length and severity? Were any of the detoxification herbs (Burbur, Parsley) effective in helping to decrease flares? And, finally, was six months adequate to treat these Lyme disease patients? We evaluated these questions using a screening questionnaire that patients filled out monthly while participating in the study.

At the end of the study, we were elated. Over 99 percent of all of my patients, who had been ill for years and were treated for MSIDS with antibiotics alone, would relapse to varying degrees once the antibiotics were stopped. Placing them on the herbal protocol once they came off

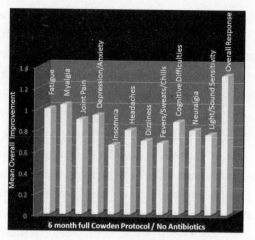

This is a graph showing the mean overall improvement in symptoms after six months of being on the full Cowden protocol, without antibiotics. Improvements were seen with fatigue, muscle and joint pains, neurological symptoms (light sensitivity, dizziness, headaches, and cognitive problems), as well as with sleep and moods.

GRAPH COURTESY OF THE AUTHOR.

antibiotics controlled the majority of their symptoms and enabled up to 70 percent to remain well for months to years. What's more, the patients in all four groups reported that they were feeling better. The graph above shows the mean overall improvement in symptoms after six months of the full Cowden protocol, without antibiotics.

Improvements were seen in fatigue, muscle and joint pains, neurological symptoms (light sensitivity, dizziness, headaches, and cognitive problems), as well as with sleep and moods.

There were differences between using the limited and full Cowden protocol. A larger number of patients showed significant improvement with the full protocol. This was because the full protocol also treated mineral deficiencies and biofilms, and assisted with detoxification, and as we've learned, these factors can be important in helping the MSIDS patient to recover. The full protocol also helped patients with their disturbed sleep patterns and underlying anxiety, since valerian root is a potent herbal therapy for these conditions. We found both the limited and the full protocols to be both safe and efficacious. There were, however, no significant effects on associated co-infections, like *Babesia* and *Bartonella*, and there was no significant effects on removing heavy metal burdens with just *Chlorella* and zeolite. Some patients had Jarisch-Herxheimer flares, requiring lowering the dosages of the antispirochetal herbs (Samento, Banderol, Cumunda). Burbur and parsley were effective in approximately 30 percent of the patients for decreasing flares.

I presented these results at various scientific conferences, including a Lyme disease symposium at the University of New Haven in Connecticut, in 2008. Dr. Eva Sapi had a particular interest in the efficacy of the herbs, as she knew of the problem of persistent *Borrelia*, despite seemingly adequate antibiotics. She decided to take our results and test them out in the laboratory. Dr. Sapi found, as we did, that these herbs were useful. Samento and Banderol in the test tube were effective in killing the Lyme-carrying spirochetes. We had confirmation of our success, not just in the clinical setting, but also in the laboratory.

Although that was gratifying, what was even more rewarding was that one of my successes was Aaron, the ten-year-old wrestler. He enrolled in the Cowden trial. We were able to taper him off antibiotics, and several months later he was symptom-free while remaining on the herbs. He was able to participate in wrestling and finish the school year with good grades. It seemed as if we had hit a home run.

Yet I was faced with the same dilemma. With each herbal protocol, we had about a 70 percent success rate, and 30 percent were relapsing when they were off the herbs. Some patients also found that the herbs worked for a while, but then, as with Dr. Zhang's regimen, relapsed while still taking them. Some of those symptoms were bad enough that they needed to go back on antibiotics.

I went back to the drawing board. Over the next several years we tried using combinations of other herbs, such as the ones discussed by Stephen Buhner in his book, *Healing Lyme*. He suggested using Samento in combination with other herbs, such as *Andrographis, Polygonum* (Japanese knotweed/resveratrol), *Stephania* root, and *Smilax* in patients with Lyme disease. I liked that these herbs had been studied extensively, and the results were published in the scientific literature. These are the primary actions for these herbs:

1. ***Andrographis paniculata***: antibacterial, antiviral, antispirochetal, antifilarial, antimalarial, anti-inflammatory, and analgesic. It crosses the blood-brain barrier and helps decrease inflammation in the central nervous system, as well as helping modulate autoimmune reactions.

2 ***Polygonum cuspidatum*** **(Japanese knotweed/resveratrol):** antibacterial, antiviral, antispirochetal, antifungal, immunomodulatory (affects autoimmune reactions), anti-inflammatory, and has antioxidant properties.

3. ***Smilax*** **(sarsaparilla):** antispirochetal, antiparasitic, immunomodulatory, lessens Jarisch Herxheimer reactions, binds endotoxins, anti-inflammatory, neuroprotective (crosses the blood-brain barrier), enhances cognitive function, protects the liver, and normalizes liver functions.

4. ***Stephania*** **root:** antiparasitic, anti-inflammatory, antioxidant, decreases cytokines (IL1-Beta, TNF-α, IL-6).

We find that we are able to use these herbs alone, or in combination, with patients both on and off antibiotics to help improve resistant symptomatology. For example, some patients with severe Jarisch-Herxheimer reactions have taken *Smilax* in combination with other herbs, i.e., Greenwood Herbal's Herxheimer formula, and found it to be effective, especially when alkalizing and using oral glutathione have inadequately controlled their symptoms. Green Dragon Botanicals in Vermont is another well-known source for these herbs. We have found them to be safe, but just as with classic medications, they are contraindicated under certain conditions (pregnancy, active gallbladder disease) and can have side effects, such as gastrointestinal upset, allergic reactions, or changing drug levels in the body. The use of these herbal compounds should therefore be monitored carefully by a health-care practitioner.

The last herbal regimen that we have found to be effective is the Byron White protocol. This is another Chinese-based regimen with multiple herbs in combination formulas (i.e., A-L has allicin and *Coptis* to treat Lyme disease, and includes antiparasitic herbs, such as clove, black walnut, and wormwood). There are many formulas for the co-infections found in the Lyme-MSIDS patient, including antiviral, antifungal, and antiparasitic formulas. We have used them in over one thousand patients and find them to be very promising for resistant patients who fail antibiotics, fail other herbal protocols, or continue to relapse when they are off antibiotics. They can therefore be an effective option for patients but have certain contraindications, as with the Zhang, Cowden, and Buhner protocols. They also can cause severe Jarisch-Herxheimer reactions if not used properly, as is the case with the other herbal protocols described above, and they should also be used under the guidance of a health-care practitioner.

Other herbal protocols exist for the treatment of Lyme and co-infections that may be effective, but we have not personally studied their safety and efficacy to date. However, the ones we use on a regular basis assist with many of the frequent symptoms we see in Lyme-MSIDS, including fatigue, memory problems, muscle and joint pains, sleep problems and

Table 9.2 Effective Herbal Protocols Used at Hudson Valley Healing Arts Center

Name	Regimen	Reasons
Zhang protocol (TCM)	Combination therapies including Allicin, HH, R-5081, Circulation P, *Cordyceps*, Puerarin, *Artemesia*, AI#3, Herbsom	Lyme disease and co-infections (*Babesia, Bartonella*), inflammation, sleep disorders
Cowden protocol	Samento, Banderol, Cumunda, *Quina*, Houttuynia, Parsley, Burbur, Serrapeptase, Amantilla, *Chlorella*, zeolite	Lyme disease, certain co-infections, biofilms, detoxification, sleep disorders, anxiety
Buhner protocol	Samento, *Andrographis polygonum* (Japanese knotweed), *Stephania* root, *Smilax*	Lyme disease, co-infections, inflammation, Jarisch-Herxheimer reactions
Byron White	Combination therapies, including A-L, A-BAB, A-BART, A-BIO, A-Myco, A-P, A-V, A-EB/H6, A-FNG, Detox 1 and 2, NT-Detox, A–INFLAMM, among others	Lyme disease and co-infections (including parasites, viruses, and fungus), detoxification, inflammation

mood disorders. They also can help support the detoxification pathways and relieve Herxheimer reactions, improving my patients' quality of life.

Antibiotics are useful in treating the underlying infections, but they do not clinically appear to eradicate the infections completely in late Lyme disease and MSIDS, as the vast majority of patients relapse when they're discontinued. This was the case with Aaron, and with the majority of the patients who come to see me, especially the ones who have been sick for many years without receiving a proper diagnosis. Therefore, further investigation of herbal and integrative therapies is needed as an alternative to antibiotics. We also need to incorporate the functional medicine diagnostic tools discussed in this chapter if we wish to get to the underlying causes of illness. Nutritional therapies can also be seen to play a preventive role, as they can influence our epigenetics and allow us to potentially avoid certain consequences of diseases, by preventing inherited DNA patterns from manifesting as we age. Good nutrition is not just a good idea. It is essential for all of us living in a toxic world.

TEN

Lyme and Mitochondrial Dysfunction

Many of us suffer from an "energy crisis." In fact, constant fatigue is one of the most common complaints of those with MSIDS and Lyme disease. Even when we are relatively healthy, many of us feel that our energy declines as we get older. Is this fatigue due to "normal aging," a result of a programmed deterioration of our cells, or are there other factors causing fatigue and contributing to chronic disease?

The energy that keeps us going is made in the body through a complex series of biochemical reactions known as the Krebs cycle, which takes place in the powerhouse of the cell known as the mitochondria. Adenosine triphosphate (ATP), the most important energy molecule in the body, is produced by the mitochondria. ATP transports chemical energy to help power our metabolism; however, when the mitochondria are not working properly, they cannot make enough ATP, and we experience fatigue that affects the entire body.

The energy made in the mitochondria is determined by our diet. If we do not have an adequate supply of healthy fats, carbohydrates, and proteins to feed into stage one of the Krebs cycle, we will experience fatigue. This is seen in chronic fatigue syndrome, when nutritional and enzyme deficiencies lead to poor digestion.

If we are exposed to a large load of environmental chemicals that need to be detoxified, we may use up nutrients, such as B vitamins and magnesium, that are essential for mitochondrial energy production. Again, the result is fatigue, which is seen in diseases such as chemical sensitivity and environmental illness (EI).

Finally, if our diet is deficient in the amino acids found in protein-rich foods, we will not be able to keep up with the energy requirements of our cells.

THE CAUSES OF MITOCHONDRIAL DAMAGE

Each mitochondrion has four main compartments: the outer membrane, the inner membrane, the matrix, and the intermembranous space. Any abnormal functioning in these areas will directly impact the mitochondria. The outer membrane contains the enzymes that help to transport fat into the matrix, where it can be converted into energy. The inner membrane contains the cristae, which are complex folds and tubules containing enzymes that are responsible for making ATP. If we lose cristae, we lose our ability to produce ATP. The matrix is enclosed by the inner membrane and contains mitochondrial DNA and a number of important enzymes, such ATP synthase, the enzyme that is responsible for the production of ATP.

Mitochondrial damage occurs naturally during ATP production, as free radicals are released. These free radicals cause oxidative stress when electrons are transferred in a transport chain from one molecule to the next. As each oxygen molecule is converted into water as the final acceptor of these transferred electrons, an unpaired oxygen molecule is released as a free radical. This can be harmful to the mitochondria if they are produced in excess. These free radicals damage DNA, proteins, lipids, and DNA polymerase, the enzyme responsible for mitochondrial replication, leading to mitochondrial structural and functional damage. Although cellular DNA is protected against damaging free radicals by histones, mitochondrial DNA lacks this protective barrier.

We can indirectly determine if there is damage to the mitochondria by measuring markers of oxidative stress, such as lipid peroxides. We can also check for inherited genetic conditions in which mitochondrial dysfunction has been implicated. Inherited disorders of mitochondrial dysfunction can cause some of the same symptoms we see in persistent Lyme disease, i.e., neurological symptoms, including cognitive impairment, neuropathy, encephalopathy, and musculoskeletal symptoms, and they may be among the underlying causes driving resistant symptomatology in the MSIDS patient for whom traditional therapies have failed.

A number of chemicals, toxins, and even medications, can damage mitochondrial structures, thereby complicating the diagnosis, since both the diseases and their drug treatments can cause similar symptoms, primarily fatigue. These medications include:

- Analgesics (aspirin, acetaminophen, and other anti-inflammatory drugs such as NSAIDS)
- Angina medications and antiarrhythmics (Cordarone/amiodarone)
- Antianxiety medications, such as Xanax (alprazolam)
- Antibiotics (tetracyclines)
- Antidepressants, such as amitriptyline (Elavil), SSRIs, such as Prozac (fluoxetine)
- Antipsychotics (haloperidol, risperidone)
- Bile acid sequesters (cholestyramine/Questran, colesevelam/WelChol)
- Cancer drugs
- Cholesterol medications, including the statins (atorvastatin/Lipitor, fluvastatin/Lescol, lovastatin/Mevacor, pravastatin/Pravachol, rosuvastatin/Crestor)
- Diabetes medications (Glucophage/metformin, troglitazone, rosiglitazone)
- Epilepsy medications (valproic acid/Depakote)
- Mood stabilizers (lithium)
- Parkinson's disease medications (tolcapone/Tasmar, entacapone/Comtan)
- Treatments for alcoholism (Antabuse/disulfiram)

DISEASES RELATED TO MITOCHONDRIAL DYSFUNCTION

Mitochondrial dysfunction can be a great imitator, and it can underlie the clinical symptomatology we see in patients who present with a wide variety of complaints. Apart from fatigue, there is a link between mitochondrial dysfunction and many other diseases. Mitochondria are found in all of the cells of our bodies (except red blood cells), but they are particularly abundant in those organs that are needing active and abundant sources of energy, such as the skeletal muscle, heart muscle, liver, kidneys, and brain. If mitochondrial dysfunction were to happen in the heart, it could lead to various cardiac conditions, including conduction defects, cardiovascular disease, cardiomyopathy (an enlargement of the heart that leads to poor cardiac output and congestive heart failure), and atherosclerosis. Mitochondrial dysfunction in skeletal muscles leads to weakness, low muscle tone (hypotonia), exercise intolerance, and myofascial pain. If it were to affect the liver, it could cause hypoglycemia, with low blood sugars secondary to defects in glucose production (gluconeogenesis), nonalcoholic fatty liver failure (steatohepatitis), cancer, and hepatitis C–associated hepatocellular carcinoma. In the kidneys, it can result in proximal tubular dysfunction (Fanconi's syndrome) and cause a loss of essential amino acids, electrolytes, and minerals such as magnesium.

When mitochondrial dysfunction affects the brain, it sets the stage for a host of neurological diseases, including: Huntington's, Alzheimer's disease, and Parkinson's disease; psychiatric disorders, such as schizophrenia, bipolar, and anxiety disorders; or as various dysfunctions of the central and peripheral nervous system. For example, when the optic nerve and visual systems are affected, we can experience optic neuritis and visual loss. When the eighth cranial nerve, which sends signals from the inner ear to the brain, is affected, we can experience hearing loss. When the peripheral nerves are affected, we can experience neuropathic pain, chronic inflammatory demyelinating polyneuropathy (CIDP), and problems with the autonomic nervous system, such as postural orthostatic tachycardia syndrome (POTS), which results in low blood pressure, palpitations and fainting, absent or excessive sweating, and problems with temperature regulation.

These different diseases, all caused by mitochondrial dysfunction, may also be worsened with oxidative stress, after free radicals damage mitochondrial cell membranes. We are constantly exposed to environmental toxins, and we have already discussed the effects of heavy metal burdens: mercury, lead, arsenic, cadmium, and aluminum can all increase oxidative stress. The resulting increased free radicals adversely affect many different neurological conditions. In Alzheimer's disease, for example, amyloid plaques and intraneuronal neurofibrillary tangles are affected by free radicals, and to make matters worse, once the amyloid plaques have formed and start to accumulate, they can further increase oxidative stress, leading to a vicious downward cycle.

Patients with Alzheimer's disease also have increased levels of oxidative stress, which is reflected in the increased levels of iron and copper in the brain, as well as in increased lipid, protein, and DNA oxidation and the production of advanced glycation end products (AGE).

The same situation exists for Parkinson's disease. In Parkinson's, there is oxidative damage to an area of the brain known as the substantia nigra, which produces the neurotransmitter dopamine. When there is an insufficient quantity of dopamine available, Parkinsonian tremors and difficulties with initiating movements appear. Markers of oxidative stress, such as elevated levels of lipid peroxidation, which damage mitochondria, have been well documented in Parkinson's patients in postmortem studies. Researchers have found that the mitochondria in these patients are much less efficient at generating ATP.

Oxidative stress has been implicated in a wide variety of central nervous system disorders, including Lyme disease and MSIDS. Free radicals are produced in Lyme disease patients infected with *Borrelia burgdorferi*, and these not only damage mitochondrial cell membranes, but also activate microglia in the brain, the cells that act as the main form of active immune defense in the central nervous system. This stimulates the production of proinflammatory cytokines, such as IL-1, IL-6, and TNF-α, which cause symptoms of fatigue, muscle and joint pain, neuropathy, headaches, mood disorders, and cognitive difficulties.

We frequently see many of the signs and symptoms of mitochondrial dysfunction in Lyme-MSIDS patients. For example, many experience episodes of optic neuritis and visual and hearing loss, neuropathy (present in up to 70 percent of persistent Lyme disease patients), and CIDP (chronic inflammatory demyelinating polyneuropathy), as well as POTS syndrome and autonomic nervous system dysfunction. Neuropathy is common in all of these diseases, ones in which there is a loss of myelin sheathing that protects nerve fibers. This may be the result of multiple infections, immune damage, environmental toxins, or problems with proper detoxification, all of which can produce free radicals and damage the fragile mitochondrial membranes.

MITOCHONDRIAL DYSFUNCTION
AND METABOLIC SYNDROME

Other problems arising from mitochondrial dysfunction include metabolic syndrome, diabetes, and obesity. Metabolic syndrome is defined as a cluster of at least three of the following five metabolic conditions: hypertension, truncal obesity (abdominal belly fat), abnormal glucose tolerance, elevated triglyceride levels, and low HDL cholesterol. Several scientific studies have now shown that one of the defects in metabolic syndrome and its associated diseases is excess cellular oxidative stress, with associated damage to the mitochondria.

Mitochondrial damage can also be a by-product of metabolic syndrome and insulin resistance. In metabolic syndrome, higher than normal levels of insulin are required to regulate blood sugar levels. One of insulin's primary effects in the body is to take sugar and convert it into fat, which is stored to be a source of energy. When fat is being stored abnormally in muscle and liver cells, it causes a breakdown of the cells' normal functioning, which subsequently affects the mitochondria. Researchers have also determined that vascular endothelial growth factor B (VEGFB), which is produced by skeletal muscle, heart muscle, and brown adipose tissue, also promotes the movement of fat from the bloodstream across vascular endothelial cells, and into the target organs. Researchers have seen a strong positive correlation between VEGFB and mitochondrial function.

We see metabolic syndrome frequently among our MSIDS patients. Although clinicians often rely on weight gain and abnormal lipid levels as warnings of disease risk in metabolic disorders such as type 2 diabetes and associated heart disease, we now know that fat accumulation in the metabolic organs (i.e., skeletal muscle, liver, and heart) are an even stronger predictor of morbidity and mortality.

A diet high in sugar often drives reactive hypoglycemia (blood sugar swings) and fatigue, increases the risk of fungal and *Candida* overgrowth, causes weight gain with increased abdominal obesity (which increases production of cytokines, such as IL-6), and adversely affects mitochondrial function. Lyme disease patients should therefore try and avoid simple carbohydrates as much as possible, especially since certain sugars, such as fructose and lactose (found in milk products), have approximately ten times the glycation activity of glucose, the primary body fuel. Glycation is when a sugar molecule attaches to the proteins or lipids of our body without an enzyme, causing new types of sugar molecules to form; these are known as advanced glycation end products (AGEs). AGEs bind to receptors for advanced glycation end products (RAGE), and the result is increased inflammation driving cytokine production. Diseases linked to RAGEs include: diabetes, with eye, kidney, and nerve complications (retinopathy, nephropathy, and neuropathy); atherosclerotic heart disease; peripheral vascular disease; and neurological diseases, such as Alzheimer's. Mitochondria are significant players in many complex diseases and contribute to the process of inflammation through the assemblage of a large molecular complex called the "inflammasome." This is created when mitochondrial membrane damage occurs, and the inflammasome further stimulates the production of inflammatory cytokines (IL-1, IL-18), leading to a vicious cycle of fatigue and inflammation.

ENHANCING MITOCHONDRIAL PRODUCTION RESTORES YOUTHFUL VIGOR

Mitochondria, as well as most cells in the body, eventually die, and their components are recycled. For example, red blood cells circulate in our bloodstream for about 120 days before they die, and then their components are recycled by immune cells such as macrophages. Mitochondria within the cells are particularly susceptible to damage and destruction, since they have no mechanism to protect them from environmental toxins and free radical/oxidative stress. Once damaged by dying or dead cells, they may be destroyed by macrophages and their components recycled to make new mitochondria. The new mitochondria are made by mitochondrial fusion (the redistribution of the components), mitophagy (the destruction of mitochondria), and mitochondrial fission (reproduction) inside the cell, which helps to recycle their mitochondrial components.

Since mitochondrial dysfunction is an important factor in chronic fatigue, fibromyalgia, and a host of neurological syndromes, the benefits of increasing the production of mitochondria can lead to an increased energy level, better exercise performance, increased metabolic functions in major organs, and a subsequent loss of body fat and increased lean muscle mass, less oxidative stress, and the possible reversal of metabolic syndrome. How can we accomplish this? There is a switch inside the mitochondria, called PGC-1α, which is one of the master regulators of mitochondrial development and metabolism. If the PGC-1α switch is turned off, whether through inactivity or obesity, we don't produce as many new mitochondria, or the existing mitochondria do not function as efficiently, which can lead to decreased energy production, decreased oxidation of fats, and the accumulation of lipids in skeletal muscle. And this can lead to insulin resistance, obesity, and diabetes. On the other hand, when the PGC-1α switch is turned on, we can increase mitochondrial energy production. This helps to break down fats, decreasing obesity and metabolic syndrome. This explains the well-known benefits of eating less and exercising more in order to increase longevity. Cutting back on our food intake and decreasing the number of calories we consume is one way to turn on this PGC-1α switch, which is also important for preventing chronic disease. Caloric restriction will extend the lifespan of many animals, lowering and delaying diseases of aging and lowering glucose and increasing insulin sensitivity.

There are three different types of nutritional supplements that can also positively affect PGC-1α. These are L-arginine, alpha-lipoic acid, and resveratrol.

- L-arginine is an essential amino acid. It works on increasing mitochondrial function through its effects on the nitric oxide pathway.

- Alpha-lipoic acid, through food or supplements, can turn on an enzyme called 5' adenosine monophosphate-activated protein kinase, or AMPK (AMP-activated protein kinase). AMPK acts as a metabolic master switch; it regulates several intracellular systems, including the cellular uptake of glucose for energy production and the formation of new mitochondria. When ATP levels go down with exercise, AMPK is stimulated, helping replenish it.

- Resveratrol, either through foods or supplements, activates the sirtuin genes (SIRT1) in the body, stimulating PGC-1α. The sirtuin genes appear to be responsible for preserving the lives of cells, and they influence age-related diseases such as cancer, heart disease, osteoporosis, diabetes, and neurodegeneration. Resveratrol from grapes and berries, and quercetin found in fruits, vegetables, and tea, both exhibit chemical properties that allow them to activate SIRT1 and the sirtuin genes of longevity. Resveratrol can also increase mitochondrial production and enhance exercise tolerance, as well as inhibiting AMPK in the hypothalamus and activating AMPK in the peripheral tissues. To date, it is the only supplement known to do this.

Combining alpha-lipoic acid and resveratrol (occasionally with L-arginine) to stimulate mitochondrial production may therefore be useful in certain chronically fatigued individuals with mitochondrial dysfunction. Using L-arginine may be contraindicated in certain patients with Lyme disease and MSIDS, who experience inflammatory symptoms (i.e., the sickness syndrome discussed in Chapter 7), or certain diseases, such as migraines and inflammatory bowel disease, as it can exacerbate all of these conditions.

LIPID REPLACEMENT THERAPY

Lipid replacement therapy (LRT) involves replacing unhealthy fats in the body with healthy ones at the cellular membrane level. Lipid replacement therapy is different than just the substitution of certain dietary fats with others for proposed health benefits. We are specifically referring to phospholipids, such as phosphatidylcholine (PC), which are major components of our cell membranes. They can be obtained from a variety of readily available sources, such as egg yolk or soybeans, and are also found in supplements and foods containing lecithin. As we age and accumulate toxins in our bodies, the PC layer of our cell membranes may be damaged. Lipid replacement therapy assists in exchanging damaged cellular lipids for healthy ones to ensure the proper structure and function of the cells.

This can be accomplished using supplements such as NT factor, a nutritional supplement essential for repairing damaged mitochondrial cell membranes. NT factor is most often prescribed with other supplements that support mitochondrial function, such as acetyl-L-carnitine (which transports fats into the mitochondria), CoQ10, and NADH (which are part of the electron transport chain that creates energy), and, occasionally, D-ribose (which acts as a fuel for energy production but needs to be limited in patients with metabolic syndrome and diabetes who have elevated levels of glycation). Recent clinical trials have shown that LRT plus NADH and CoQ10 can prevent excess oxidative mitochondrial membrane damage and restore mitochondrial and other cellular membrane functions, which reduce fatigue. It was shown to be safe and effective in treating intractable chronic fatigue, fibromyalgia, and unresolved Lyme disease. Patients actively treated for babesiosis with atovaquone (Mepron or Malarone), the drug of choice to treat babesiosis and piroplasmosis, should not take CoQ10 with LRT. Atovaquone's action is on the mitochondrial electron transport chain in parasites, and CoQ10 inhibits its action.

DAVID'S MITOCHONDRIAL DYSFUNCTION AFFECTED HIS HEART

David was fifty-eight when he first came to me complaining of severe fatigue, muscle and joint pains, swelling of the legs, significant shortness of breath, and worsening memory and concentration problems. His past medical history was significant for hypertension, hyperlipidemia, atherosclerotic heart disease, and a cardiomyopathy. He had already seen a cardiologist, who sent him for an echocardiogram, which showed that the muscles of his heart were weak and not functioning properly. His ejection fraction (the volume of blood pumped from the heart) was 28 percent on the echocardiogram, which is the equivalent of having severe congestive heart failure. His doctors assumed it was from a combination of heart disease and a probable viral infection, causing a viral myocarditis and cardiomyopathy. They treated him with standard cardiac regimens of Lanoxin, Lasix , Aldactone, ACE inhibitors, and a statin drug, Mevacor, for his elevated cholesterol. His cardiac function did improve a bit with this medication regimen, but he was still complaining of being quite tired with significant shortness of breath.

David remembered being bitten by a tick when he visited Saugerties, New York, years earlier. He did not notice an unusual rash but did remember feeling flulike symptoms several days after the bite. Those eventually disappeared, but he never felt the same afterward. Now that his heart issues were mostly under control, he didn't know if his fatigue, intermittent joint and muscle pain, and poor memory were just old age or something more serious.

I had David fill out the Horowitz Lyme-MSIDS questionnaire, and we administered a physical exam, which revealed a normal blood pressure and no abnormal heart sounds. I picked up some faint crackling in the lungs (signs of fluid overload) and a slight edema of the lower extremities, again consistent with his history of congestive heart failure. We sent off for a Lyme Western blot with a full tick-borne co-infection panel and a fungal and viral panel, and did a CBC, a CMP, vitamin levels with his MTFHR gene status and homocysteine levels, checked his mineral levels (magnesium, zinc, and iodine, as he was on a high-dose diuretic), as well as hormone panels for thyroid, adrenal, and sex hormone deficiencies. We also sent off bloods for a HbA1c for metabolic syndrome, did a high-sensitivity CRP, and fibrinogen levels with a full lipid panel; finally, we checked him for food allergies, gluten sensitivity, and heavy metals.

David's Western blot came back strongly positive, confirming past exposure to Lyme disease. He also tested positive for ehrlichiosis and Rocky Mountain spotted fever. His thyroid functions were fine, but he suffered from low cortisol in the morning and at midday, confirming adrenal fatigue, and he was in andropause, as his testosterone levels were low (normal is 275 or higher; his was 234). His heavy metal tests revealed significant exposure to mercury, lead, arsenic, and cadmium, as well as to small amounts of uranium. We asked him about any prior environmental toxin exposure, but he couldn't recall any. His food allergy tests revealed IgG delayed food hypersensitivity reactions (antibodies involved in delayed immune reactions against foods) to dairy, wheat, and corn, and his mineral levels were low. He had a normal serum magnesium but a low red blood cell magnesium level (implying total body magnesium deficiency) and a low zinc level. His CRP was high, consistent with inflammation, and his HbA1c was 6.0, confirming that he was prediabetic and suffered from metabolic syndrome. His hyperlipidemia was controlled on his statin drug, as he had an LDL of 72, and now he was diagnosed with elevated blood sugars and inflammation, which were all separate risk factors worsening his underlying cardiovascular disease. He was also found to be MTHFR positive, with an elevated homocysteine level, at 16. This is another cardiac risk factor that could have been responsible for the development of his atherosclerotic heart disease.

I told David that, based on these test results, there were multiple reasons why he was not feeling energetic. They could also explain why he continued to suffer from muscle and joint pains and memory problems. David was placed on Plaquenil and minocycline for his Lyme and co-infections. He was given adrenal support with low-dose Cortef and adrenal supplements, and mung bean extract to raise his free testosterone. We recommended that he follow a low-carbohydrate diet, having small frequent meals that would treat his metabolic syndrome, and told him to avoid his allergic foods. He was given a multivitamin with B_6, methyl B_{12}, and activated folic acid for his elevated homocysteine level and MTHFR status, and nystatin tablets to control yeast overgrowth.

We also discussed trying mitochondrial support. I suggested using four different types of supplements that together would hopefully improve his energy level and help treat the cardiomyopathy. His high CRP alerted us to chronic inflammation, and since mitochondrial cell membranes have no protection against free radical stress, there was a high likelihood that they had been damaged. The first supplement used was enzyme CoQ10, which is an essential nutrient in the mitochondrial pathway and for heart muscle function (statin drugs, like the one he was taking, have been shown to deplete CoQ10 from the body). The second supplement was acetyl-L-carnitine, which provides a transport mechanism to get fatty acids into the mitochondria to make ATP. The third was NT factor, which may indirectly help heart function by helping the muscles of the heart function more efficiently. Finally, he was given adequate amounts of minerals, such as zinc and magnesium, which he was deficient in. The zinc could help decrease his cytokine levels and improve his immunity, and the magnesium would help support his heart muscle function.

David came back a month later. He reported that his energy level and his joint and muscle pain were better, and he was thinking more clearly. His stamina had increased, and his shortness of breath had decreased, and I suggested that after six months on this regimen, he recheck his echocardiogram to see if his heart muscle function had improved. He agreed, and after six months of rotating through several antibiotic regimens, chelating his heavy metals, taking hormonal support for his adrenals and low testosterone, shoring up his mineral deficiencies, and giving him mitochondrial support, he returned to see us with his new echocardiogram report in hand. His ejection fraction had increased to 42 percent, roughly a 30 percent increase. He was no longer winded with exertion and wasn't waking up in the middle of the night with shortness of breath. His lungs were clear, and the edema of his lower extremities had improved, all signs that his congestive heart symptoms and cardiomyopathy were resolving. In short, David was not suffering from old age with simple cardiac disease. He also had Lyme disease and MSIDS with mitochondrial dysfunction, which, when treated, improved his energy, cardiac functioning, and overall well-being.

ELEVEN

Lyme and Hormones

A s we continue to search for clues as to why many patients with Lyme-MSIDS remain ill, we are faced with one of the most important factors in the Horowitz sixteen-point differential diagnostic map for explaining ongoing symptoms: endocrine, or hormonal, abnormalities. Hormone deficiencies and imbalances are some of the most commonly overlooked causes for the failure of antibiotics in MSIDS, and I often find that by treating them I can restore my patient's health.

Many of the patients I see have hormonal imbalances. Sometimes their adrenal function is low, and they aren't producing enough of the hormones necessary for an adequate response to stress, i.e., cortisol. Others have abnormal patterns of cortisol secretion. They can also have antithyroid antibodies and associated clinical hypothyroidism, or they may have low levels of sex hormones; I often see young men, even those in their twenties and thirties, who I diagnose with andropause (low testosterone) with significant drops in testosterone levels. Women occasionally present with amenorrhea (lack of menstrual cycles), irregular cycles, or early menopause, in their late thirties or early forties. A large percentage of American men and women have insulin resistance, with hypoglycemia and metabolic syndrome. Often several endocrine abnormalities coexist, which can increase the severity of symptoms and contribute to the patient's underlying disease process.

Most often, patients who have clinical hormone imbalances complain of an increase in fatigue and a lack of stamina. Low adrenal and low thyroid hormones (T3, T4), low growth hormone and sex hormones (testosterone, affecting men and women), and insulin resistance with low blood sugars can all cause fatigue. Fatigue is one of the most common symptoms that my patients complain about. They may have been diagnosed with fibromyalgia, chronic fatigue syndrome, Gulf War syndrome, environmental illness, or Lyme disease, but they all share one symptom in common: fatigue.

Fatigue can also be caused by other conditions. These include:

- Autoimmune disorders and rheumatological diseases
- Cancer
- Co-infections with bacteria and parasites
- Deconditioning
- Depression
- Environmental toxins
- Food allergies
- GI disturbances
- Heart disease
- Metabolic syndrome—diabetes
- Mitochondrial dysfunction
- Sleep disorders
- Viruses
- Vitamin and mineral deficiencies (with anemia)
- Yeast and mold

It is therefore up to the health-care practitioner to look into all of these possibilities and to figure out which one, or which combination of factors, may be contributing to ongoing fatigue.

Hormonal imbalances also cause problems with maintaining or losing weight. With hypothyroidism (low thyroid function), patients gain weight, and in hyperthyroidism (high thyroid function), they tend to lose weight. Polycystic ovarian syndrome (PCOS) is characterized in women by: multiple ovarian cysts; irregular menses; high levels of male hormones, causing acne and/or abnormal hair growth (often with associated obesity); high cholesterol; and type 2 diabetes, with high insulin levels and insulin resistance. These women will gain weight and have great difficulty taking it off, despite following a low-carbohydrate diet. Insulin resistance is a precursor to type 2 diabetes, in which cells do not respond to the normal action of insulin, causing blood sugar levels to rise, and it is a factor in metabolic syndrome. Resistance to Leptin (the hormone from fat which regulates appetite and metabolism) can occur simultaneously with high levels of insulin, further increasing the difficulty in losing weight. Women with there conditions usually require a medication such as Glucophage to stop gluconeogenesis—the production of sugar in the liver—and to help with insulin resistance.

Cushing's disease (an overactive adrenal gland) and high cortisol secretion will increase weight, whereas low cortisol with adrenal insufficiency (Addison's disease) usually results in a loss of weight. Low testosterone levels can contribute to weight loss through the loss of muscle mass, and it may cause body fat to shift toward the abdominal region, increasing abdominal girth, as it may with insulin resistance. Low testosterone, elevated levels of the hormone prolactin (one with many functions, including milk production), and slightly elevated levels of cortisol can also be seen in weight loss syndromes, such as in AIDS patients, who lose weight rapidly.

Pain and inflammation are also part of the symptom complex of endocrine conditions. Various chronic inflammatory conditions, autoimmune diseases, such as rheumatoid arthritis, lupus, chronic fatigue syndrome, and fibromyalgia, can all result in immune disorders and neuroendocrine abnormalities. In medicine we usually do not think of hormones as necessarily playing an important role in driving autoimmune reactions, but they demonstrably can. Autoimmune diseases are more common in women than in men, and in the case of the autoimmune diseases rheumatoid arthritis and lupus, estrogen levels can accelerate, and androgens, such as DHEA, can inhibit the development of the disease. For example, underlying lupus is exacerbated during pregnancy. This is not just due to a predominance of estrogen, since other hormones, such as prolactin, may also contribute to the autoimmune manifestations. Elevated prolactin levels have been associated with a number of autoimmune diseases in addition to lupus: autoimmune thyroid disease, Addison's disease (adrenal insufficiency), and an eye inflammation called iridocyclitis. By lowering the prolactin levels with a drug such as Parlodel, we can lower the autoantibody titers in related autoimmune eye diseases, such as uveitis and iridocyclitis. Hormonal manipulation in this case can lead to the remission of autoimmune symptoms.

Growth hormone and prolactin also play important roles in regulating inflammatory reactions. Scientific studies have shown that they both increase resistance to bacterial infection, and therefore may be important factors in fighting the chronic infections we find in patients with MSIDS. This could explain, in part, the resistant symptoms seen in patients with growth hormone deficiency.

Other hormonal abnormalities that may contribute to autoimmune diseases are caused by defects in the hypothalamic-pituitary-adrenal (HPA) axis. The hypothalamus and the pituitary gland are located in the brain, and the adrenal gland is located right above the kidneys. The HPA axis is the master controller of hormones, via a feedback loop. The hypothalamus monitors the levels of hormones in the blood, and then sends out a message to the pituitary gland (via hypothalamic releasing hormones) to increase or decrease its secretion of hormones. The pituitary then secretes "stimulating" hormones, which affect the production of other hormones, such as: thyroid hormones (TSH, thyroid stimulating hormone); adrenal hormones (ACTH, adrenocorticotropic hormone); sex hormones (LH, luteinizing hormone, and FSH, follicle-stimulating hormone, which affect testosterone and estrogen levels); growth hormone (GH); hormones associated with autoimmune diseases and pregnancy (prolactin); and influences melanocyte-stimulating hormone (MSH), which affects melanocyte production (darkening of the skin) and appetite and sexual arousal.

The hypothalamus has many other roles, including controlling body temperature and sleep, and regulating hunger and thirst, as well as having an effect on our immune system. For example, animal models show that deficiencies in the HPA axis directly affect a broad range of autoimmune conditions. When functioning well, the HPA axis helps suppress excessive cytokine production and inflammation through the same feedback loop. However, cytokines themselves can also affect the HPA axis, and thereby affect hormone levels, especially the production of stress hormones, such as cortisol. Cortisol is the main brake in the production of inflammatory cytokines. Although cortisol production is enhanced by cytokines, shutting down the production of cytokines will only take place if there is no cortisol resistance, and cortisol resistance can be seen in painful musculoskeletal syndromes such as fibromyalgia and Lyme disease. Defects in the HPA axis due to trauma, infections, and stress all have been reported in the medical literature in patients with both fibromyalgia syndrome and Lyme disease. Similarly, defects in the functioning of the HPA axis show up in autoimmune diseases such as rheumatoid arthritis, where the immune and inflammatory reactions are supposed to raise the levels of steroids in the blood to control inflammation, but do not, due to dysfunction in the secretion and function of hormones from the pituitary gland. These abnormalities lower adrenal, thyroid, and sex hormone production by decreasing the pituitary hormones ACTH, TSH, and HCG. This causes abnormal growth hormone and prolactin secretion, with decreased activity of prolactin, higher basal levels of insulin, which leads to metabolic syndrome and diminished serum levels of endorphins, adversely affecting pain control. The cytokines produced in rheumatoid arthritis are therefore able to lower endorphins and multiple hormones simultaneously through their effect on the HPA axis. The result is an increase in fatigue and joint pain.

The endocrine abnormalities that are seen in chronic fatigue syndrome and fibromyalgia, as well as in Lyme disease, are also linked to cytokine production affecting the HPA axis. It is therefore not sufficient to just treat the symptoms, or to just treat the infections in MSIDS. The underlying problem with cytokine production must be addressed, and the hormones must be rebalanced, by either getting the HPA axis to work correctly or through hormonal support.

It is important to identify all of the endocrine problems present in the MSIDS patient, since addressing one without the others will often lead to an unsatisfactory result. For example, adrenal problems are often associated with thyroid dysfunction, and vice versa. If we try treating the thyroid without addressing the adrenal dysfunction, the thyroid may not function as effectively, contributing to ongoing symptoms.

ISSUES WITH THYROID HORMONES

Thyroid problems are commonly found in my Lyme patients. Some of these problems are from an overactive or underactive adrenal gland affecting thyroid function, but many patients have an overlapping autoimmune thyroid problem, such as Hashimoto's thyroiditis. In this disease, the thyroid is attacked by antibodies made by an unbalanced immune system, causing bouts of hyperthyroidism (elevated thyroid hormones) and/or hypothyroidism (low thyroid hormones). Here antithyroid antibodies are produced, such as antithyroglobulin antibodies (anti-TG ABs) and, less frequently, antithyroid peroxidase antibodies (anti-TPO ABs), which may or may not be associated with clinical hypothyroidism.

It is important to test for these thyroid antibodies, and for all of the thyroid functions when doing the initial MSIDS workup, as MSIDS patients frequently complain of fatigue, and the thyroid regulates our general metabolism and energy levels. The two main types of thyroid hormones, T4 and T3, are made when TSH (thyroid stimulating hormone) is produced by the pituitary gland and then travels in the bloodstream to the thyroid, stimulating it to increase thyroid hormone production. It does this by taking the amino acid tyrosine and adding four molecules of iodine, to make T4, then removing one molecule of iodine with a specialized enzyme, making the active form of the hormone, T3 (tyrosine with three molecules of iodine), or occasionally an inactive form of the hormone, reverse T3. These thyroid hormones then leave the gland and are bound in the blood to carrier proteins, such as thyroxine-binding globulin (TBG) and albumin, before reaching their final destination. The bound hormone, however, is not metabolically active, and cannot do its job. Only the free, unbound hormone has metabolic activity. It is therefore important to check the total and free thyroid hormone levels in patients with resistant symptoms, and to not just rely on standard tests of thyroid function, such as T4 and TSH levels. It is also important when evaluating thyroid functions to use the new reference ranges that were established by the American Association of Clinical Endocrinologists (AACE) in 2002. These ranges are usually not included on the standard laboratory reports sent to most medical offices. The new range for TSH is 0.3 to 3.0, and, in some patients, TSH levels need to be on the lower end of the spectrum, i.e., a TSH close to 0.3, to see a significant clinical improvement.

TSH and T4 also may not be reliable predictors of the other thyroid hormone levels, since both of them may be suppressed by cytokines. Also, levels of cortisol elevated by stress may prevent T4 from converting to more active forms of the hormone, T3 and free T3. The initial screening thyroid panel should therefore include tests for anti-TG and anti-TPO antibodies, T4, T3, free T3, and reverse T3 with a TSH. I also usually include a serum iodine level on the initial workup since we have found that roughly 25 percent of all of our chronically ill patients are deficient in iodine and other trace minerals. Iodine is necessary in the production of T3 and T4, so low iodine may contribute to low thyroid function, and in certain predisposed individuals, iodine deficiency may also lead to a goiter. Also, iodine deficiency is now considered to be an underlying cause of fibrocystic breasts. For example, my patient Melissa required over eight breast biopsies and surgeries over the years for her severe fibrocystic breast condition. The surgeons wanted to rule out breast cancer, as her breasts were so severely cystic that imaging studies couldn't determine if the masses that were identified by mammography were benign. Once we determined that she was iodine deficient, we treated her with one drop of Lugol's Solution every day (a concentrated solution of high-dose iodine). Her cystic disease significantly improved, and she no longer required multiple surgical evaluations. Her low thyroid function also improved, and she saw an improvement in her stamina.

The classic symptoms of hypothyroidism include fatigue, weight gain, dry skin, dry hair, constipation, cold intolerance, and memory and concentration problems. These symptoms may not improve until the levels of T3 and T4 are in the top third of the reference range, with a TSH below 1. Reference ranges are usually established for healthy populations and may not reflect the needs of chronically ill individuals. Some patients require a TSH level just above the lower range of normal (reflecting improved thyroid function) before they notice a clinical improvement.

Clues that you may be suffering from a low thyroid, apart from the above clinical symptoms, include loss of the external third of the eyebrows, swelling around the ankles (nonpitting edema of the lower extremities), swelling around the eyes/orbits (periorbital edema), scalloping of the tongue, and a delayed Achilles tendon reflex on physical examination. Basal body temperatures may also be low upon awakening in the morning (around 96 degrees to 97 degrees Fahrenheit) in some patients with hypothyroidism.

Hyperthyroidism that accompanies Lyme-MSIDS is usually due to an acute thyroiditis (inflammation of the thyroid from an infection), Graves's disease (autoimmune hyperthyroidism), or hyperfunctioning thyroid nodule(s) with a multinodular goiter, in which independent nodule(s) on an enlarged thyroid gland oversecrete thyroid hormones. It is not as frequently seen as hypothyroidism but should always be considered in patients who report sweating, anxiety, tremors, palpitations, and diarrhea with weight loss. Some of these same symptoms are seen in Lyme disease with co-infections like babesiosis or brucellosis and should always be considered in the differential diagnosis with other hormonal problems, such as the carcinoid syndrome or a pheochromocytoma. Carcinoid tumors can produce a variety of biologically active messenger molecules, such as prostaglandins, serotonin, and histamine. They commonly produce flushing and diarrhea, which can be confused with hyperthyroidism. A pheochromocytoma is usually a benign tumor of the adrenal gland that can also mimic the symptoms of hyperthyroidism through the production of elevated levels of catecholamine hormones, such as epinephrine and norepinephrine.

It is important to keep all of these differential diagnoses in mind with symptoms of what may appear to be an overactive thyroid. Evaluating the patient with a full thyroid panel, checking urinary VMAs and metanephrines in the urine to rule out a pheochromocytoma, and assessing urinary 5-HIAA levels to rule out carcinoid syndrome will help to differentiate among these illnesses.

ADRENAL DYSFUNCTION

The next most common endocrine abnormality that occurs for MSIDS patients is adrenal dysfunction. In medical school I was taught that there were two main forms of adrenal disease: Addison's syndrome, which is adrenal failure, and Cushing's syndrome, which is due to an overactive adrenal gland. One could recognize Addison's disease by its major clinical features of fatigue, weight loss, anorexia (loss of appetite), gastrointestinal complaints of nausea, vomiting, and occasional diarrhea, with hyperpigmentation, low sodium (hyponatremia), and mildly elevated potassium levels. Cushing's disease, on the other hand, is due to elevated levels of cortisol and is responsible for obesity, hypertension, diabetes, hyperpigmentation (similar to the pigmentation seen in Addison's disease), acne, hirsutism (increased hair growth), memory problems, and decreased resistance to infection. Yet we now know that there is a spectrum of adrenal dysfunction that lies between these two diseases, which is what typically presents in Lyme disease patients with MSIDS.

During times of extended or extreme stress, the adrenal glands go into a "fight or flight" mode and secrete high levels of hormones, such as DHEA, aldosterone, and cortisol. Cortisol's main functions include a proactive mode, in which it helps coordinate circadian rhythms, such as sleeping and eating, and processes involved in attention, learning, and memory. But it also has a reactive mode, which enables us to adapt to and cope with stress. We know that Lyme disease patients are under huge amounts of stress, both mentally and physically. The stress can be caused by the multiple infections that they are dealing with as well as by the illness and its consequences on their jobs, families, and friends. Our patients often have elevated levels of cortisol, either throughout the day or at night, when they are desperately trying to get to sleep. These interfere with their already disturbed sleep patterns, worsening their insomnia. Giving the patients phosphatidylserine at night (and up to three times per day) with adaptogenic herbs during the day, such as rhodiola, ashwagandha, and ginseng, and B vitamins, vitamin C, and pantothenic acid will help lower the stress response and support and rebalance the adrenal glands.

Cortisol receptors are found throughout the central nervous system and are especially abundant in the limbic system and hippocampus, the parts of the brain involved with mood, learning, and memory. Chronically elevated levels of cortisol eventually may lead to adrenal fatigue and burnout. When cortisol levels are chronically too high or too low, the hippocampus, the center for memory and attention, is affected. Some research suggests that severe stress can even cause atrophy of the hippocampus, which is associated with recurrent clinical depression, posttraumatic stress disorder, and mild/moderate cognitive impairment, and may be associated with the breakdown of the blood-brain barrier. We know, for example, that severely stressed Vietnam veterans and women who are sexually abused display an 8 percent shrinkage in the hippocampus. Patients like these will experience fatigue, food cravings, mood changes, and memory problems, many of the same symptoms commonly seen in those with non-Lyme-MSIDS (especially with *Mycoplasma spp.* and other intracellular infections) and Lyme-MSIDS. Chronically low cortisol levels also interfere with immune functioning, and the MSIDS patient may have chronic infectious symptoms that are resistant to antibiotics when they suffer from low cortisol levels.

Patients progress through various phases of adrenal gland fatigue when they are chronically ill. Phase I is when there is the acute fight or flight response associated with elevated levels of cortisol and early adrenal fatigue, with an elevated or high-normal cortisol level in the morning. Phase II is when there is evolving adrenal fatigue, with a normal or low morning cortisol level, and phase III is when there is established adrenal fatigue, with low cortisol levels. During these stages we often see decreased functioning of the HPA axis, when the hypothalamus and pituitary gland are unable to secrete enough releasing hormones to compensate for the low adrenal function, leading to varying levels of fatigue and increased susceptibility to infections.

Symptoms of adrenal fatigue overlap those of Lyme disease and MSIDS, including nonregenerative sleep, salt craving, hypoglycemia, decreased libido, fatigue, low blood pressure with dizziness standing (postural hypotension), depression/irritability, decreased memory/focus, and an increase in the time needed to recover from illness, injury, or trauma. We often need to give our patients adrenal support and rebalance their adrenal hormones, or their chronic symptoms may persist.

Testing and Treating Adrenal Gland Issues

There are several methods for testing adrenal hormones, and they each have their advantages and disadvantages. Blood tests, such as an 8:00 A.M. fasting cortisol level (checking the adrenal hormones first thing in the morning), may give a rough indication of the patient's adrenal status, but it is only a snapshot of the hormone level, which changes throughout the day. The other problem with blood tests are that they don't measure the tissue levels of the hormone, and the population used to standardize the tests may have included many people with some level of adrenal fatigue. Laboratory tests are defined and standardized based on statistical norms, not on physiologically optimal norms. A twenty-four-hour urinary cortisol test would be a better indicator of the total production of cortisol throughout the day, and if the levels are in the bottom third of the "normal" range, we would suspect decreased adrenal functioning.

The most specific method of testing for low adrenal function is to do an ACTH challenge. Adrenocorticotropic hormone (ACTH) is the hormone produced by the pituitary gland that stimulates cortisol secretion (as well as other adrenal hormones, such as aldosterone and DHEA sulfate). We can give a patient ACTH and measure the amount of cortisol that is produced. It is considered to be a positive test for low adrenal function if the cortisol levels are less than two times normal after the patient receives a bolus of ACTH. The easiest, simplest, and most practical method, however, is to conduct a DHEA/cortisol salivary test. This procedure has been validated as a reliable marker of cortisol levels, and it is reflective of tissue levels of the hormone in the body. We perform this test routinely on patients during their first consultation. There are many good laboratories performing the tests, including Aeron, Metametrix, Genova, Labrix, and Diagnostek. At least 40 percent to 50 percent of my patients coming in for an initial consultation have adrenal dysfunction, which explains in part their resistant symptoms. They will not completely recover from their illness if this is not adequately addressed.

In phase I of adrenal gland fatigue, or at times when cortisol levels are elevated, such as at night, when it interferes with sleep, we can use phosphorylated serine mixed with melatonin. Vitamins B_5, B_6, and C are also useful, in combination with lifestyle modifications that help reduce stress, such as meditation, yoga, deep breathing, exercise, and a healthy diet.

In phase II, we can add adaptogenic herbs to the B and C vitamins, such as rhodiola, ashwagandha, ginseng, and *Cordyceps* (a medicinal mushroom), and consider an adrenal glandular supplement while continuing to try and achieve better stress management. Finally, in phase III, when adrenal fatigue is established by low cortisol levels and a decreased functioning of the HPA axis, Cortef needs to be added. We have seen remarkable improvements in some patients who were in phase III of adrenal gland fatigue when we give adrenal supplementation. The hormone DHEA may also be added at this stage, or at any time when levels are low, as DHEA does not just function as a precursor for testosterone and estrogen, but also plays a role in stress management. It is secreted in response to ACTH stimulation, as is cortisol, and has been shown to help with mood stability during stressful events. DHEA elevates mood, calms emotions, increases alertness, and helps improve memory. Pregnenolone, the DHEA precursor helping to make cortisol and sex hormones, is also sometimes necessary at this stage. Adrenal balancing with pregnenolone,

DHEA, adaptogenic herbs, and cortisol is an important foundation for endocrine balancing, and is often necessary in the Lyme-MSIDS patient.

Larry Was Affected by Low Adrenal Hormones

Larry was forty-five years old when he first came to my office. He had a past medical history significant for allergies (allergic rhinitis) since childhood, osteitis pubis (inflammation of the pubic bones, requiring pelvic surgery), a torn meniscus of his left knee, and a history of Lyme disease. He had been sick for nearly thirteen years and had seen multiple physicians for his illness, which started with grand mal seizures; his initial workup at a major medical center in New York City did not reveal a cause for his seizures. Instead, he was told that they were "idiopathic," meaning no clear cause could be discovered. He was placed on Depakote to control them, but would still have occasional breakthrough seizures, despite the medication.

Larry suffered several tick bites on Cape Cod shortly afterward, at which point he developed a host of other symptoms. These included drenching night sweats, teeth-chattering chills, recalcitrant insomnia with associated restless leg syndrome and nocturia (getting up to urinate at least five times per night), irritable bowel symptoms, with alternating constipation and diarrhea, light and sound sensitivity, fatigue, joint pain and low-back pain, with associated neuropathy, and severe memory and concentration problems, with overwhelming depression.

He then went to see a host of specialists. For his insomnia, he saw a sleep specialist, who tried him on multiple medications without significant help. For his GI and urinary complaints, he saw a urologist and a gastroenterologist. The urologist scoped him and told him that he had a "shrunken bladder" and interstitial cystitis, for which they tried bladder instillations and stretching, with Elmiron. It was unfortunately only partially effective. The gastroenterologist also scoped him and couldn't find a cause for his bowel symptoms. He was placed on drugs for irritable bowel syndrome that did not provide any relief. Then he saw a psychiatrist, who wrote prescriptions for many different antidepressants and antipsychotic drugs, all of which were ineffective in relieving his depression.

Larry was completely homebound due to his illness, as he was in the bathroom for up to four hours a day trying to relieve his bowels, and constantly urinating. He became so forlorn over his resistant symptoms that his depression worsened, and led to thoughts of suicide. He finally sought out the advice of a Lyme-literate physician. This doctor diagnosed him with Lyme disease based on his history of multiple tick bites preceding his illness, his symptom complex, and prior testing that ruled out other disease processes. His Lyme ELISA was negative, and his Western blot was not CDC positive, but it tested positively for outer surface protein C, a specific band showing prior exposure to *Borrelia burgdorferi*, the agent of Lyme disease, which can be considered confirmatory in the right clinical setting. The physician initially prescribed high-dose amoxicillin, which only gave him minimal improvement in his physical symptoms. However, his memory and concentration symptoms were so severe that he was then prescribed IV Rocephin to get better penetration into the central nervous system, along with Flagyl and Zithromax.

He had a severe Jarisch-Herxheimer reaction two weeks into the IV medication, but then started to feel better. His bowel symptoms improved, as did his memory and concentration. Yet despite these medications, he was still severely affected by his illness. He continued to have drenching sweats; severe fatigue and cognitive problems; severe depression and mood swings, including paranoid episodes and occasional hallucinations; as well as double and blurry vision; facial twitching; almost constant nausea; intractable constipation, and nocturia, which compounded his poor sleep patterns. That's when he decided to get another opinion.

When Larry came to see me his vital signs were stable. His blood pressure was normal, but after standing for five minutes, his pulse rate went up by twenty-four beats per minute, and he experienced dizziness. His physical examination was otherwise completely within normal limits, except for some sinusitis stemming from his allergies. We sent off for a full range of blood tests, including a CBC, a CMP with mineral levels, a PSA, vitamin levels (B_{12}, folate, methylmalonic acid, and homocysteine), a co-infection panel (testing for *Babesia microti* and *duncani*, and *Bartonella*, *Mycoplasma*, *Chlamydia*, RMSF, Q fever, tularemia and *Brucella*, EBV, CMV, HHV-6, and West Nile). We also tested his immunoglobulin levels and subclasses, with complement studies, an antigliadin antibody and TTG with a food-allergy panel (IgE and IgG), an ANA, RF, ESR (sedimentation rate), cytokine panel and high-sensitivity C-Reactive protein (HS-CRP), and studies to evaluate the thyroid, growth hormone, and sex hormones. He was also sent home with a salivary adrenal test kit to check his adrenal hormones, and a six-hour urine DMSA challenge, to check for heavy metal exposure.

The tests clearly showed that he continued to suffer from multiple tick-borne infections, including Lyme disease, with severe neurological involvement, and babesiosis. There was also laboratory evidence of probable brucellosis (which may have been responsible, with *Babesia*, for the drenching sweats and teeth-chattering chills), possible *Bartonella* (which might explain his seizures and severe neurological involvement), and evidence of very low white cell counts, which may have contributed to his low immune status. We also suspected autonomic nervous system involvement causing his constant nausea, constipation, and bladder difficulties (implying possible vagal nerve problems), and postural orthostatic tachycardia syndrome (POTS). His symptom complex also pointed to a diagnosis of low adrenal function. At the end of his history and physical, when I reviewed the stacks of records he had brought in from prior physicians, I noticed an adrenal test done years earlier showing a low cortisol level that had never been repeated.

We then designed an initial antibiotic regimen and herbal protocol to help him with his resistant symptoms. A round of oral medications had already failed, as had IV Rocephin, so I asked him if he had ever had Bicillin injections. He said no. I then asked him if he liked pain. He smiled and said no, but he was willing to do whatever it took to get better. Since Bicillin is one of my most effective regimens for persistent Lyme disease, with twenty-four-hour killing power, we put him on it as my cell wall drug, and on grapefruit seed extract to address the cystic forms of *Borrelia*. We waited on starting other cystic drugs, such as Plaquenil, until he had an eye exam for his history of blurry vision and double vision, and didn't start Flagyl or Tinidazole right away, as he had a history of GI problems and severe Jarisch-Herxheimer reactions. I gave him minocycline with Zithromax as a double intracellular regimen and added nystatin tablets with meals to keep down yeast in the gastrointestinal tract. This was on top of a sugar-free, yeast-free diet with three different probiotics. He was told to order the herb cryptolepis to treat his babesiosis, and Florinef was prescribed for his POTS, with a high-salt diet, drinking at least two to three liters of fluid per day to help increase his blood pressure. He was too ill to go to the hospital and do a tilt-table test (the diagnostic test for POTS), so we treated him presumptively for ANS dysfunction, as untreated POTS could interfere with positive clinical results from other regimens. Zofran was prescribed for his nausea, Lyrica at bedtime to help him sleep, as well as Detrol LA, a drug used for urge incontinence. He was also to add herbs such as valerian root if he still had difficulty falling asleep or frequent awakening.

Finally, we asked him if he had ever had a shot of glutathione. He asked if it was as good as a shot of whiskey. (I saw a glimmer of humor come out after he had been in our office for three hours and we had worn him down.) He read and signed the consent form, and we started him on a glutathione trial.

The next morning Larry called to schedule another shot. He let us know that his response to the glutathione was no less than a miracle. Within several hours of getting home from our medical office, his energy level started to improve, he felt much calmer, and his mind had started to clear up for the first time in years, with greatly improved mental clarity. Prior antibiotic regimens had been ineffective in helping these resistant symptoms. Glutathione had probably helped remove some of the neurotoxins that were responsible for his symptoms, and Larry had hope for the first time in years.

During his next visit one month later, I realized that I hadn't received the results from his adrenal test. I was also disappointed to learn that Larry's positive results from the glutathione did not last. He complained again of bad nausea and constipation, and his urinary problems had worsened. Since his constipation was still severe, we stopped the Detrol and increased his fluid intake and magnesium, to try and enable him to move his bowels more regularly. Zofran did not significantly help the nausea, so I took him off that regimen. We changed the minocycline to rifampin with Zithromax for his low positive *Brucella* titers, and subsequently increased his Depakote dosing, since the rifampin could lower his seizure drug levels. The only positive clinical improvement we saw after the first month was in his drenching night sweats and chills: They were significantly better on the cryptolepis for the *Babesia*, which was interesting, because he was not yet taking the classical drug regimen for babesiosis. Otherwise Larry was still feeling extremely ill, and very depressed. I decided to add Deplin to his drug regimen. This is a form of activated folic acid that helps to augment the efficacy of other antidepressants. On the way out the door I gave Larry a hug and told him not to give up, and to please send off the adrenal saliva test. I told him that we would solve this mystery together.

The next month was still quite rocky, as Larry felt mood changes on the rifampin, and despite raising his Depakote level initially, he dropped below the therapeutic range several weeks into the rifampin. We therefore changed the rifampin to Septra DS with the Zithromax, since Zithromax and Septra would also cover possible bartonellosis, and that combination can be particularly effective in resistant babesiosis. We also added Mepron with a high-fat meal to the regimen, since he had not yet had a drug for babesiosis, and *Babesia* is known to cause an overall worsening of Lyme symptoms. We represcribed his Detrol LA in an attempt to help his resistant insomnia by decreasing the frequency of his urination. Finally, before leaving and getting his monthly hug and pep talk, I encouraged Larry again to please send off his adrenal testing. Except for the positive response to glutathione and the lessening of his *Babesia* symptoms with the cryptolepis, Larry was still quite ill, and I was searching for any clues to help explain the severity of his symptoms.

After the third month of treatment, Larry was seizure-free, had a normal Depakote level, his white cell count had stabilized, and his neutrophil count was improving. Neutrophils are the cells responsible for fighting bacterial infections. I had referred him to a hematologist to evaluate the low white cell counts, who thought that it was probably due to familial neutropenia and not to any of the drugs that he was taking, which was my major concern. He no longer had major sweats or chills with the addition of the Mepron for the babesiosis, and he was finally sleeping for longer periods at a time, probably due to the Detrol. His gastric issues were also starting to resolve. His memory and concentration were slightly better, and continued to improve each time he had a glutathione injection. His wife also reported that for the first time in years he laughed at a social gathering at his home. That might not sound like much, but from someone in the throes of deep despair and depression for years, that was my first clue that we were finally starting to make some significant progress.

But Larry still hadn't sent off his adrenal test! He also had stopped the Florinef on his own, because he was worried about the side effects, so I let him know in no uncertain terms before he left the office that there would

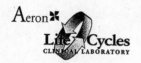

Adrenal Function Panel

Richard I Horowitz MD
Hudson Valley Healing Arts Center
4232 Albany Post Road
Hyde Park   NY   12538

2AL166

274984	11:00 am	0.09 ng/ml	Collection Date	06/13/2012
274985	02:00 pm	0.21 ng/ml	Received Date	06/18/2012
274986	06:00 pm	0.22 ng/ml	Report Date	06/21/2012
274987	01:30 am	0.18 ng/ml		

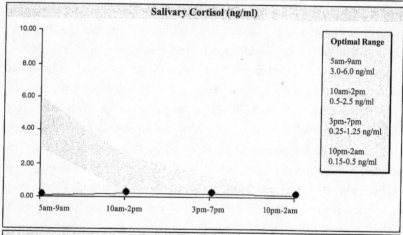

Salivary Cortisol (ng/ml)

Optimal Range

5am-9am
3.0-6.0 ng/ml

10am-2pm
0.5-2.5 ng/ml

3pm-7pm
0.25-1.25 ng/ml

10pm-2am
0.15-0.5 ng/ml

Reference Guide

Hypocortisolism: Results show low morning cortisol suggesting an under active adrenal cortex. Primary adrenal insufficiency, prolonged stress, post traumatic stress disorder, chronic fatigue syndrome and insomnia have been associated. Glucocorticoid or cortisol stimulating intervention should be considered.

Aeron LifeCycles Laboratory   1933 Davis Street #310 San Leandro CA 94577 (800) 631-7900

Evaluation of adrenal function with a 24-hour DHEA/cortisol test.

be "no more hugs for you" if I don't see that test on my desk in the next several weeks, and if you are not compliant with our protocols. I guess my threat must have worked. I got the DHEA/cortisol salivary test result back two weeks later, and I nearly fell off my chair when I saw the results.

Larry had virtually no cortisol production in the morning, and his cortisol graph was essentially flat for the rest of the day. His only minimally normal cortisol level was at night. The normal range for this test is 0.15 to 0.5 ng/ml nanograms per milliliter between 10:00 P.M. and 2:00 A.M. and he was just above the low-normal range in the evening. I'd seen low cortisol levels before, but I had never seen anything like this. Larry was clinically in full-blown adrenal insufficiency, which would explain his resistance to standard treatment regimens.

I hurriedly got on the phone with him and his wife to explain the results and discuss treatment options. My first choice was Cortef. It is the bioidentical equivalent to the cortisol naturally made in the adrenal gland, and it is the standard treatment for adrenal insufficiency. He let me know that he had tried steroids one time when he was in the hospital while they were attempting to treat his low back pain, but he didn't like it, because it made him confused and agitated. That reaction was so severe that he refused to take a steroid like hydrocortisone (Cortef) ever again. It became obvious that there was no way I was going to convince him to take the medication, so I thought for a moment, and then realized that he might be willing to take a natural supplement. I suggested a product called Adrenal Complex, which is a glandular adrenal extract from New Zealand I had used in the past with good results. Larry agreed to take the Adrenal Complex at the maximum dosage, and made an appointment to see me two weeks later.

The next time I saw Larry he had a big smile on his face. He looked like a new person. Within one week of starting the adrenal supplements he started feeling so well that he stopped his antibiotics (I almost didn't give him a hug for that one), and he let me know that he had more energy than he had felt since the beginning of his illness thirteen years earlier. If that wasn't enough, his bowel movements were now normal for the first time in years! His bladder symptoms had also improved—80 percent! He no longer was getting up at night, and his sleep was better. His joint pain had completely resolved, as well as his chronic low back pain, and he no longer had any neuropathic symptoms. His memory and concentration were also much better, and he was happy. There were no more mood swings. This was the same man who had been close to suicide several months before, when he felt he had no hope.

I was close to tears as he described his newly found good health. I have seen patients respond to adrenal support in a positive fashion, but what he told me was certainly one of the most telling stories regarding the importance of the adrenal gland with Lyme-MSIDS. For Larry, his low adrenal function had interferred with his body's response to the antibiotics used to treat the Lyme disease and co-infections. We see this problem in at least 40 percent of our patients with Lyme-MSIDS. Without properly addressing the underlying adrenal issues, patients with MSIDS will not fully recover from their illness.

TESTOSTERONE REPLACEMENT THERAPIES FOR MEN

Treatment resistance can also occur in some patients because of low levels of sex hormones. My view of hormone replacement has changed radically over the years, as I have learned more about hormone replacement therapy from colleagues at major medical centers. They essentially debunked most of the scientific information that I learned in medical school or throughout my clinical practice. I had learned, for example, that testosterone replacement was dangerous in men. In fact, it is the opposite. For example, at the 2012 Integrative Healthcare Symposium conference in New York City, at which I was a speaker, I learned about the importance of hormone levels for adult health. In an article published in 2006 in the *Archives of Internal Medicine*, I learned that mortality levels are 88 percent higher in men with low testosterone (low T) compared to men who had normal levels of testosterone. Low testosterone contributes to degenerative diseases of aging that involve chronic inflammation, and testosterone is cardio-protective. Men who receive testosterone replacement therapy have a slower progression from metabolic syndrome to diabetes or cardiovascular disease. This is because testosterone increases insulin sensitivity and helps to regulate blood pressure and lipid levels in the body. Declining levels of testosterone are also linked to rises in markers of inflammation, such as CRP. This elevated level of CRP is due to low levels of testosterone that, in conjunction with other stress hormones (epinephrine and cortisol), alter protein synthesis in the liver, increasing the production of inflammatory cytokines such as IL-6. As we have discussed, inflammation and cytokine production are responsible for many of the symptoms of MSIDS and are also crucial in the development of insulin resistance, obesity, and type II diabetes, which increases cardiovascular risk. Abdominal obesity, which results from testosterone deficiency, actually pumps out increasing levels of inflammatory cytokines, which is one of the reasons why low testosterone has been shown directly, in multiple scientific studies, to increase the risk for atherosclerosis.

Similarly, when pregnenolone and DHEA sulfate (DHEA-S) levels drop with age, we also see an increase in cardiovascular mortality. Pregnenolone is the precursor to DHEA production in the body, which subsequently is converted into androstenedione and then into testosterone. Chronic stress can initiate a "pregnenolone steal," which is when the body begins to make more cortisol from pregnenolone instead of making sex hormones, thereby lowering DHEA and sex hormone levels. A low serum DHEA(-S) level has been shown to be associated with a higher death rate from all causes, including cardiovascular disease and ischemic heart disease. This association remained after adjusting for the CRP, circulating estradiol, and testosterone levels. Testosterone use in men is not associated with significant cardiovascular risks, although we still need large clinical trials to be completed to evaluate its long-term effects. We certainly see that the men with unresolved Lyme disease who also have low T feel significantly better with hormone rebalancing.

Testosterone is necessary for energy, mood, libido, sexual functioning, prostate growth, muscle and bone mass, muscle strength, red blood cell production, proper sleep, and cognitive health. Its deficiency is associated with a decline in energy, lethargy, anemia, insomnia, a decreased sense of well-being, low mental energy, difficulties in short-term memory, depression and anxiety, loss of muscle mass, an increase in abdominal fat (increasing the risk of metabolic syndrome), osteoporosis, an increase in prostate size with Benign Prostatic Hyperplasia (BPH), and decreased sperm production. These symptoms are usually associated with "normal" changes in aging. However, the question is, are these really normal events?

Testing and Treating "Low T"

The symptoms of andropause in the aging man have been well validated in the scientific literature, and they have been correlated with all of
the above symptoms. The problem for my practice is that we see these
same symptoms in many young men with Lyme disease, co-infections,
and MSIDS. Therefore, our physical examination for men focuses on the
amount of body hair, muscle mass, breast enlargement or tenderness,
and the size and consistency of the testicles, as well as the size of the
penis. Preliminary testing includes an LH (luteinizing hormone), total
testosterone level, bioavailable and free testosterone level (unbound
hormone), estrogen level, SHBG (sex hormone binding globulin, the carrier protein for testosterone in the blood), and DHEA-sulfate. Although
serum total testosterone levels of 300 ng/dl to 1,000 ng/dl are considered
normal, these can vary between laboratories. What's more, normal values are based on statistical values of healthy individuals. Many men
with symptoms of low T may be in the bottom third of the normal range.
Morning measurements around 8:00 A.M. are recommended, when levels
are usually the highest, but certain medications, poor nutrition, and illness can temporarily reduce levels.

Laboratory tests showing a total testosterone level of less than 300 ng/
dl, bioavailable testosterone of less than 70 ng/dl, and free testosterone of
less than 50 pg/ml are considered proof of andropause. Screening tools
such as the ADAM questionnaire (androgen decline in the aging male),
the AMS (aging male's symptoms) scale, and the MMAS (Massachusetts
male aging study) questionnaire can also be used to assist in evaluating
symptoms.

There are four basic medications that can be used to increase testosterone: beta-human chorionic gonadotropin (β-HCG) and Clomid (clo-
miphene) in the younger male, and testosterone replacement by cream or
injection in men over forty, with or without aromatase inhibitors. β-HCG
and Clomid will preserve sperm generation, and are therefore preferred
for younger men who may wish to have families. Testosterone cream is
easy to administer, but absorption through the skin may decrease over
time, and injections may yield more consistent blood and tissue levels.
Aromatase inhibitors, such as Arimidex, stop the conversion of testosterone to estrogen (and are therefore also used in women with estrogen-
receptor-positive breast cancer) and help maintain testosterone levels.

Elevations of estrogen levels are not uncommon while trying to replace testosterone using the above medications, and also happens in men who are overweight, so following estrogen levels is important when placing men on hormone replacement therapy.

There are also natural ways to increase testosterone. Cardiovascular exercise in both younger and older men, as well as strength training, can increase levels of testosterone and free testosterone. It is essential that men exercise regularly, lifting weights or using other forms of strength training, to maintain hormone levels. Since some men are also deconditioned (as are the majority of MSIDS sufferers), starting an exercise regimen slowly and gently is fine, gradually increasing the level of difficulty.

Getting proper sleep is also crucial to maintaining proper testosterone levels. Sleep reduction drastically reduces the levels in healthy young men, according to a study published 2011 in the *Journal of the American Medical Association*. The effects of sleep loss on testosterone became apparent after only one week without adequate sleep. Researchers found that getting only five hours of sleep per night decreased testosterone levels by 10 percent to 15 percent. That is a big drop, and unfortunately, the majority of my Lyme patients do not sleep well. Their significant insomnia may raise cytokine levels (such as IL-6) and increase fatigue and cognitive difficulties, as well as affect the HPA axis, decreasing hormone production. We will discuss this issue further in Chapter 13, which is on sleep disorders and Lyme disease.

Certain nutraceuticals, such as vitamin D, mung bean extract, zinc, high-protein diets, soy, and fish oils will also have a positive effect on increasing testosterone levels. This increase in testosterone is due either to increasing its internal production (using vitamin D), decreasing its conversion to estradiol (from zinc, DIM, increased soy intake), or decreasing binding to sex hormone–binding globulin (related to using mung bean extract, EPA, DHA, and a high-protein diet).

All hormone therapies need to be carefully monitored, especially for men taking testosterone. Side effects to watch for include:

- Testicular atrophy (due to decreased luteinizing hormone production)
- Benign prostatic hypertrophy (BPH) with lower urinary tract symptoms (LUTS)

- Gynecomastia (breast enlargement due to increased aromatization to estrogen)
- Increased edema in those with preexisting cardiac, hepatic, or renal disease
- Worsening of sleep apnea
- Polycythemia (an increase in red blood cells)

Follow-up testing should include CBCs, liver functions, PSAs, LH, total and free bioavailable testosterone levels, estradiol levels, SHBG, dihydrotestosterone, androstenedione, and DHEA-S levels after the first month of treatment. These tests should be repeated every three months afterward for several cycles, until the target goals are reached, or more frequently, if any abnormalities are found. Then, testing CBCs, liver functions, and hormone levels every four to six months are usually adequate, while also checking PSAs twice a year, with intermittent prostate exams.

John Was Too Young to Have Low T

John was just twenty-four when he came in for a medical evaluation. His past medical history was significant for labile hypertension, and his review of systems was positive for moderate fatigue, decreased libido, a forty-pound weight gain over an eight-month period, sweats, joint pain in the knees, tingling and numbness of the extremities, significant memory and concentration problems, and chronic anxiety. After performing a history and physical examination and sending off blood tests, we diagnosed him with: Lyme disease, with a CDC-positive IgM Western blot; babesiosis, with a positive titer to *Babesia microti*; adrenal dysfunction, with high cortisol levels on a DHEA/cortisol adrenal test; and elevated levels of heavy metals, including very high levels of lead, with some evidence of cadmium. He also had low levels of immunoglobulins, consistent with an immunodeficiency syndrome, and he told me that throughout his childhood, he frequently had infections. His testosterone level was 300 (very low for a twenty-four-year-old), his free testosterone level was low, and he also had low leuteinizing hormone levels. Normally the leuteinizing hormone level from the pituitary gland should be much higher with a low level of testosterone, and this was consistent with an HPA axis abnormality caused by Lyme disease.

I treated John with a rotation of antibiotics for his Lyme disease and antiparasitic drugs for his babesiosis. He had his heavy metals chelated, was given adrenal support, including phosphatidylserine at bedtime to help control the high cortisol levels that were interfering with his sleep, and referred him for IVIG therapy for his immunodeficiency. Even though we had the Lyme symptoms under control, we now had to treat his low T. I first prescribed Clomid to try and boost his testosterone production naturally, since his leuteinizing hormone levels were low (Clomid and B-hCG both increase leuteinizing hormone production). I opted not to give him testosterone shots or a cream, as he was young, and this could negatively impact his sperm production. John was engaged and wanted to have a family later on in life.

A month later his repeat testosterone level was over 1,000 ng/dl, and although he felt somewhat better, he told me that he was concerned, because his aggressiveness had increased. We stopped the medication, and his mood became calmer, but his testosterone level dropped all the way back to 202 off the Clomid, so we tried β-hCG shots instead. His testosterone level the following month increased to 1,013 ng/dl. There was no aggressiveness, and he felt better. His energy increased, and his mood was a lot more even. His estradiol level, however, was slightly elevated, implying increased testosterone to estradiol conversion (he also had metabolic syndrome, with significant weight gain and abdominal obesity, increasing estrone synthesis), so I prescribed zinc with DIM (di-indol methane). His follow-up estrogen levels were within normal range.

Over the next four months we decreased the frequency of his testosterone β-hCG injections to once every five days instead of twice a week, and eventually we tried him off the shots, to see if his testosterone levels would stay in the normal range. Unfortunately, his testosterone levels dropped back into the low range again, to 372 ng/dl. We therefore increased his exercise, had him follow a low-carb diet for his metabolic syndrome, gave him vitamin D and fish oils (which naturally help maintain testosterone), and restarted him on lower doses of Clomid than he had taken in the past. The Clomid had been effective but caused mood changes with normal dosing (25 mg, three times a week), so we decided to try much lower doses. With just 12.5 mg of Clomid twice a week we were able to maintain his testosterone levels in the mid-to-upper range of normal (751 ng/dl, normal range 348–1,197). On that dose, his moods remained stable, his energy level and libido increased, his weight decreased, and his metabolic syndrome improved. Lyme disease had affected his HPA axis, lowering his leuteinizing hormone levels and causing premature andropause. However, antibiotics alone would never treat testosterone deficiency. Getting John to a sustainable level of testosterone, at which he was feeling well all the time, required a delicate balancing of medications. This is why it is so important to routinely check men with Lyme disease for low T, even at a young age, especially when it would not normally be suspected. We have seen many cases like John's over the years, in which hormone replacement therapy helped with a range of resistant symptoms.

WOMEN AND HORMONES

Women also are affected by a lowering of DHEA, cortisol, and testosterone, but it is of course estrogens and progesterone that play the major roles in maintaining a woman's health. It is easier to see the effects of hormones in women, as Lyme symptoms are frequently affected during the fluctuations in estrogen and progesterone that take place during the menstrual cycle. Many women report that right before, during, or after their menses (when estrogen and progesterone levels drop off), their Lyme symptoms flare up and get much worse, and subsequently improve as they move into the first part of their cycle. The menstrual cycle and hormonal changes clearly affects their underlying Lyme symptoms.

There are three major estrogens—E1, E2, and E3—present in women, and the ratios change as they get older. In younger women, the predominant estrogen is estradiol (E2), but that changes to estrone (E1), which is not as biologically active, during menopause. E1 converts to both estradiol and estriol (E3) in the body. Estradiol (E2) is the most biologically active estrogen, and it is produced in the ovaries and in the peripheral tissues (fat) by the enzyme aromatase, which converts testosterone into estrone. Estriol (E3) is the weakest of the estrogens, but estrogen receptors are more sensitive to E3 than to estrone (E1) or estradiol (E2). There are many E3 receptors in the vaginal mucosa, and E3 vaginal suppositories may therefore be useful to help restore and support the vaginal tissue during menopause.

Natural estrogens stimulate the growth of breast and endometrial tissue and sex characteristics, encourage the body to store fat, produce the brain chemical serotonin, stimulate the receptors for the neurotransmitter GABA in the brain, aid in glucose transport across the blood-brain barrier, sensitize neurons to nerve growth factor, and decrease thyroid function by increasing thyroid-binding globulin (TBG).

There are other estrogens that we are exposed to that are not as beneficial. These include chemical xenoestrogens (foreign-based estrogens), such as PCBs, dioxins, plastics, pesticides, heavy metals, and bisphenol A. These xenoestrogens are artificially produced, and due to their chemical structure, may act like estrogen in the human body. They have been associated with various forms of cancer, in the breast, ovaries, uterus, prostate, lung, thyroid, and colon. These chemicals may also explain why in some countries the age of puberty is getting lower.

Progesterone, like estrogen, is also produced in the ovaries, and it is especially abundant during the second half of the menstrual cycle. Small amounts are also produced in the adrenal glands. Their positive effects are to balance out the stimulatory/growth effects of estrogens and help differentiate tissue, reduce cholesterol, inhibit spasm in the coronary arteries, promote glucose utilization, promote sleep by affecting GABA receptors, improve mood by acting like an antidepressant, and act as a diuretic. Progesterone also enhances thyroid hormone activity by increasing the conversion of T4 to T3 and decreasing thyroid-binding globulin, which is the opposite effect of estrogens, which increases TBG. Like sex hormone–binding globulin (SHBG), thyroid-binding globulin binds thyroid hormones and prevents free hormone levels in the blood from increasing. Estrogens and progesterone are therefore on the opposite sides of the seesaw: one without the other creates an imbalance.

Women who suffer with MSIDS often have an estrogen dominance or estrogen deficiency with or without early menopause. Estrogen dominance refers to an excess of estrogen with insufficient levels of progesterone, causing a poor estrogen/progesterone balance. Signs and symptoms of estrogen dominance include irregular and/or heavy menses, increased ovarian cysts, fibrocystic breasts with breast tenderness, uterine fibroids, weight gain, bloating, irritability, anxiety with mood swings and hypersensitivity. It is also associated with an increased risk of blood clots, gallstones, breast cancer, and metabolic syndrome with high triglycerides. Causes include a poor diet, stress, adrenal fatigue, luteal-phase deficiency with lack of ovulation, erratic cycles, and, in postmenopause, a decline in estrogen production by as much as 60 percent, with levels of progesterone dropping to nearly zero and causing the imbalance of estrogen to progesterone.

Iodine deficiency and xenoestrogens will also contribute to estrogen dominance. Lack of adequate levels of iodine, apart from affecting thyroid function, result in increased estrogen receptor activity in the breast. As discussed in Melissa's case, we have found that replacing iodine helps to reverse fibrocystic breast disease in women who are estrogen dominant.

Estrogen dominance is now common in many women because of the load of xenoestrogens that regularly enter the body from industrial pollution. Unless we make a conscious effort to avoid plastics, eat organic foods, and avoid pesticides, we are exposed to a regular diet of estrogen-containing compounds every day. This would explain the significant lowering of men's sperm counts over the last fifty years. Detoxification of xenoestrogens can be accomplished through the regular use of far-infrared saunas (FIR). Eating cruciferous vegetables, such as broccoli, cauliflower, brussel sprouts, kale, and garlic, with the use of broccoli-related compounds such as DIM and sulforaphane (broccoli sprouts) can also help to transform unhealthy estrogens into healthy estrogens in the body. It can also be beneficial in trying to reduce the risk of breast cancer and prostate cancer. In addition, they support the phase I and phase II detoxification enzymes necessary to remove these foreign-based chemicals.

Many women in perimenopause and menopause complain of symptoms of estrogen/progesterone imbalance, such as fatigue, low libido, hot flashes and sweats, and memory and concentration problems, with brain fog. These symptoms of hormonal deficiency also overlap those symptoms of Lyme disease with babesiosis, and they should be differentiated with proper blood testing. Apart from tick-borne testing, we will check FSH, LH, estradiol, progesterone, testosterone, and DHEA levels in women complaining of these symptoms. It is also advisable to check a CBC, a CMP, salivary hormone levels, serum iodine levels, 25 (OH) vitamin D levels, thyroid functions, HbA1c, and a lipid panel in appropriate patients to evaluate them for associated hormonal dysfunction, metabolic syndrome, and increased cardiovascular risk. Since Lyme disease can affect the HPA axis in women just as it does in men, younger women should also be evaluated for hormonal imbalances if presenting with low libido (which may be due to testosterone deficiency), symptoms of estrogen deficiency, such as unusual sweats, fatigue, or brain fog, or symptoms of estrogen dominance.

PMS can also be due to estrogen dominance, and the symptoms of fatigue, headaches, joint pain, depression, and irritability (with bloating and breast tenderness) can also overlap with symptoms of unresolved Lyme disease. Again, it is necessary to check a full hormone panel for these women, because of the effects of Lyme disease on the HPA axis, which can cause an imbalance in the sex hormones. Overlapping factors can include adrenal fatigue and mineral deficiencies. Diet and life-style changes, with progesterone supplementation, can sometimes help to balance the effects of the excess estrogen in PMS, and occasionally SSRIs like Prozac are necessary to help patients with severe mood disorders and associated depression.

Hormone replacement therapy (HRT) needs to be considered for some women who suffer from severe symptoms of estrogen deficiency, progesterone deficiency, and/or testosterone deficiency. Women who experience vaginal dryness and atrophy can be treated with estriol cream, an estriol suppository, or vaginal DHEA. If a woman complains of severe fatigue, unrelenting night and day sweats, worsening brain fog, mood swings, and evidence of osteoporosis, which are symptoms of severe hormone deficiencies, then she should be treated more aggressively. Various treatment options exist, but many integrative practitioners use compounded Biest or transdermal patches, such as Climara or Vivelle-Dot. Oral estradiol is also available but is not used as commonly. Since these treatments have both benefits and risks, they should be discussed with your healthcare practitioner.

DHEA supplementation can also be considered when levels are low. Since approximately 50 percent of DHEA converts into testosterone, this is another way to boost hormone levels. It is important to follow the levels of DHEA, estrogen, and testosterone in these patients, since it converts differently in individuals, and this may significantly elevate levels of estrogens in overweight women. Both blood and salivary levels may be used. Finally, progesterone at bedtime, in either a cream or orally, may help women who have severe insomnia as part of their clinical picture of Lyme disease and MSIDS. Progesterone stimulates GABA receptors in the brain and helps to put these women to sleep.

Both men and women often feel much better with the treatment of hormonal deficiencies, and hormone imbalances are frequently found in the patient with persistent Lyme disease. It is therefore important to use the MSIDS diagnostic map with appropriate testing to rule out endocrine abnormalities as one of the underlying causes of the patient's symptoms. You should never assume that symptoms of "normal aging" cannot be treated, as hormone deficiencies and hormonal imbalances are some of the most commonly overlooked causes for the failure of antibiotics in MSIDS.

TWELVE

Lyme and the Brain

yme disease frequently affects the central nervous system (CNS), as *Borrelia* travel from the site of the initial infection into the bloodstream, past the blood-brain barrier and into the brain and surrounding tissues. This causes inflammation in the various sites of infection. When this happens we refer to the associated symptoms as neurological Lyme disease.

Neurological symptoms of Lyme disease include memory and concentration problems, difficulties with processing new information, word-finding problems, mood disorders (such as depression), anxiety, as well as a host of psychiatric manifestations, including the potential for mental health disorders such as obsessive-compulsive disorder (OCD) and even schizophrenia. It can also include neurodegenerative problems, when *Borrelia* affects various nerves in the body. The central nervous system and peripheral nervous systems are preferred sites for *Borrelia* to establish an infection, and Lyme disease can cause both subtle and severe neurological complications. For example, Adam, who was featured in the last chapter, had both severe neuropsychiatric symptoms from the Lyme disease that invaded his central nervous system, as well as autonomic neuropathy, which caused fatigue, dizziness, constipation, and urinary difficulties.

The list of neurological Lyme symptoms includes:

- Autonomic nervous system disorders (such as POTS)
- Bell's palsy or pain disorders affecting the face
- Changes in hearing
- Changes in vision
- Dizziness and balance problems
- Headaches and migraines
- Insomnia
- Light and sound sensitivity
- Memory and concentration problems
- Mood disorders
- Neurodegenerative disorders (with associated motor neuron diseases, such as ALS)
- Psychiatric disorders
- Seizures

The brain is attached to the body through the spinal cord. It floats in a cushion of cerebral spinal fluid, which is encased in the meninges, a sac that encloses the brain and the spinal cord. When the sac surrounding the brain is affected, it causes meningitis-type symptoms to appear, and patients may complain of a stiff neck, a headache, and light and sound sensitivity. When *Borrelia* invades the brain tissue, it can cause encephalitis, which manifests as memory and concentration problems, a broad range of psychiatric symptoms, and in rare cases, levels of decreased consciousness. When it affects the cranial nerves it can cause abnormalities in the function of each of these nerves, resulting in optic neuritis (loss of vision), vestibulitis and hearing loss (due to effects on the eighth cranial nerve, which controls balance and hearing), and Bell's palsy (when the seventh cranial nerve controlling facial muscles is affected).

The spinal cord connects to the rest of the body through the peripheral nervous system. These nerves begin at the spinal cord and end in your extremities: arms and legs, fingers and toes. Affected peripheral nerves lead to symptoms of a radiculitis (inflammation in the nerve root coming out of the spinal column) and/or peripheral neuropathy, which causes symptoms such as tingling, numbness, burning, and hypersensitivity of the skin. There are four principal patterns of peripheral neuropathy that we see when Lyme disease invades the brain and peripheral nervous system:

- Mononeuropathy: A single nerve is affected.
- Mononeuritis multiplex: Multiple nerves are affected in varied parts of the body, asymmetrically (i.e., left arm and right leg). This leads to a loss of sensory and motor function in the individual nerves.
- Polyneuropathy: Many nerve cells in the body are affected, often in a symmetrical fashion (i.e., both hands and/or feet). It can affect the axons (distal axonopathy), the myelin sheath surrounding the nerves (which help conduct electrical impulses for proper nerve function), or the cell body of the neuron, and therefore the sensory nerves (sensory neuropathy) or motor neurons that control voluntary muscle activities, such as walking, speaking, swallowing, and breathing. In severe cases, this type of neuropathy causes motor neuron diseases (MND) such as progressive bulbar palsy (PBP), in which patients have difficulty with speech and swallowing, primary lateral sclerosis (PLS), in which only the upper motor neurons are affected, causing balance problems and spasticity, with associated speech and swallowing difficulties, and Amyotrophic Lateral Sclerosis (ALS, or Lou Gehrig's disease), which is caused by the degeneration of both the upper and lower motor neurons. This is the most severe of the motor neuron diseases and often leads to severe disability and death. While we can't say that Lyme is the sole cause of these motor neuron diseases, this severe type of neuropathy is occasionally seen in the Lyme-MSIDS patient.
- Autonomic neuropathy: a form of polyneuropathy that affects the involuntary nerves of the autonomic nervous system. This affects the functioning of internal organs, such as the digestive tract (causing constipation), bladder muscles (causing difficulties with urinating, such as incontinence or urinary retention), and the cardiovascular system (causing problems with blood pressure control and heart rate). One form of autonomic nervous system (ANS) dysfunction is postural orthostatic tachycardia syndrome (POTS), in which low blood pressure occurs when standing (postural orthostasis) with compensatory high heart rates (tachycardia),

often causing resistant fatigue, dizziness, anxiety, and cognitive problems. This will be further discussed in detail in Chapter 14.

NEUROPSYCHIATRIC COMPLAINTS

Apart from physical symptoms, many of my Lyme disease patients complain of mood disorders, especially severe anxiety, depression, and posttraumatic stress disorder. Typically, their previous physicians have told these patients that these feelings and emotions are psychiatric in nature and unrelated to their physical health, since their physicians were unable to find a cause for their illness. This pronouncement is often devastating for the patient to hear. And truthfully, I find it to be equally upsetting, because I've found that treating their Lyme disease and associated coinfections often improves their psychiatric symptoms.

As we've discussed, Lyme disease is a multiple systemic disorder, and it can therefore affect any part of the body, including the brain. Lyme disease can mimic every psychiatric symptom and can cause numerous psychiatric and neurological presentations. In fact, it is often underdiagnosed in the psychiatric community. Lyme disease has been discussed in the psychiatric literature as being "the great imitator" just as it is in other medical specialties. Psychiatric case reports have linked Lyme disease to paranoia, thought disorders, delusions with psychosis, schizophrenia, with or without visual, auditory, or olfactory hallucinations, depression, panic attacks and anxiety, obsessive-compulsive disorder, anorexia, mood lability, with violent outbursts, mania, personality changes, catatonia, and dementia. Other psychiatric disorders in adults due to Lyme disease include atypical bipolar disorder, depersonalization/derealization, conversion disorders, somatization disorders, atypical psychoses, schizoaffective disorder, and intermittent explosive disorders. In children and adolescents, Lyme disease can also mimic specific or pervasive developmental delays, attention-deficit disorder (inattentive subtype), oppositional defiant disorder, mood disorders, obsessive-compulsive disorder (OCD), anorexia, Tourette's syndrome, and pseudopsychotic disorders.

A 2010 review of the medical literature by Dr. Brian Fallon, published in the journal *Neurobiology of Disease*, suggests that psychiatric problems can be a prominent feature of Lyme borreliosis. For example, in one

U.S. study, 33 percent of patients with Lyme disease were clinically depressed, and controlled studies show much more depression among patients with late Lyme disease than among normal controls. It is therefore incumbent on mental health professionals to always keep MSIDS in the back of their mind, since patients may well have it in the back of theirs.

Some physicians do their best to treat psychiatric manifestations by placing patients on a range of psychiatric medications and recommending a course of psychotherapy. However, by treating complaints without finding a common root cause, these physicians have overlooked the fact that psychiatric manifestations are often the result of a physical health problem. Microbes as well as toxins, free radical stress, and mitochondrial dysfunction can all impair mental health. For example, one young man came to see me with a history of schizophrenia, which started suddenly in his early twenties. His test came back positive for Lyme disease, and we were able to improve his psychiatric functioning and, by working with his psychiatrist, eliminate his antipsychotic drug (Risperdal) and replace it with the antibiotic doxycycline. When he stopped the antibiotic, his thought disorder and hallucinations returned.

With these severe types of psychiatric symptoms, Lyme disease treatment should be closely monitored and coordinated with a psychiatrist. Without understanding MSIDS and the map of chronic illness, it would be impossible to discover the multiple causes for psychiatric symptoms in a chronically sick individual, as they can occur in the following conditions:

- Autoimmune disorders (such as *Lupus cerebritis*)
- B_{12} and/or folic acid deficiency
- Carcinoma of the brain or pancreas
- Chronic inflammation resulting from infection with *Borrelia burgdorferi* and co-infections such as *Mycoplasma*
- Defects in mitochondrial function, which can cause disorders of the central nervous system, such as schizophrenia, bipolar disorder, and anxiety
- Endocrine abnormalities
- Endogenous toxins, such as quinolinic acid from *Borrelia*
- Environmental toxins, including mercury, lead, and aluminum

- Inadequate detoxification systems, which allow neurotoxins to accumulate in the brain (chloral hydrate, ammonia, quinolinic acid)
- Temporal lobe epilepsy
- Viral encephalopathies
- Wilson's disease with copper overload

If you are experiencing psychiatric disturbances along with the multisystemic signs of Lyme disease, then the odds are that the Lyme disease has or is also affecting your brain. The following features have helped to make or support a diagnosis of Lyme disease:

1. Atypical features of a psychiatric disorder (e.g., absence of typical early signs or symptoms, unusually acute onset without new traumas or life challenges, and an uncharacteristic constellation of symptoms)
2. Absence of a family history of psychiatric disorders
3. Presentation of a psychiatric disorder at an older or younger age than is typical (e.g., autistic behavior at age six, forgetfulness at age thirty-five, first manic episode at age forty-five)
4. Lack of expected response to psychotropic medication
5. Adverse response to previously well-tolerated psychotropic medication
6. Lack of expected correlation of symptoms to psychological triggers (e.g., mood lability without apparent cause)

Signs that a tick-borne infection could be the cause of a psychiatric disorder would include symptoms of meningitis, encephalitis, cranial neuritis, and radiculoneuropathy early in the illness. We also know that *Borrelia burgdorferi* can rapidly disseminate to the central nervous system, and antibiotics given early in the illness are not necessarily curative. The organism may then lie dormant and reemerge months or even years later, producing neuropsychiatric symptoms at any point in the life span, regardless of when the initial tick bite occurred. Patients may also be exposed to new tick bites, and sudden neurological deterioration or new psychiatric symptoms should be evaluated with repeat tick-borne titers and PCRs with culture as appropriate, understanding the limitations of the tests.

Cognitive issues can manifest as mild, moderate, or severe memory and concentration problems that can be mistaken for early Alzheimer's disease or other forms of dementia, especially if other illnesses have been ruled out, such as B_{12} deficiency, gluten sensitivity, or hypothyroidism. Patients with these deficits will frequently reverse numbers and letters and have word-finding problems, and occasionally be so confused that they get lost driving, unable to remember familiar streets and signs.

Other common complaints of patients with later stage Lyme include insomnia, which contributes to their already profound fatigue. This may be accompanied by light and sound sensitivity, headaches, with a stiff neck, dizziness, visual difficulties, with blurry vision, and an associated neuropathy or radiculopathy. Women may experience an exacerbation of psychiatric symptoms around their menstrual cycle (when the estrogen and progesterone levels drop, women often experience Jarisch-Herxheimer flares), and their mental health symptoms may be exacerbated while taking antibiotics for another infection (i.e., sinusitis, upper respiratory infection), which then subsequently improves.

We see a similar improvement in psychiatric symptoms in children who have been exposed to group A beta-hemolytic streptococcal infections who subsequently develop pediatric autoimmune neuropsychiatric disorders associated with streptococcal infections (PANDAS). These children develop obsessive-compulsive disorders and/or tic disorders after being exposed to a bacteria (beta hemolytic strep), and these symptoms improve when the streptococcus is treated, but the children often relapse when the antibiotics are stopped. Microbes, toxins, detoxification problems, and mitochondrial and endocrine disorders are just some of the physical causes of psychiatric symptoms. Combined with the enormous stress of being diagnosed with a long-term illness, and consequently losing your job, social status, and home, and being mistreated by a skeptical medical community, these physical and psychological stressors often result in significant anxiety and depression. Yet there is hope, for when we treat all of the underlying physical and emotional causes of the illness, patients often get better.

Determining the Medical Causes of Neuropsychiatric Illness

Failure to recognize a medical illness causing psychiatric symptoms is not uncommon in medicine. In one study, nearly 20 percent of psychiatric outpatients had a medical condition causing their symptoms, and these conditions had been missed by the referring physician in approximately one third of the cases. There are some scans and other tests that can be performed to help confirm that the brain has been affected. These include functional brain imaging, using MRI studies, SPECT scans, and PET scans, as well as performing a spinal tap and administering neuropsychiatric testing. Unfortunately these are not sensitive or specific enough to confirm a diagnosis of Lyme disease, or that Lyme has caused these problems. For example, MRI scans of the brain can reveal nonspecific white matter abnormalities that are commonly found in Lyme patients, although it is not specific enough for establishing a diagnosis or causation. Similarly, an abnormal SPECT scan result simply tells us that there are problems with the blood flow to parts of the brain, but these defects can result from a variety of causes, including vascular problems (vasculitis), metabolic problems, and cellular dysfunction due to the indirect effects of cytokines. We see an increase in brain cytokines in many inflammatory diseases, such as autoimmune, Alzheimer's, and neurological Lyme disease, so we cannot use the SPECT scan as a stand-alone test to make an accurate diagnosis.

The typical PET scan is more specific, and in the right clinical circumstance, it can be more useful, since it reflects changes in the brain's regional metabolism. PET scans are valuable to neuropsychologists as a tool to evaluate the effect of various drugs on cerebral metabolism. Lyme disease is known to cause changes in the brain's metabolic pathways, which can affect memory, concentration, and moods. This was demonstrated in the NIH clinical trial conducted by Dr. Brian Fallon at Columbia University, where Lyme disease patients with chronic encephalopathy were re-treated with antibiotics to see if their cognitive problems improved. PET scans did show an increased metabolism in the brain in the group treated with antibiotics, with associated improved physical symptoms of fatigue and pain, and improvements in physical functioning as well as cognition. Rocephin improved patients' physical and neuropsychiatric symptoms as compared to their matched controls, and this improvement was verified via PET scan.

In 2012 the FDA approved a new radiopharmaceutical agent to be used during PET scans to assist clinicians in differentiating the cognitive impairments caused by Lyme disease from other diseases such as

Alzheimer's. This drug, Florbetapir F18, is different than the one used in Dr. Fallon's study to evaluate the metabolic changes in the brain with Lyme disease. It binds to amyloid plaques in the brain, a specific finding commonly seen in Alzheimer's, and it helps determine the amount of amyloid present. A negative Florbetapir scan would help rule out AD, and would inform the clinician that he or she should intensify efforts to look for another cause of the cognitive decline. This test should be considered for patients with an undetermined cause for their neurocognitive impairment after an extensive workup has been performed.

Since MRIs, SPECT scans, and PET scans of the brain are not able to definitively determine if a patient has neurological Lyme disease, physicians will occasionally perform a spinal tap and look at markers in the spinal fluid to determine if *Borrelia burgdorferi* has invaded the CNS. Unfortunately, spinal taps also have their limitations. Although increased antibody production in the spinal fluid can be seen in early Lyme disease with a lymphocytic meningitis or encephalitis, late-stage neurological Lyme patients can have normal cerebrospinal fluid (CSF) antibody studies. For example, Dr. Coyle and Dr. Schutzer studied thirty-five patients with the specific Lyme antigen (Osp A) in their cerebrospinal fluid, which would be indicative of neurological Lyme disease. Of these patients studied, although the Lyme antigen was positive, 43 percent had no evidence of antibodies to Lyme in their CSF testing, and 47 percent had otherwise normal routine CSF analyses. Sixty percent of these patients were also seronegative for Lyme disease when tested with standard blood tests, implying that a patient can have Lyme disease despite a negative blood test and a negative spinal tap. The authors concluded that "neurologic infection by B. burgdorferi should not be excluded solely on the basis of normal routine CSF or negative CSF antibody analyses."

Dr. Alan Steere, a well-known researcher in Lyme disease, has also shown that local antibody production in the cerebrospinal fluid is an inconsistent finding in American patients with late neurologic manifestations of the disorder. Thirty-nine percent to 54 percent of the patients in his study with late neurologic Lyme were found to be antibody negative in the CSF; his results were published in the *New England Journal of Medicine*.

If these antibody tests in the spinal fluid are so unreliable, what about conducting a PCR study on the spinal fluid to demonstrate the existence of the Lyme disease spirochete by DNA analysis? In children with known Lyme meningitis, Lyme CSF-PCR had a sensitivity of only 5 percent and a specificity of 99 percent. This means that we will only be able to diagnose Lyme meningitis by PCR in five out of one hundred children who have contracted the disease. So we see there are obvious limitations to these tests. A positive test can make the diagnosis, but a negative test result cannot rule it out.

One test performed on the spinal fluid that may be useful in differentiating patients with neurological posttreatment Lyme disease (nPTLS) from patients with other illnesses, such as chronic fatigue syndrome (CFS), is to look at certain specific proteins in the spinal fluid. A recent study performed by Dr. Steven Schutzer and colleagues used a technique known as proteomics, which examines the entire complement of proteins in the cerebral spinal fluid. They found specific protein profiles in Lyme patients that varied from patients with CFS, supporting the hypothesis that these are two distinct disease processes. As we have shown, many of the cytokine profiles increasing inflammation in CFS, FM, Alzheimer's, and Lyme disease are similar, yet there are still distinct differences between these disease processes.

Since laboratory testing for tick-borne disorders is imperfect, and neuroimaging studies are nonspecific, the last commonly used test to help establish the diagnosis of neurological Lyme disease is neuropsychiatric testing. This is usually administered by a psychologist who has been trained in administering a specific battery of tests—including the Minnesota Multiphasic Personality Inventory (MMPI), Patient Health Questionnaire-9 (PHQ-9), Beck Depression Inventory, Mini-mental State Examination (MMSE), Alzheimer's Disease Assessment Scale–Cognitive Subscale (ADAS–Cog), and Severe Impairment Battery, for example—that determine the severity of mood and cognitive disorders present. Neuropsychiatric testing can help determine the extent of a patient's disability, as well as how much their underlying depression and anxiety is interfering with their cognitive processing. Fifty percent to 60 percent of patients with chronic neurological Lyme disease have objective evidence of impairment on neuropsychological tests. There are patterns seen in neurocognitive testing that are often found in patients suffering from Lyme disease. These include verbal fluency and word-finding problems, memory and concentration problems, dyslexia, with number and letter reversals, problems with executive functioning, with an inability to make decisions, and problems with perceptual motor functioning, with spatial disorientation. These objective cognitive deficits can be seen on neuropsychiatric testing, while other studies, such as an MRI of the brain, EEG, or cerebrospinal fluid results are completely normal. These patterns of neurocognitive deficits help the clinician to determine the likelihood that a patient's neurocognitive disorders are caused by Lyme disease, as opposed to depression, which has a different profile, especially when other disease processes have been ruled out.

Lyme Can Make Psychiatric Problems Worse

Lyme disease can exacerbate underlying psychiatric symptoms, no matter what the cause. The increase in neuropsychiatric symptoms seen with Lyme disease is due in part to lipoproteins on the outer surface of the organism causing ongoing proinflammatory cytokine production. These cytokines contribute to MSIDS patients' frequent complaints of fatigue, pain, depression, anxiety, and cognitive problems that tend to come and go in severity. Symptoms often remit and then relapse again when the lipoproteins that stimulate cytokine production change over time. Some appear on the surface of the organism (up-regulation) and others disappear from the surface of the organism (down-regulation), depending on environmental conditions, such as the temperature and pH of the host. Certain lipoproteins are also more inflammatory than others, contributing to an increase in the severity of symptoms. An increase in neuropsychiatric symptoms also takes place when a patient has contracted co-infections, such as babesiosis, where *Babesia* can exacerbate underlying Lyme disease symptoms, including depression.

Other co-infections also can influence psychiatric symptoms. Ehrlichiosis can cause central nervous system symptoms, as can viruses and intracellular infections with *Mycoplasma spp.* and *Chlamydia pneumonia*, which are frequently found in MSIDS patients. Often the patients with the worst neurological symptoms have Lyme disease, *Mycoplasma*, and/ or *Bartonella* simultaneously, with or without other co-infections. This is especially true in patients who present with severe neuropathy and encephalopathy. *Bartonella henselae*, the organism that causes cat scratch fever, exacerbates many of the neurological and neuropsychiatric symptoms we see with Lyme disease, and has been linked to anxiety disorders and depression, as well as various central nervous system abnormalities. These include: encephalomyelitis (involving inflammation in both the brain and spinal cord, leading to difficulties with cognition and motor function); transverse myelitis (inflammation and demyelination of the spinal cord, leading to difficulty walking); spastic paraparesis (stiffness and spasm in the lower extremities, affecting walking); seizures, with hemiparesis (weakness on one side of the body); cerebellar syndromes (primarily defined by symptoms of dizziness and poor balance); and movement disorders (which can cause a variety of symptoms, including spasms, twitching, and involuntary movements). Like Lyme disease and babesiosis, *Bartonella* can also be transmitted to the fetus. Therefore, resistant neuropsychiatric symptoms in children might be linked to maternal transmission of the organism, and it should be suspected if the patient is living in a Lyme-endemic area, or has cats at home.

Some patients with *Bartonella* have other severe neurologic manifestations with ophthalmologic involvement, i.e., inflammation of the eye manifesting as optic neuritis, episcleritis, conjunctivitis, uveitis, or iritis. *Bartonella* can also cause an oculoglandular syndrome with preauricular adenopathy and conjunctivitis, neuroretinitis, branch retinal artery occlusion, and vision loss. *Bartonella* should therefore be considered when patients present with particularly severe ophthalmological symptoms.

The profile of cognitive deficits, depression, headaches, ongoing muscle and joint pain, poor sleep, and persistent marked fatigue is also seen in chronic fatigue syndrome (CFS), also now known as myalgic encephalomyelitis, because it is affecting brain function and the musculoskeletal system. Even symptoms of light and sound sensitivity, with symptoms of ANS dysfunction, such as low blood pressure, tachycardia (rapid heart rate), and digestive disturbances have been reported with CFS. If we look at the symptom complex used to define CFS, we see that the symptoms overlap those seen in Lyme disease and associated co-infections, and it explains why Lyme disease is frequently misdiagnosed. Apart from the results of a spinal tap, one of the primary differences is that the symptoms of persistent Lyme disease tend to come and go, fluctuating with good and bad days, and the symptoms tend to migrate, improving or worsening with antibiotics.

Barbara's Anxiety Was Both Tick-Borne and Traumatic

Chronic stress markedly increases a patient's vulnerability to poor medical outcomes across a wide variety of mental and medical conditions. Most of my patients notice that when they are under increased stress (psychological/emotional, physical, contracting a new illness such as an upper respiratory tract infection or sinus infection), their underlying Lyme symptoms often come out of hiding, or significantly worsen. I see this in my office almost every day, but Barbara's story is particularly interesting to share.

Barbara was from Martha's Vineyard and had a past medical history significant for a seizure disorder, which started in her early twenties. She had seen multiple neurologists and was diagnosed with grand mal seizures with atypical features. She was tried on multiple antiseizure medications but they had either failed or had significant side effects, and she was still breaking through with intermittent seizures when she came to see me for the first time.

Barbara had been ill for the past twenty-two years. She had a sudden onset of flulike symptoms in the summer of 1996, followed by deep exhaustion, during which she was unable to get out of bed. This was accompanied by intermittent night sweats, severe joint and muscle pain, unremitting headaches, light and sound sensitivity, dizziness with episodes of vertigo, intermittent tingling and numbness of her extremities with burning pain, severe memory and concentration problems, chest pain and shortness of breath, palpitations, recalcitrant insomnia, and episodes of anxiety with panic attacks that would often wake her up at night. She had been to multiple physicians, including her general practitioner; two rheumatologists for her joint pain; three neurologists for her seizure disorder, headaches, and vertigo; a cardiologist for the chest pain and palpitations; and ultimately a psychiatrist, since all of the other physicians were unable to find the cause of her illness. The psychiatrist diagnosed her with an anxiety disorder and placed her on the antidepressant Paxil, as well as an antianxiety medication, Xanax, at a high dosage three times per day, along with Ambien at night to help her get to sleep. Yet even on this regimen, Barbara was not getting better.

Her social history was significant for having been married and divorced. She divorced her first husband after fifteen years of living in an abusive marriage, and she had since remarried and stated that she was happy in her present marriage of eighteen years. Barbara also had three children, one of whom had been diagnosed with Lyme disease (she lived in a very Lyme-endemic area). Her family history was significant, because many of her family members suffered from seizure disorders. There were no significant toxic exposures, and her only other complaint was regarding menstrual irregularities, with a worsening of her symptoms around her menstrual cycle. Her physical examination revealed a well-nourished, well-developed, thin, white female in no apparent distress. Her examination was within normal limits, except for some painful anterior and posterior cervical lymph nodes, mild swelling of the joints in the hands, and raised, red, warm nodular areas over her fingers, elbows, lower extremities, and back.

We sent off for laboratory tests that included a CBC, a CMP, an ESR, and a high-sensitivity CRP, hemoglobin A1c, mineral levels, food allergy panel, with antigliadin/TTG antibodies, an autoimmune panel with complement studies, antiganglioside antibodies, VEGF (vascular endothelial growth factor), hormone studies, including thyroid functions, sex hormones, and an IgF-1 (to test for growth hormone deficiency), a viral panel (EBV, CMV, HHV-6, and West Nile), and a tick-borne panel, which included an IgM and IgG Western blot and *Babesia* panel, which was sent to IGeneX, as well as local titers for *Ehrlichia/Anaplasma*, *Bartonella henselae*, *Mycoplasma*, *Chlamydia pneumonia*, Rocky Mountain spotted fever, Q fever, typhus, tularemia, and *Brucella*. She also went home with a DHEA/cortisol test to check her adrenal function, as well as a six-hour urine DMSA challenge to check the levels of her heavy metals. Finally, we asked her to see a dermatologist to evaluate the lesions on her hands and a neurologist to evaluate her seizure disorder, since she was still breaking through with intermittent seizures.

Barbara returned one month later. Her CBC showed a mild microcytic anemia due to iron deficiency, her zinc levels were low, her food allergy panel revealed multiple allergies, to dairy, wheat, and corn, she had a borderline antigliadin antibody with negative TTG antibodies, a low-positive antinuclear antibody (1:80 positive), positive exposure to Epstein-Barr virus, CMV, and HHV-6 (low positive), an elevated sedimentation rate of 28 with an elevated CRP at 5.6, consistent with ongoing inflammation, and she had a positive IgM Western blot, positive *Babesia microti* IFA and positive *Babesia* FISH test, and positive titers to *Bartonella henselae* and *Mycoplasma*. Her adrenal test showed borderline low levels of cortisol in the morning and at noon, with elevated levels at night, and her heavy metal test was positive for elevated levels of mercury, lead, arsenic, and cadmium. She was also seen by the dermatologist, who made a diagnosis of granuloma annulare, a benign condition of the skin. The neurologist sent her for a repeat EEG to evaluate her seizures, which returned negative, and tried her on phenobarbital to help control them, which was effective.

We sat down and discussed a comprehensive regimen to address all of the abnormalities that were found in her lab tests. She was started on Plaquenil, doxycycline, nystatin, and Malarone for the Lyme and babesiosis, iron and zinc supplements for her mineral deficiencies (away from the antibiotics), adrenal supplements, with phosphatidylserine at night for the adrenal dysfunction, which was interfering with her sleep, as well as a low-carbohydrate diet that also avoided her food allergens, with acidophilus and saccharomyces boulardii to prevent yeast and diarrhea. We also placed her on DMSA every third night for her heavy metals, with antioxidant and mineral replacement, and I discussed meditation and stress reduction techniques for her chronic anxiety.

Barbara was only getting about five hours per night of interrupted sleep. She kept waking up with nightmares and anxiety attacks. We therefore added Topamax at bedtime for the history of seizures and resistant headaches (Topamax is an antiseizure drug also used for migraine prophylaxis), as well as Trazodone for her sleep and anxiety, with the supplements valerian root and GABA-L-theanine to help calm her down. She was also instructed to use low doses of valerian root during the day to help with her anxiety, which she was still experiencing, even though she continued to take the Paxil and Xanax.

Barbara came back a month later. She had flared badly on the new regimen, with severe Jarisch-Herxheimer reactions. Her fatigue, joint pain, headaches, cognitive problems, and anxiety were much worse, and although her night sweats had improved, they were still present and interfering with her sleep. We discussed using oral glutathione with Alka Seltzer Gold for the flares, and rotated the regimen to a different Lyme and *Babesia* regimen, using Omnicef, Plaquenil, Zithromax, and Mepron with the herb artemisia. Unfortunately, the same scenario unfolded month after month. She remained chronically ill and was in bed most of the time, due to the severity of her fatigue. The joint pain was also intolerable, and she wasn't sleeping well with ongoing anxiety attacks. We tried rotating her through different regimens, including high-dose amoxicillin, Bicillin shots, and double intracellular regimens for the Lyme and *Bartonella*. She also was tried on various herbal regimens, including Samento, Banderol, Cumunda, and traditional Chinese herbs. She was anxious about IV medications and would not try them.

The only regimen that seemed to help significantly, though for a short period of time, was Levaquin, which addressed the Lyme and *Bartonella*, but even after feeling better on the medication, she would end up flaring again, with severe fatigue, intermittent seizures, and joint pain. We would have to stop the antibiotics temporarily to let the flare die down, but her symptoms would return shortly afterward. We therefore sent off for repeat tick-borne testing, including a *Bartonella* PCR and Lyme PCR, after she had completed over nine months of my antibiotic rotations. The *Bartonella* PCR ended up being positive in her blood. This was significant, because even though she had been taking antibiotics for nine months, the infection was still lingering in her body. *Bartonella* has been described in the medical literature as a cause of seizures. I also knew from my own studies that persistent *Bartonella* might explain her resistant symptoms. It looked like Barbara may have had a genetic predisposition to seizures, but the *Bartonella* was exacerbating this neurological condition.

I turned to Barbara and discussed our options. We decided to stop the antibiotics and try a different approach. I discussed using the Byron White protocol. There were herbs to address the Lyme, *Babesia*, and *Bartonella*, as well as herbs to help control the Herxheimer reactions. So we placed her on SyDetox to help with the flares, as well as A-L for the Lyme, A-Bab for the *Babesia*, and A-Bart for the *Bartonella*. I also discussed with her the necessity to see a specialized therapist who dealt with anxiety disorders. She had not been helped by classical psychotherapy and was denying that there was anything at this point that was making her anxious. She certainly wasn't happy about her present health situation, but we couldn't identify a cause for her anxiety disorder that was interfering with her treatment. So I referred her to a therapist who did deep emotional healing work, including eye movement desensitization and reprocessing therapy, known as EMDR. This type of therapy can be useful for those with a history of posttraumatic stress disorder, and I thought Barbara would benefit because of her previous marital abuse. I also asked her to read the book *The Journey* by Brandon Bays. A patient of mine had given it to me after she had an amazing healing experience using Bays's techniques. She agreed to do so, and we scheduled a follow-up visit six weeks later to evaluate the results of the herbs.

When Barbara came in, she looked like a new person. She was beaming, and she had a sense of wellness and calm that I had not experienced in our prior visits. When I asked her what had happened, she said that coming off the antibiotics and starting the Byron White protocol was definitely helpful. She was having a much better response to the herbs, without the Herxheimer reactions. The fatigue, joint pain, headaches, and sweats were much better. She was also sleeping through the night, and her anxiety was almost gone. When I asked her about the anxiety, she confided in me that she had seen the new therapist that I had suggested and undergone several sessions of EMDR. She also started doing the *Journey* technique and a significant event came up during her sessions with the EMDR and *Journey* work. While she was in a state of deep relaxation with her therapist, a prior memory emerged that she had completely blocked out. She had been describing to her therapist the recurring dreams that would wake her at night, in which a man was holding her down, bruising her arms. Every time that she tried to pull away, he pinned her down and told her that he would hurt her if she told anyone about the experience. While she was in a state of deep relaxation, she remembered the rest of the dream. She had been raped when she was twelve years old. When she tried to tell her family about the trauma, they didn't believe her, and subsequently she had completely blocked out the experience. She had been living with this trauma for the last thirty-four years, and she believed, as I do, that this traumatic event had never been dealt with properly, and therefore was preventing her from deeper healing. All the medications in the world would not allow Barbara to get better until she dealt with this event, which was why she was still breaking through with panic attacks, despite taking antidepressants and antianxiety medications, and why she was not responding to the Lyme and *Bartonella* prescriptions. Once she began the EMDR therapy, the majority of her symptoms began to clear. The emotional trauma was interfering with her ability to properly deal with her tick-borne infections, and the tick-borne infections were clearly exacerbating her anxiety. Once both of these issues were addressed, Barbara was able to finally improve with her treatment.

Treating Lyme and Psychiatric Symptoms

The primary modes of treatment for the Lyme patient that presents with neuropsychiatric illness involves a combination of antimicrobial therapies, psychotropic medications, herbal and vitamin therapies, and various forms of psychotherapy and stress reduction techniques, including yoga and meditation. Antimicrobial therapies do not differ from what has been previously discussed, but certain guidelines should be observed in the patient with severe CNS symptoms. IV Rocephin should be strongly considered in patients with severe neuropsychiatric manifestations from Lyme disease who have failed oral therapy. IV Clindamycin should be considered in patients with severe overlapping babesiosis who have failed oral *Babesia* regimens, and we have found that IV vancomycin is surprisingly effective in a small group of patients who have failed other treatment regimens. Some of these treatment-resistant patients require several months of IV and oral antibiotics, rotating the regimens, to achieve a significant clinical improvement.

Macrolides such as azithromycin or clarithromycin may be used alone or in combination with these drugs, but caution must be exercised in patients being treated with certain psychiatric medications, such as carbamazepine (Tegretol) or SSRIs, such as Celexa, Prozac, and Paxil. In the case of SSRIs, macrolides may increase the levels of the psychiatric drugs and subsequently increase the risk of mania, delirium, and serotonin syndrome (a potentially life-threatening drug reaction affecting the autonomic nervous system), so SSRIs, which have the least effect on the cytochrome P450 3a/4 enzymes, would be the safest choices, such as Zoloft. Rifampin, a useful drug for intracellular infections such as *Bartonella*, can change the drug metabolism in the body of many medications, so caution needs to be taken with its use. Quinolones (Cipro, Levaquin, Avelox, and Factive) can also be very helpful in cases of resistant neurological Lyme disease with associated bartonellosis, but again, attention needs to be paid to possible drug interactions and side effects (including tendon problems with fluoroquinolone toxicity). Patients with encephalopathy, neuropathy, and severe musculoskeletal pain who have failed other regimens may respond to a quinolone, and the higher the generation, usually the better the clinical effect.

Psychotropic medications may be needed if a mood disorder does not improve on antibiotics or professional therapy. Medications that are commonly found to be of benefit in our practice include herbs such as St. John's wort, and SSRIs, such as Lexapro, Celexa, Paxil, Prozac, and Zoloft. Paxil is particularly useful in treating severe anxiety disorders. Cymbalta may be a better choice if there is a weight problem with low libido associated with depression, since those are more common side effects of the other class of SSRIs. Cymbalta also has effects on associated fibromyalgia symptoms that include neuropathy, which makes it a very useful drug in the MSIDS patient who suffers simultaneously from those two symptoms.

Augmentation therapy with Wellbutrin, which stimulates dopamine receptors, may be useful in patients not adequately responding to an SSRI. It is also weight neutral, and can be helpful as an activating agent in the morning for patients with significant fatigue and ADHD (attention-deficit hyperactivity disorder). Activated folic acid with a medication such as Deplin can also help to augment the mood effects of other antidepressants. Deplin is essential for detoxification of certain hormones and heavy metals, as well as for improving neuronal cell health and regeneration. Some resistant patients, for whom traditional therapies have failed, will respond to nutritional approaches. S-adenosinemethionine (SAMe) is useful as a nutritional supplement, because it both decreases joint pain and increases mood.

Other treatments to be considered for severe and resistant neuropsychiatric symptoms include the use of oral and IV glutathione, which assists detoxification, LDN and other pharmaceuticals and nutraceuticals that decrease the production of cytokines or help eliminate neurotoxins from the body (bile acid sequestrants such as Questran or WelChol, supplements such as *Chlorella*, Pekana drainage remedies, lymphatic drainage). We occasionally see miraculous results using these treatments, especially when we use glutathione.

Glutathione may remove some other toxins that affect mood and brain function, although this line of thinking has not been researched directly. However, we do know that while *Borrelia* increases inflammation in the brain, microglial cells (immune cells of the central nervous system) are activated by free radicals and proinflammatory cytokines. These in turn release more proinflammatory cytokines (IL-1-β, IL-6, TNF-α), which leads to increasing fatigue and reduced physical activity, muscle pains (myalgias), joint pain (arthralgias), enhanced perception of pain, impaired learning, and depression. This inflammation, created by oxidative stress, damages our cell membranes, mitochondria, and nerve cells. It is therefore crucial that we have an adequate antioxidant reserve to protect the brain and nerves from this free radical stress (using supplements such as alpha-lipoic acid, which is water soluble and fat soluble and penetrates the brain well), shut down the production of these inflammatory cytokines, and open up the detoxification pathways to remove the toxins that may cause neuropsychiatric symptoms such as depression.

The vast majority of my patients are suffering from acute and chronic anxiety. Some handle it better than others, but I have seen many cases where anxiety levels are as high as those experiencing posttraumatic stress disorder. Some of it is due to simply dealing with their physical symptoms. Other times I notice that they are anxious to get better and are continually worrying about their health status, which in turn makes them more anxious. Lyme and co-infections actually exacerbate underlying anxiety issues. Finally, Jarisch-Herxheimer reactions are also known to cause anxiety, as well as the lack of sleep, which in turn increases anxiety. Whatever the reason, my patients often benefit from learning how to relax, and I typically prescribe stress reduction techniques such as a mindfulness-based meditation, Shamatha (calm-abiding meditation), deep breathing techniques, and/or yoga.

Drugs such as the benzodiazepines (Valium, Ativan, and Xanax), BuSpar, SSRIs such as Paxil, and Trazodone at bedtime can be helpful when relaxation techniques are insufficient. If the anxiety symptoms are mild, drugs may not be necessary, and certain herbs can be used instead. They also can be used in combination with pharmaceuticals, and are known to augment the efficacy of antianxiety medications. For example, valerian root is helpful for anxiety during the day, with associated insomnia at night. GABA and L-theanine, a green tea extract, can also be useful for anxiety and assisting with sleep. Inositol helps with obsessive-compulsive disorder symptoms in adults and children. Some patients will also respond to Bach flower remedies such as Rescue Remedy, or an individualized homeopathic remedy, such as Kali Phos, or Psystabil, which is a combination of different homeopathic remedies in varying dilutions.

Although antibiotics, psychotropic medications, meditation, and herbal treatments are often useful in patients with neuropsychiatric symptoms associated with Lyme disease, patients will occasionally need to see a therapist to help them deal with significant depression, anxiety, trauma, and PTSD. I have found that my patients with a history of trauma and abuse will have an exceedingly difficult time healing from Lyme disease. Severe trauma and abuse can affect the immune system. The mind and body do not function separately, and when patients have had trauma or been abused, or if they suffer a loss with unresolved grief, the unresolved conflict usually has a deleterious effect on their immune systems. Some people (often on an unconscious level) feel that they are somehow responsible for the event, and have often lost the will to be well, believing that they need to suffer. It is as if the guilt, shame, and grief that are experienced from their emotional trauma acts as a signal to the immune system to fail. These people require deep emotional healing and must be willing to gently confront their trauma and learn to transform it, by identifying their own capacity for coping and healing. Skilled psychotherapy and techniques of restructuring memories and painful emotional experiences through EMDR, the *Journey* technique (Brandon Bays), the emotional freedom technique (EFT), cognitive behavioral therapy (CBT), and body-centered therapies (i.e., Rosen Method Bodywork) can also be helpful in shifting frozen emotional memories that are stuck in the body, affecting our mood and immunity. Family systems therapy and couples work may also be necessary, as the stresses of chronic illness can take a toll on relationships. A compassionate and empathetic ear, one that is fully present to validate the patient's experience, is healing in itself, no matter what drugs, antibiotics, or herbs are used in the healing process.

NEURODEGENERATIVE DISORDERS: ALS AND LYME

Amyotrophic lateral sclerosis, or ALS, is a disease of the nerve cells in the brain and spinal cord that control voluntary muscle movement. ALS is also known as Lou Gehrig's disease, and it is the most common motor neuron disease. This is one of the most devastating illnesses, as it leads to progressive weakness and atrophy of the muscles of the extremities, leading to difficulty walking, speaking, swallowing (associated bulbar palsy), and, ultimately, death. As the illness progresses and the respiratory muscles are affected, there are also problems with breathing. Early physical examinations often reveal fasciculations (twitching) of the muscles of the extremities and tongue, with slurring of speech and difficulty walking and grasping objects: A common early sign is the loss of muscles in the thenar eminence, at the base of the thumb.

Approximately 2 percent of ALS cases are linked to genetic factors. A mutation in the superoxide dismutase enzyme (SOD 1) that helps control oxidative stress has been identified as one possible cause of familial ALS. Other factors may include systemic mycoplasmal infections and higher than normal levels of glutamate in the blood and spinal fluid, which might play a role in motor neuron degeneration. However, none of these factors has been shown to adequately explain the cause of the disease or its progression.

Of the twelve thousand patients I have treated in the last twenty-six years, I have seen approximately forty to fifty ALS patients. A combination of genetics, chronic infections, environmental toxins, inadequate detoxification pathways, and oxidative stress with free radical damage may all be implicated. Many of my ALS patients have told me of significant environmental exposures, especially to pesticides and volatile organic solvents. Furthermore, a 2006 study by the Centers for Disease Control and Prevention showed that over 116 different environmental toxins can be found in over 50 percent of Americans, including pesticides, heavy metals, and volatile organic solvents, and each one of these can affect the brain. Perhaps ALS patients are more sensitive to these environmental chemicals.

Lyme and associated co-infections also seem to be associated with neurodegenerative symptoms. *Mycoplasma fermentans*, the organism associated with Gulf War syndrome and found in ticks carrying Lyme disease, has also been implicated with several neurological diseases, such as MS and ALS. Garth Nicolson, PhD, chief scientific officer and research professor at the Institute for Molecular Medicine, has published extensively on this topic. *Mycoplasma* infection might increase demyelination in patients who have been exposed to Lyme disease and mercury, another cofactor known to cause demyelination. What's more, anecdotal evidence that I have seen firsthand strengthens my convictions. This was made clear to me after speaking with one of my colleagues, Dr. David Martz. He was diagnosed with ALS, and then discovered he had Lyme disease. He is still alive more than ten years after the diagnosis, having treated himself for Lyme disease with long-term IV antibiotics, even though he still has neurological symptoms, with some weakness of the lower extremities and balance problems. However, they have not progressed, and he is still able to function after being diagnosed years ago with what should have been a life-threatening illness. I am treating another physician with the same diagnosis and presentation who continues to show slow clinical improvement year after year. Yet if Lyme disease and co-infections were the sole cause of ALS, I would expect to see even more of these patients coming in with the disease.

It is possible that patients with a genetic predisposition to ALS are exposed to the same wide array of environmental toxins affecting all of us, and also contract Lyme disease and associated co-infections, which then exacerbate their original neuronal insults. As we know, Lyme disease and co-infections cause inflammation and free radical stress in the central nervous system, which certainly may exacerbate and quicken the neuronal cell death seen in this disease. A small percentage of ALS patients do respond positively to antimicrobial therapies combined with antioxidants, detoxification, and mitochondrial support, lending an endorsement to the theory that there may be a multiplicity of factors at work underlying the pathology of the illness.

It is clear that a lot more research needs to be done in this area. In the meantime, it seems prudent that we test ALS patients for multiple environmental toxins, check their detoxification pathways and environmental loads, look for oxidative stress driving inflammatory pathways, and determine if Lyme disease and co-infections, including *Mycoplasma*, *Bartonella*, and *Babesia*, are present.

Was Robert Suffering from Lyme or ALS?

Robert was thirty-five when he came to my medical office. Robert had been diagnosed with ALS two years earlier and already had symptoms consistent with some of the advanced stages of the disease. When I entered the exam room to meet with him, the first thing that I noticed was a good-looking, tall, lean man sitting on the exam table in a short-sleeve shirt in the middle of winter, and his wife sitting in the corner with a tight smile on her face and clenched hands. Robert's muscles were twitching all over, especially in his forearms, hands, and thenar eminence (the group of muscles on the palm of the hand at the base of the thumb). He had an almost certain death sentence hanging over his head, and they both knew it as I approached the examining table to shake his hand.

"Hi Robert, I'm Dr. Horowitz, nice to meet you."

He lifted his hand to meet mine, but barely had enough strength to grasp it. However, a large smile beamed on his face as his eyes met mine. "Hi, Dr. Horowitz," he said with great difficulty, his speech slurring. "It's a pleasure to meet you."

Now, one of the first things that I look for in patients who have been diagnosed with a life-threatening disease is how they are handling their illness. Are they depressed? Anxious? Upset? The remarkable thing about Robert was that he appeared genuinely happy. He had a smile that literally lit up the room. He seemed to radiate peace and joy despite having such a serious diagnosis. If I have a bad meal in a restaurant, I'm likely to be grouchy for the rest of the day. I was intrigued by his spirit and attitude.

"How can I help you?" I asked. "I understand you're here for a Lyme consultation."

Robert and his wife took turns describing his history and symptoms. He was living in Connecticut in a wooded area and shared that three years earlier he suddenly noticed that his fingers had started twitching. This was followed by a general weakness in his left hand, which then progressed slowly and moved to his right side. He finally saw a neurologist, who did an EMG and diagnosed him with ALS. He was given Rilutek, the only drug approved for ALS, but stopped taking it after a short time, as it was no help. Robert continued to progress with other systemic symptoms, and a year later he was referred to a doctor in New Jersey for an evaluation for tick-borne diseases. He was diagnosed with Lyme disease after his blood tests came back with a positive Western blot. He was also diagnosed with ehrlichiosis and babesiosis. His physician placed him on a rotation of antibiotics, including doxycycline, Ceftin, and Augmentin and rotations of intramuscular Bicillin shots and intramuscular Rocephin shots. He also took two courses of Mepron for his babesiosis and noticed that on this drug he felt the best he had in a while: His energy, speech, and walking improved. (Sound familiar?)

I asked Robert to walk. He shuffled without striking his heels to the ground but still had reasonably good strength in his lower extremities. He had brisk tendon reflexes in his arms and legs (hyperreflexia), and his sensory examination (light touch and vibration sense) was intact. His speech was slurred but intelligible. I then asked him what symptoms he still had after two full years of treatment. He replied, "Well, Dr. Horowitz, I still have night sweats and feel cold often. I get tired during the day, and I can't sleep because of the sweats and cramps in my muscles. I can't walk well, and often fall over." When I asked Robert why he kept falling over, he said, "I usually trip over my dog."

Now, I've heard a lot of reasons over the years why people may fall, but this was a new one. Dogs are said to be man's best friend. They usually aren't implicated in schemes to try and break their master's hip. So I asked the logical question, "Doesn't your dog move when he sees you coming?"

Robert replied, "He's old, blind, and partially deaf. I don't think he sees or hears me, and he often runs in front of me." So here was a man with a life-threatening illness who smiled at death and would rather risk a hip fracture than get rid of his family dog.

As I went through his history, the main clue that surfaced as to why he may have developed an ALS-type response to Lyme was his history of toxic environmental exposures. Robert had worked in a chemical factory for ten years and never worn a mask or other protective gear in an environment where he was frequently exposed to toxic paints and volatile organic solvents. Standard lab tests were negative, including a normal CBC, CMP, thyroid functions, vitamin levels for B_{12}, folic acid, methylmalonic acid, and homocysteine. His magnesium levels were also normal, which were checked because they can be associated with muscle spasms. We repeated his Western blot as well as his tick-borne co-infection panel with a *Babesia* IFA and a FISH test, a *Bartonella* IFA and PCR, a *Mycoplasma* IFA, a *Chlamydia* IFA, Rocky Mountain spotted fever titers, and viral titers. We also gave him a six-hour urine DMSA challenge to check for heavy metals at home.

When I got the tests back I noticed other clues that would explain his medical situation. His tests returned with an elevated lead level of 11 (normal is less than 5) and an elevated mercury level of 3.1 (normal is less than 3). These levels were high enough to add a few more free radicals to an already damaged and strained central nervous system. His Western blot was still positive, and so was his *Babesia* FISH test. He had already done one and a half months of Mepron, and his *Babesia* was still active, consistent with the ongoing sweats that kept him up at night. His CPK (creatine phosphokinase) levels also were slightly elevated, at 388 (normal less than 320). CPK is a muscle enzyme that can come from the brain, muscle, or heart. It was probably elevated because of the muscle loss associated with ALS, or because he kept tripping over his dog. I started getting suspicious about the dog story and could see that he had a good sense of humor, so when I received the lab report I threw out a line to see what I would catch. If I didn't engage in some type of humor, I might actually cry.

"How do you know when you fall that it isn't your wife that is pushing you from behind?" I asked. Robert had a sly grin on his face. "Good point, Dr. Horowitz. I think you're right. I'll have to watch her more carefully." And it was from that moment on that Robert and I bonded. Wife- and dog-tripping jokes would clearly be part of our medical shtick.

We then discussed putting in an IV line and starting him on IV Rocephin. I explained how Rocephin was not only beneficial for neurological Lyme disease, but had been found to up-regulate the production of the glutamate transporter, leading to less glutamate in the intersynaptic space (the space between neurons). This was important, because glutamate is an excitatory amino acid that could damage neurons. Robert agreed to the Rocephin, and we also tried him on IV glutathione before he left the office. With a neurodegenerative disease, I didn't want any free radicals causing oxidative stress to his neurons, and up to 70 percent of Lyme sufferers have reported benefits with glutathione, with improved fatigue, headaches, joint and muscle pain, and cognitive functioning.

On Robert's next visit we placed him on a regimen of: IV Rocephin as his cell wall drug against *Borrelia*, which would also help decrease glutamate levels; Plaquenil for the cystic forms of *Borrelia* (and also to alkalize the intracellular compartment); Minocin and Zithromax, for the intracellular location of *Borrelia*; and IV glutathione three times per week. Since the medical literature reports an association of *Mycoplasma fermentans* in neurodegenerative disorders such as ALS, and we had patients fail to improve while using single intracellular drugs for *Mycoplasma fermentans* with positive PCRs up to one year posttreatment, we opted to use two intracellular drugs simultaneously. This regimen would also help cover the frequent intracellular co-infections often seen in our Lyme patients, including *Chlamydia* and *Bartonella*. *Bartonella* can also cause severe neurological manifestations in Lyme patients, including encephalopathy, radiculitis, and transverse myelitis, and we have seen positive PCRs for *Bartonella* after months of single intracellular drug treatment. We also added Mepron to treat the babesiosis.

Ten days into the new regimen, Robert returned to our medical office feeling much better. He especially noticed improvements after the IV glutathione and Rocephin. He had good and bad days, but the good days were outnumbering the bad ones. "So how are your basic symptoms?" I asked.

"Well, Dr. Horowitz, my muscle twitching has decreased all over, except in my hands. I feel more energetic, and my overall strength is better. But I'm still having night sweats."

The information was interesting, but what was more remarkable was the clarity of Robert's speech. He was no longer slurring words as badly as just one month earlier. I added magnesium sulfate to his IV bag for his muscle cramps and twitching, and gave him vitamin B_{12} injections with N-Acetylcysteine and alpha-lipoic acid to help open up his detoxification pathways. We also increased his IV glutathione, since I would be unable to use classical chelating agents such as EDTA or DMSA to pull out his heavy metals. Other ALS patients I had tried this on reported a worsening of their symptoms within one dose of those chelating agents. It was probably due to their inability to handle moving the heavy metal burden through their bodies with the associated increased free radical load. We also added a supplement of high-dose phosphatidylcholine to help support his nerve function and move neurotoxins out.

Robert's follow-up visits over the next few months were generally encouraging; he reported improvements in his energy and mental clarity. This latter symptom was especially better after receiving the IV glutathione. I added lithium carbonate to his IV treatment: I had come across a study from Rome in which patients on Rilutek for ALS had a much lower mortality rate when lithium was added to their regimen. These were patients with the most aggressive form of the disease, known as bulbar palsy, which is characterized by severe speech and swallowing deficits. The hypothesis was that lithium could accelerate the mechanism removing proteins and altered mitochondria and promote the growth of new mitochondria, helping neurological symptoms.

Despite these medication changes, however, he would relapse after several months on the same regimen. So we started to rotate his antibiotics each time he plateaued. First we added Septra double strength to try and make the Mepron more effective, since Septra helps with some cases of resistant babesiosis. I had presented an abstract at the 12th International Scientific Conference on Lyme Disease and Other Spirochetal and Tick-Borne Disorders on the role of Septra: I reported that I had found it to be particularly useful in some patients for whom standard therapies with Mepron or Malarone were failing. It is also a useful drug in patients with overlapping *Bartonella*. The Septra helped decrease his dizziness and twitching. It also definitely decreased his joint and muscle pain, increased his energy, and decreased the slurring of his speech. But the Septra's positive effect would wear off after a month or two, and we were forced to continuously rotate his intracellular drugs over the next two years. The Zithromax would be changed to Levaquin with Minocin. Then the Levaquin would be changed to rifampin, or a different intracellular drug, and the same scenario would unfold. It would help for one or two months, and then he would plateau and have a return of certain symptoms.

Four years after his initial ALS diagnosis, and a full year under my care, he had stabilized and improved in certain areas, especially in his musculoskeletal strength, balance, and speech, and he had demonstrated increased energy. He still was not completely well but had definitely improved. I then sent out for a new set of tests to see where we were. All laboratory results were fine. He had no gallbladder problems on the Rocephin, and his IV line was clean. We then added low-dose naltrexone (LDN) at bedtime. This was to try and help modulate his immune system and decrease his musculoskeletal complaints. There has been anecdotal evidence of LDN helping patients with neurological syndromes. I had found that many of my patients who complained of frequent Jarisch-Herxheimer flares and musculoskeletal pain started to improve with LDN when other therapies had been ineffective. L-theanine, a green tea extract that has been shown to decrease glutamate naturally in the central nervous system, was also added to his regimen, since lowering glutamate and up-regulating its transport appears important in patients with ALS.

ALS patients typically live for only a few short years once bulbar symptoms appear. I had already lost several ALS patients despite my best efforts. Robert was one of the few whom I was able to stabilize with IV medication by hitting Lyme, decreasing glutamate, detoxing with IV glutathione, and hitting *Mycoplasma*, *Babesia*, and other possible co-infections. But how long could I realistically prolong his life with this treatment?

Many health insurance companies only allow one month of IV Rocephin, since they follow the practice guidelines of the Infectious Diseases Society of America (IDSA). This guideline insists that Lyme disease can be "cured" after thirty days, and therefore doesn't require long-term therapy. I had a long discussion on the telephone with the medical director of Robert's insurance company: I thought Robert would benefit from a longer course of IV Rocephin, since it would address both the Lyme and the ALS. Afterward I sent him scientific articles on the use of Rocephin to up-regulate the glutamate transporter in ALS patients, with evidence that it helps to stabilize their neurological symptoms. The compassionate heart of this particular medical director allowed Robert to continue IV Rocephin for an additional two years, as I made a case that we had nothing else to offer him, and his prognosis was, indeed, grim without it. Besides ongoing clinical trials with IV Rocephin for ALS, I know of at least two other individuals who have been diagnosed with Lyme disease and ALS symptoms, like Robert, and are still alive years later, after receiving long-term therapy with IV Rocephin.

Robert is still alive, and his neurological functioning has improved, even though he still has an ALS diagnosis. By all accounts he should have passed away years ago. Studies have shown that more than 90 percent of ALS patients will not be as lucky as Robert. Yet in a clinical study of ALS patients treated by Dr. David Martz in his Colorado clinic, approximately 10 percent of the participants in his study either stabilized their illness or improved their symptoms by using long-term antibiotic therapy, including IV Rocephin.

Even while treating Robert, I still had many questions left unanswered. Was it the Rocephin up-regulating glutamate transporters that led to his improvements? Can Rocephin stabilize ALS and neurological Lyme disease? Did the glutathione and phosphatidylcholine play an additional role by helping remove neurotoxins and protecting against further free radical damage of the nerve cells? Will new innovative therapies, such as tamoxifen (a neuroprotectant) and ketogenic diets (high fat, very low carbohydrate diets), have an effect on altering the clinical course and progression of ALS? Will stem cell therapy be helpful in stopping and reversing some neuronal degeneration? These are some of the next scientific areas of research that need to be explored.

What is clear to me is that some patients with ALS who have Lyme with co-infections as well as heavy metals and environmental toxins can improve with antibiotics, especially when Lyme, *Babesia*, and *Mycoplasma* are present. Some of them also respond to IV glutathione, which is a strong antioxidant and detoxifier of environmental chemicals. I've also learned that by following the MSIDS model and identifying all possible causes of symptoms, I can provide some answers for patients with neuropsychiatric and neurodegenerative disorders for whom classical treatment regimens have failed.

THIRTEEN

Lyme and Sleep Disorders

hose who suffer from Lyme disease with MSIDS do not sleep well. Severe insomnia is by far one of the most common complaints I hear during patients' office visits. My patients either have problems falling asleep or complain of frequent awakenings during the night. They also complain of hypersomnolence: sleeping for twelve to fourteen hours. Yet despite sleeping for long periods of time, they often report that they are still extremely fatigued. Worst of all, they often experience these problems despite using classical sleep remedies like over-the-counter Benadryl, or prescription Ambien, or Lunesta. I hear over and over that these sleep aids just don't work for many of my patients: The medication doesn't put them to sleep as it is supposed to, and/or it can take several hours to work, or they aren't able to stay asleep. Resistant insomnia is one of the hallmarks of MSIDS in the context of an associated multisystemic illness.

Sleep deprivation is one of the primary reasons that you may remain chronically ill. It is difficult to improve the overall functioning of those with MSIDS without adequately addressing this essential piece of the medical puzzle. Getting to the source of a sleep disorder is crucial, whether it is a direct effect of *Borrelia burgdorferi* and co-infections or due to overlapping medical problems, such as associated sleep apnea, restless leg syndrome, mood disorders, medications, diet, nocturia (getting up to urinate), or hormonal dysregulation.

Poor sleep is particularly problematic, because impaired sleep directly correlates with impaired immune function. As we've discussed, a healthy immune system is our body's basic line of defense; it helps keep chronic bacterial, viral, parasitic, and yeast infections under control. Most MSIDS patients notice that when they are under increased stress for any reason (psychological/emotional or physical triggers, as is the case when they contract an upper respiratory illness, for example) their Lyme symptoms often worsen significantly. A poorly functioning immune system that is already affected by multiple infections or diseases cannot easily handle new illness or stress, and it worsens their symptoms.

We have already discussed the effects of stress on the adrenal gland, and how it can impair immunity. We also know that *Borrelia* alone can suppress the immune system: The longer lymphocytes remain in contact with *Borrelia* in the laboratory setting, the stronger their effect on immune suppression. I often find that the longer my patients have Lyme disease, especially if it has been undiagnosed or untreated, the more difficult it is to for them to get better. Similarly, parasites such as *Babesia* may further suppress immune functioning, and the medical literature doesn't adequately reflect the simultaneous effects of multiple co-infections on an individual's chronic illness.

Unfortunately, when you add poor sleep on top of the burden of infections and hormonal imbalances such as adrenal fatigue, the resulting immune dysfunction is worsened, and all existing symptoms can significantly increase. Insomnia can cause fatigue, daytime sleepiness, increased pain perception, as well as irritability and memory and concentration problems. These same symptoms occur both for those sleep-deprived "normal" healthy individuals and for those with unresolved Lyme disease. What's more, they mimic the disease states of fibromyalgia and chronic fatigue syndrome, making it exceedingly difficult to differentiate which symptoms are due to one particular disease and which are caused by the resulting sleep deprivation. This may be one of the reasons why so many Lyme sufferers are misdiagnosed with chronic fatigue syndrome and fibromyalgia.

We also know that elevations in inflammatory cytokines are seen both in Lyme-MSIDS and FM, as well as other rheumatologic disorders, such as rheumatoid arthritis. These elevated levels of cytokines cause an increase in pain. To add insult to injury, a lack of sleep can further increase the production of inflammatory cytokines, as well as increasing the perception of pain. Luckily, once my patients are able to sleep, they usually report less pain: One study of rheumatoid arthritis sufferers who used a sleep medication (a benzodiazepine) reported less joint pain, even though their illness was still active.

Aside from inflammation and immune disorders, there are a host of medical conditions associated with significant insomnia. These include:

- Acute viral illnesses and HIV
- Adrenal hormone imbalance, in which cortisol is high at night and low in the morning
- Chronic bacterial infections
- Chronic fatigue syndrome
- Chronic pain conditions
- Depression and anxiety
- Endocrine disorders, such as hypothyroidism and acromegaly
- Fibromyalgia
- GI reflux (from coughing, acid brash, or choking)
- Lyme-MSIDS
- Menopause (secondary to hormonal changes)
- Nocturia (having to get up several times per night to urinate)
- Non-Lyme-MSIDS
- Obstructive and restrictive lung diseases
- Renal disease
- Restless leg syndrome

Medications can also interfere with sleep. Over-the-counter stimulants such as Sudafed can be a problem, especially if it is taken as a twenty-four-hour slow-release preparation (also, Claritin D 24 hr, Allegra D 24 hr, Zyrtec D 24 hr). If you have to take Sudafed for sinus congestion, I recommend the short-acting form (30 mg) taken up until 5:00 P.M., at a maximum dose of 120 mg per day, or a maximum of one twelve-hour slow-release formulation per day (120 mg total of Sudafed, as in Claritin D-12 hour, Allegra D-12 hour), taken early in the morning. This way the effect of the drug wears off before bedtime. Individuals with ADD/ADHD may also be taking stimulants to help them concentrate, which may interfere with sleep. These include medications such as Vyvanse, Ritalin, and Adderall XR. Vyvanse is particularly problematic for those with sleep disorders, due to its long half-life. Other stimulants that may interfere with sleep are Provigil and Nuvigil, which are medications taken in the morning to help with resistant fatigue from sleep apnea, or from shift worker syndrome (working abnormal shifts, i.e., 3:00 P.M. to 11:00 P.M., 4:00 P.M. to midnight), in which their sleep cycles are affected by getting to bed late every night.

Certain foods can also have a stimulant effect. For example, some people cannot tolerate caffeine, or even chocolate, especially in the afternoon, since the stimulant effect may keep them up at night. These varied conditions, and the effects of drugs and diet, show the importance of evaluating all the possible sources of sleep disruption, and not just prescribing sleep medications.

SLEEP APNEA AND THE IMPORTANCE OF A SLEEP STUDY

If it is unclear which factors may be responsible for causing insomnia, a sleep study can be useful. Sleep studies (also known as polysomnography) are now performed at many hospitals, where the patient stays overnight and their sleep patterns are monitored, evaluating brain wave patterns (EEG), eye movement patterns (EOG), changes in heart rhythm (EKG), as well as the quality and duration of sleep. Sleep studies are particularly useful for determining a condition known as sleep apnea, which typically is thought of as affecting overweight individuals who snore. We have been surprised at the number of individuals diagnosed with sleep apnea in our practice who don't fit these criteria: This included young, thin women who were not overweight and denied snoring.

Obstructive sleep apnea (OSA) is typically first noticed by bed partners, who are kept awake with loud snoring or witness their spouse or partner stop breathing at night. Epidemiological evidence has shown that approximately 6 percent of the U.S. population suffers from sleep apnea, and it can contribute to the daytime fatigue and headaches that we often see in the MSIDS patient. This is particularly important to diagnose, because while poor sleep is taxing on the brain, it also takes a toll on your total health. Disturbed sleep patterns have effects on cardiovascular morbidity and mortality, increasing cardiovascular risks. Sleep debt, which is defined as the amount of sleep required for optimal functioning less the amount actually obtained, has been linked to an increased risk of cardiovascular disease. Specifically, low oxygen levels in the blood during sleep apnea can adversely affect the heart, leading to heart attacks and arrhythmias in those with underlying heart disease.

During a sleep study the individual is observed for the number of times they stop breathing during the night (number of apneic events), have decreased breathing (hypopneic events), or if their sleep is interrupted due to the occurrence of restless legs. The severity of the apnea is also evaluated by monitoring decreases in oxygen saturation in the blood during the event. A patient with severe sleep apnea, for example, may have many episodes during the night where they stop breathing for several seconds at a time, while simultaneously the oxygen saturation in their blood drops.

Some MSIDS patients may also suffer from narcolepsy, where they fall asleep suddenly in the middle of the day, have excessive daytime sleepiness (EDS), and/or cataplexy, where there is a sudden loss of voluntary muscle control. In cataplexy, the signs can be obvious (dropping objects, dropping to the knees, or falling down with sudden strong emotions, such as laughter, anger, fear, or orgasm), or there can be more subtle manifestations, such as a slackening of the facial muscles and a dropping of the head or jaw. These different conditions are best evaluated with a different type of sleep study, known as a MSLT (multiple sleep latency test). Although cataplexy is rare, it happens in about 70 percent of those with narcolepsy, and can also be present as a side effect of the discontinuation of an SSRI like Prozac.

DECONSTRUCTING POOR SLEEP

There are two major sleep patterns: rapid eye movement (REM) sleep and non-REM (NREM) sleep. When we first start to fall asleep, we enter non-REM sleep, which is further divided into four stages of progressively deeper, quieter sleep. Stage 1 is sleep onset. Stage 2 is a deeper state characterized by changes in brain wave activity, where sleep spindle patterns can be seen on an EEG. Stages 3 and 4 are stages of deep sleep characterized by slow wave activity on the EEG, and are therefore known as slow wave sleep (or delta sleep).

We then enter REM sleep, which is primarily when we dream. REM begins about ninety minutes after falling asleep, and it happens between four and five times per night and occupies approximately 25 percent of our sleep time. REM sleep is important for many brain functions, and it is critical for consolidating memories.

The length and type of sleep we get in each of these stages depends on our biological clocks. We have biological rhythms in the body known as circadian rhythms, which affect our appetite, level of alertness, and sleep. Our biological clocks control our circadian rhythms. People with circadian rhythm sleep disorders are unable to get to sleep at normal times at night and are unable to wake up at times required for work and school schedules. This is frequently the case in MSIDS. Getting MSIDS patients to sleep at the proper time and normalizing their circadian rhythms is essential for improving their health.

A sleep deficit occurs when we don't sleep well for long periods of time and become sleep-deprived. Because the brain and the body need sleep to function properly, the brain can bypass the earlier stages of sleep, and shift into Stage 3 and REM sleep more quickly, in order to make up for the sleep deficit. However, a good night's sleep really must include all of the stages of sleep. Limited amounts of sleep during each stage, as well as a lack of depth and intensity of sleep during REM and NREM stages, correlates with impaired immune functioning. This has been well documented in the scientific literature for multiple disease states. An important scientific study published in 2006 showed that disturbed sleep has an effect on chronic age- and stress-related disorders, and increases cytokine levels, worsening symptoms of chronic inflammatory diseases such as rheumatoid arthritis, FM, and chronic fatigue syndrome.

Certain cytokines not only affect inflammation, but also can have deleterious effects on sleep, affecting our endocrine function. Stress hormones (cortisol) and growth hormone secretion are both affected by sleep. Some studies have reported persistently elevated levels of cortisol in people with chronic insomnia, particularly insomnia related to aging and psychiatric disorders, with high levels of cortisol reducing REM sleep. However, a 2003 study of people with chronic insomnia reported that cortisol levels were high, especially when their sleep was of poor quality. When they slept well, cortisol levels were lower. This study and other research suggest that high levels of stress hormones can be caused by poor sleep, rather than just being the cause. This sleep deprivation then results in higher levels of interleukin-6 and TNF-α during the day, increasing fatigue, while significantly reducing cortisol secretion the next day, which can have deleterious effects on our immune functioning. Growth hormone (GH) secretion is also affected by aging and poor sleep. There is a blunting of regular, cyclical surges of growth hormone as we get older, and GH is associated not only with growth, but also with deep, slow wave sleep. GH deficiency is related to reduced muscle mass and strength, increased fat stores, and a weakened immunity to infection. There are complex interactions between cytokines, sleep, endocrine function, and immune function, which must all be accounted for in the MSIDS patient.

Cytokines also directly disturb sleep patterns through their effect on the hypothalamus, which controls hunger, thirst, body temperature, hormone production, sleep, and circadian cycles. The mechanism by which this works is also complex. Cytokines alter the synthesis of nitric oxide on the cellular level, where products of the nitric oxide pathway, such as peroxynitrite, stimulate inflammatory cytokine release; this also happens through changes in growth hormone production. Cytokines also signal the brain by blood-borne routes and/or peripheral nerves to activate the HPA axis and sympathetic nervous system, leading to altered sleep patterns. And when we don't sleep, we naturally produce higher levels of the inflammatory cytokine IL-6, which further increases inflammation and contributes to ongoing symptoms of the sickness syndrome. High amounts of IL-6 are also associated with insomnia, narcolepsy, obstructive sleep apnea, chronic fatigue syndrome, fibromyalgia, and obesity. This vicious cycle of inflammation contributes to our sleep deprivation.

There are other specific cytokines involved with the different stages of sleep. First, interleukin-1 and tumor necrosis factor help regulate NREM sleep. IL-1 is critical for going to sleep, and it also helps to induce the onset of Stage 3 slow wave sleep. Too much IL-1 produced during an infection will induce a large increase in NREM sleep and reduce the duration of REM sleep. This is one of the reasons why, when we don't feel well due to an infection, like Lyme disease, we tend to have more restless sleep.

The balance of REM and NREM sleep is also crucial for maintaining hormonal systems and a control of inflammatory processes. An overproduction of the cytokines IL-1 and TNF-α interferes with this balance and affects NREM sleep. IL-1 and TNF-α act on the neurons in the brain and their sensitivities to inhibitory neurotransmitters, such as glutamate and GABA, which are essential for shutting down the brain for sleep. We also find that TNF-α plays a critical role in regulating many other important neurotransmitters in the central nervous system that are involved in sleep-signaling pathways. These include the stimulating, or excitatory, brain chemicals norepinephrine, serotonin, and dopamine. TNF-α modulates the production of these substances through neurotransmitter-coupled G protein–signaling, which promotes sleep.

These two mechanisms, therefore, enable IL-1 and TNF-α to both induce and promote sleep, and if they are produced in abnormal quantities during the day, they can cause drowsiness and fatigue. Patients will not feel well until we decrease levels of these inflammatory molecules during the day and enable them to produce the molecules in the proper amounts for sleep later at night. Getting patients to balance their REM and NREM sleep is crucial to shutting down the abnormal production of these inflammatory cytokines.

Whereas IL-1 has an effect in inducing slow wave sleep early on in the sleep cycle, IL-6 has a direct action in the central nervous system, and it has been shown to increase slow wave sleep in the second half of the night, during NREM sleep. IL-6 levels are negatively correlated to the amount of sleep we get each night. We need lower levels of IL-6 to get a good night's sleep and feel well the next day. Both plasma IL-6 and TNF-α levels also peak at different times in normal, healthy adults. Plasma IL-6 levels normally decline at 8:00 A.M. and 9:00 P.M., and peak between 5:00 P.M. and 7:00 P.M. in the evening. The strongest peak is between four and five o'clock in the afternoon, when many patients feel drowsy. If we have increased levels of IL-6, or it peaks at the wrong times of the day, it will interfere with sleep and increase fatigue as well as pain.

Controlling and balancing inflammatory cytokine levels are essential if we are to feel energetic and get a good night's sleep. An analogy that I often use with my patients to explain this process is that of a faucet and a sink. If we have a running faucet (the ongoing production of cytokines) as well as a clogged drain (poor detoxification pathways), we are going to accumulate abnormal levels of these inflammatory molecules in our body. We therefore need to control cytokine production by "shutting down the faucet" (i.e., decreasing their overproduction) and "opening up the drain" (eliminating them from the body), as well as eliminating associated toxins, if we are to feel well. This is crucial in getting chronically ill patients back into balance.

SLEEP MEDICATIONS THAT WORK FOR MSIDS

Many sleep medications share the same liver detoxification pathways, so it is important to check for drug interactions, as they may have additive effects and cause excessive daytime drowsiness if one drug interferes with the excretion of another from the body. Since we often use combination therapy to get sufferers with resistant insomnia to sleep, I find it essential to use the trusty *Physicians' Desk Reference* (known as "the PDR") to check for drug interactions when combining medications.

General treatment guidelines to deal with resistant insomnia and fatigue include using activating agents, which are drugs with a stimulating effect in the morning, and sleep-promoting agents in the evening, especially those that encourage Stage III/Stage IV sleep. Activating agents include medications such as Provigil and Nuvigil, stimulants like Ritalin, Vyvanse, and Adderall, and Wellbutrin, noradrenergic agents, and the SSRIs. Provigil and Nuvigil have been approved for narcolepsy, shift work sleep disorder, and OSA/hypopnea syndrome.

Provigil can be effective for those who are unable to stay awake during the day, and for whom classical therapies for insomnia have failed. It must be used with caution if there is an associated anxiety disorder and/or heart palpitations, since it can increase these symptoms, and also interfere with sleep if taken late in the day or in too high a dose. Wellbutrin, on the other hand, is a much easier drug to use. It augments the efficacy of other antidepressants, such as SSRIs, improving patients' moods, and inhibits the neuronal uptake of the excitatory brain chemicals dopamine and norepinephrine. This helps patients be more alert in the morning. I have generally found Wellbutrin to be a very well-tolerated medication with fewer drug interactions than many of the commonly used antidepressants on the market.

344 • RICHARD I. HOROWITZ, MD

Sleep agents that promote deep, slow wave sleep include Lyrica, Trazodone, Gabitril, Seroquel, and Xyrem. These are drugs that are typically used for other conditions (except Xyrem) but have been proven very effective for getting people to sleep. However, a typical internist would not normally consider them, since we are primarily taught in medical school to use sleep drugs such as Ambien, Lunesta, and benzodiazepine derivatives (Valium, Restoril). Yet these other drugs have certain distinct clinical advantages. For example, Lyrica is commonly used for neuropathic pain in both diabetics and in postherpetic neuralgia (pain experienced after getting shingles). Up to 70 percent of persistent Lyme disease patients have peripheral neuropathy, so although this is an off-label use of the drug, we have found it to be very helpful in patients with neuropathy and sleep problems. Similarly, Lyrica is approved for use in fibromyalgia. I have therefore found that my patients suffering from insomnia, neuropathy, and FM may benefit from the use of this drug if standard sleep medications have failed. Since the drug can cause the side effects of drowsiness, dizziness, visual changes, and confusion, we generally need to keep the doses of this medication on the lower side during the day, since the side effects mimic the same symptoms seen in our MSIDS patients. Many of our patients are also on antidepressants, and the combination of Lyrica and antidepressants may increase the risk of central nervous system depression, leading to a decreased level of consciousness, so this also needs to be kept in mind.

Gabitril, like Lyrica, is an antiseizure medication. It is effective because it stimulates the brain's GABA receptors, which help induce sleep. Gabitril has also been shown to be effective in inducing deeper stages of sleep, i.e., Stage 3 and Stage 4 NREM sleep. Like Lyrica, it can cause central nervous system depression, as well as other possible side effects, including fatigue, dizziness, and impaired concentration. It can be used alone or in combination with other drugs that hit GABA receptor sites, such as the benzodiazepines like Valium. Some patients who have failed trials of standard sleep medications, such as Ambien (which also interacts with GABA-benzodiazepine receptors), find that they finally fall asleep taking Gabitril, with or without benzodiazepines. Since benzodiazepines are addictive, their use should be limited if possible, as their effect will wear off over time and require higher and higher doses to be effective. We find the same problem regarding certain pain medications and narcotics, which, apart from their addictive potential, can also interfere with sleep.

Trazodone is also helpful in treating resistant insomnia. This is especially true if there is significant overlapping depression and anxiety. I find it to be a helpful addition to standard sleep medications such as Ambien or Lunesta. It has been a very safe medication in my experience, but the common reactions present in the other drugs apply here, since it may cause drowsiness, fatigue, headaches, and dizziness. It also can cause a rare and serious reaction known as the serotonin syndrome, or neuroleptic malignant syndrome. Serotonin syndrome is a potentially life-threatening drug reaction, affecting the autonomic nervous system and leading to high temperatures (hyperthermia), sweating, nausea, diarrhea, elevated heart rates (tachycardia) with elevations in blood pressure (hypertension), tremors, and muscle twitching (myoclonus). It can also affect cognition, causing agitation and confusion, and can even lead to a coma. Careful attention, therefore, needs to be paid to using drugs that affect serotonin pathways simultaneously. I have never seen a case of serotonin syndrome in all of my years of practice, but it should always be kept in mind, as MSIDS patients also often suffer from autonomic nervous system dysfunction.

Another atypical sleep drug is Seroquel. Seroquel is used by many Lyme-literate psychiatrists as an adjunct for sleep, especially for those with overlapping psychiatric problems such as schizophrenia or bipolar disorder. I have tended to avoid it because of my concern that it may cause extrapyramidal symptoms (movement disorders) and that it may affect the endocrine functioning of the thyroid (hypothyroidism) and pancreas (increased risk of diabetes).

The last and most infrequently used uncommon sleep medication that addresses disrupted Stages 3 and 4 sleep is Xyrem. It is my last choice among sleep medications, but I use it in patients for whom all other drug and herbal regimens have failed. It is indicated for use with patients with excessive daytime sleepiness (EDS), cataplexy, and narcolepsy, or shift work sleep disorders. One of the advantages of Xyrem is that it is metabolized in the liver but primarily excreted through the lungs as carbon dioxide, with a very short half-life of thirty to sixty minutes. The short half-life is why the drug needs to be given twice a night, right before bedtime and then four hours later. The pharmaceutical manufacturer insists that doctors provide an instructional DVD on its use and have their patients participate in a specialized Xyrem educational program before they are allowed to use this medication.

Other medications for sleep that we have found to be useful include some of the older tricyclic antidepressant drugs, such as Elavil, muscle relaxers such as Flexeril, and antidepressants such as Remeron. Elavil has similar indications as Lyrica, as it is a neuroleptic drug that can be used for neuropathic pain and postherpetic neuralgia. Therefore, it can be useful for those with Lyme disease and *Bartonella* who suffer from an associated neuropathy. Elavil was a commonly used drug for depression until SSRIs emerged.

Many who suffer from Lyme-MSIDS with associated insomnia also experience muscle pain and spasm that in turn may further interfere with sleep. A calcium-magnesium supplement at bedtime may be helpful. Flexeril is the drug that is classically used for muscle spasm. I have generally avoided its use during the daytime because of its significant side effect of drowsiness, but if it used as a nighttime aid for sleep, it may be effective, even in low doses.

Remeron is an antidepressant that I did not frequently prescribe prior to treating patients with Lyme disease. Although its exact mechanism of action is unknown, it seems to increase the efficacy of serotonin receptors and block excitatory neurotransmitters, such as norepinephrine and epinephrine, therefore allowing the brain to quiet down and induce sleep. At its lowest dose it has the greatest effect on putting patients to sleep. Therefore, patients with overlapping depression and insomnia may benefit from the use of this drug. Although the *PDR* lists a whole range of possible side effects for Remeron, we generally have found the drug to be well tolerated with minimal side effects.

Frequently prescribed sleep drugs such as Ambien were created and approved for the short-term treatment of insomnia; however, some patients need it for longer periods of time if no other medications have been effective. One of the serious side effects of Ambien is that it can cause complex sleep-related behavior, such as sleepwalking. There are stories in the medical literature of people eating or even driving their car and not remembering their actions the next morning. Similarly, it can cause memory loss, not a desired side effect in the Lyme patient who may already suffer from severe neurocognitive deficits. Taking patients off medications for a drug-free holiday may be important when it is difficult to determine whether certain symptoms are due to the disease or to the drug that they are taking.

Lunesta is a frequently used medication that has been approved for longer-term use. We have generally not seen significant side effects in our patients who use Lunesta. However, as with Ambien, side effects of drowsiness, hallucinations, and confusion have been reported. Once again, it is important to be sure that the patient is not having a drug side effect that resembles the symptoms of their disease.

I have also found certain herbs and nutraceuticals to be useful for treating insomnia, and many have been studied scientifically. These include valerian root, melatonin, GABA and L-theanine (taken separately or together), phosphatidylserine, certain herbal formulas with schizandra (i.e., Herbsom, by Dr. Zhang) as well as Bach Flower Remedies and other homeopathic aids. If one regimen is ineffective, these herbs and nutraceuticals can be combined, helping to increase their efficacy.

Valerian root is the subject of hundreds of published studies, and has been extensively reviewed by the German Commission E, a governing body in Germany that created a therapeutic guide for licensed medical professionals prescribing herbal medicine. It has been shown to have a relaxing effect, and can be used for the treatment of anxiety and stress-related disorders during the day and at night to help patients get to and stay asleep. It comes in drops (Amantilla, NutraMedix) and capsules. I generally prefer the drops, as the dosage can be adjusted much more easily and because (according to my patients) the capsules smell like old socks. GABA-L theanine comes in creams, powders (Xymogen), and capsules. L-theanine is a derivative of green tea, which has a relaxing effect on the body, and also affects glutamate reuptake in the brain. The GABA-L theanine cream can be applied to the temples and on the back of the neck before bedtime, and when combined with inositol, can be helpful in treating obsessive-compulsive disorder for those who can't shut off their thinking at night. I have used this combination in both adults and children with OCD, and it has definitely been effective without the associated side effects of certain OCD drugs, such as Anafranil.

Melatonin is also a supplement commonly used by patients with sleep disorders. It is an essential hormone produced by the pineal gland that elicits sleep, and whose production tends to decrease as we age. When it is used at bedtime, it helps regulate sleep. There are controlled release, long-acting formulations (Xymogen) that may also help decrease frequent awakening in the middle of the night. The dosage needs to be properly adjusted, however, because too much melatonin can cause a hangover effect in the morning.

Phosphatidylserine (PS) is also used frequently in our practice, as it has an effect on the dysregulated hormone systems of the body. When patients have an overstimulated adrenal gland—excess production of cortisol—this effect can contribute to the sleep problems seen in MSIDS patients. PS helps to decrease the overproduction of ACTH from the pituitary gland, which subsequently leads to lower levels of cortisol, helping to regulate the stress response and relax the body at night. It is insufficient as a stand-alone supplement to regulate sleep, but it can be helpful when excess production of cortisol is identified as one of the causes of poor sleep.

Some of the Bach Flower Remedies, such as Rescue Remedy, and homeopathic remedies like Kali phos have been prescribed as sleep aids by naturopathic doctors with whom I work, and have occasionally been useful when patients wake up in the middle of the night and can't fall back asleep. Chinese doctors who treat Lyme disease with traditional Chinese herbs also have herbal formulas that include herbs such as *Ziziphus jujuba*, Schisandra Chinensis, *Paeonia lactiflora*, and Rehmannia glutinosa. All of them have been shown to be helpful with sleep. The advantage of combining herbs and medications is that less prescription medication can be used, with generally less drug interactions and side effects.

MICHELLE COULDN'T SLEEP

Teenagers are some of the best sleepers, yet my patient, Michelle from Vermont, couldn't get to sleep. At just eighteen years old she started complaining of severe fatigue, migraines with light and sound sensitivity, dizziness, joint pain in multiple joints that would migrate around her body, GI problems, vaginal itching and discharge, day sweats, chills, flushing, lack of a regular period for years, anxiety and palpitations, moderate to severe memory and concentration problems, and severe insomnia: She had difficulty falling asleep and also was complaining of frequent awakening. She was diagnosed with Lyme disease a year before she came to see me, after suffering with these symptoms for years, and was referred to a Lyme-literate doctor for treatment. She underwent one year of antibiotics before coming in, but she was still only functioning at about 30 percent of normal. A gynecologist also placed her on birth control pills, as her estrogen and progesterone levels were all found to be in the very low range, yet she still was not having regular periods when she came to see me. She had also been seen by a cardiologist and an endocrinologist, because of her palpitations. She had a negative workup, including a negative echocardiogram and Holter monitor, with normal norepinephrine and VMA levels in her urine.

Michelle's physical examination showed a blood pressure of $^{108}\!/_{62}$, with a resting pulse rate of 92 per minute while she was sitting on the examination table. When I stood her up, within one minute her blood pressure dropped to $^{90}\!/_{54}$ with an increase in her heart rate to 110 beats per minute, and she complained of feeling dizzy, with associated palpitations. This was consistent with possible POTS and autonomic nervous system dysfunction. Otherwise there were no abnormal findings on her physical exam.

We sent off for a CBC, a comprehensive metabolic profile, B_{12}, folate, methylmalonic acid, and homocysteine levels with a MTHFR test, as well as a comprehensive co-infection panel, which included a *Babesia* FISH test, *Bartonella* titer and PCR, *Mycoplasma* titer and PCR, rickettsial panel for RMSF, typhus, and Q fever, and tularemia and *Brucella* titers for her chronic fatigue, sweats, joint pain, and severe memory problems. We also performed hormonal studies and checked vitamin D levels, sex hormone levels, thyroid functions (T3, free T3, T4, TSH with antithyroid antibodies), adrenal function (DHEA/cortisol levels by saliva), and an IgF-1 level to rule out growth hormone deficiency. We also tested for mineral deficiencies (magnesium, iodine, and zinc), checked autoimmune markers to rule out an autoimmune disease, and completed her GI workup by sending off for an *H. pylori* test, an antigliadin antibody and TTG with an IgE and IgG food allergy panel (for her chronic digestive complaints), with a Metametrix gastrointestinal effects panel and a comprehensive digestive stool analysis (CDSA). After drawing blood, we gave her an injection of 2 gm of IV glutathione, since it has been effective in so many patients who we see with fatigue, muscle and joint pain, and cognitive problems. Michelle felt better within fifteen minutes of the injection, with a significant decrease in her fatigue, headache, and cognitive problems.

We saw Michelle in our office one month later. Her tests came back positive for babesiosis, *Bartonella*, very low adrenal function, with cortisol levels below range in the morning but high at night (which may have interfered with her sleep), a low free T3, other thyroid functions within range, low sex hormone levels (low estradiol and progesterone levels), a positive antigliadin and negative TTG, positive food allergies by both IgE (shrimp, hazelnuts) and IgG (milk, wheat, beef, and eggs being the highest) with a low vitamin D3, at 8 (normal range is greater than 30), and a slightly low B$_{12}$ level. Her comprehensive digestive stool analysis showed infections with two parasites. In other words, not only did Michelle suffer from Lyme disease, she had MSIDS. The overlapping factors that were contributing to her illness included several other tick-borne co-infections with *Babesia* and *Bartonella*, intestinal parasites, various hormonal abnormalities, including adrenal dysfunction, with probable POTS, gluten sensitivity with food allergies, vitamin deficiencies, and detoxification problems. This was on top of her severely resistant insomnia.

Due to the yeast and the severity of her GI symptoms, Michelle did not want to try antibiotics nor antiparasitic drugs right away. We started her on supplementation with adrenal essence and complex in the morning, to treat her adrenal fatigue, with low-dose Cortef and Florinef, which would help support her low blood pressure and clinical POTS. She did not feel well enough initially to go to the hospital for a tilt-table test. PS (phosphatidylserine) was also prescribed for her elevated cortisol and her difficulties with sleep, and pregnenolone cream, to give her further hormonal support for low adrenals and sex hormones.

She was placed on a strict hypoglycemic diet, avoiding her allergic foods (many of her symptoms were worse after eating carbohydrates, especially the wheat products she was allergic to), and she was given digestive enzymes. She was also asked to follow a yeast-free diet as much as possible, and was given nystatin, as she had developed GI symptoms of gas and bloating, with vaginal itching and discharge after stopping the last round of antibiotics before coming to see me. It was important that she follow a strict yeast-free diet, since *Candida* symptoms can mimic Lyme symptoms.

We started her on an herbal protocol for Lyme disease with Samento and Cumunda instead of antibiotics, which would have exacerbated her *Candida* problem, and gave her Malarone with *Artemisia* for the babesiosis. She was also given NAC, alpha-lipoic acid, and glycine to help support her own glutathione production after we saw how effective the IV glutathione was in relieving her headache and brain fog. Finally, she was given Amantilla (valerian root in liquid form) for her anxiety, palpitations, and difficulty sleeping.

At her next visit she reported that her energy swings were more stable with a hypoglycemic/yeast-free diet, and her migraines and GI symptoms had improved once she stopped eating gluten and her allergic foods. Her joint pain initially flared from the herbs that she was taking to treat the Lyme disease, but it eventually improved; the sweats and chills decreased with the antimalarial therapy for *Babesia*. However, she still complained of resistant fatigue, brain fog, and insomnia. We reviewed the sleep medications she had tried and that had failed. Standard sleep medication such as Lunesta and Ambien had failed, as well as benzodiazepines, such as Valium, Xanax, and Restoril, before coming to see me. She had seen a Lyme-literate doctor, who had tried to rotate her through some of the more atypical sleep medications, and especially the ones that have the potential to help with non-REM and deep sleep. She had tried Lyrica, Trazodone, Gabitril, Elavil, Flexeril, and Remeron, and multiple natural products, including melatonin, and now she was on valerian root and phosphatidylserine. Every one had failed. Michelle was sleeping barely four hours per night and couldn't go to school, as she was exhausted most of the time.

At this point we discussed having her go for a sleep study to further evaluate the sleep difficulties and to rule out sleep apnea. We also discussed referring her back to her ob-gyn to adjust her birth control pill, as she was still having irregular and very painful periods, with severe PMS. During this visit I also discussed having her try Xyrem. I gave her a DVD that instructed her on how to take it. She would have to be in bed when she took the initial dose, then wake up four hours later to take the next dose. I told her to call if she had any side effects. We started with 3 gm (6 ml) twice a night, as I had found that the lower doses can cause confusion and disorientation. If 3 gm didn't work after a week, and she tolerated it without side effects, she was instructed to try increasing the dose to 4 gm (8 ml) twice per night, four hours apart.

Michelle returned a month later. She was sleeping soundly for the first time in years! Xyrem was the answer. She had no side effects from the drug and felt a sense of wellness that she had not experienced in a long time. She was now sleeping eight hours per night and was able to start going back to school. Over time she eventually tolerated antibiotics and antiparasitic drugs for her Lyme and *Bartonella*, and her GI symptoms continued to improve. She required the addition of Catapres, which significantly stabilized her POTS, and was able to start LDN to help regulate her inflammation and fibromyalgia symptoms, now that she was finally sleeping.

Michelle believes that without getting her to sleep none of the other interventions would have made a difference. Even though they were all beneficial—balancing the hormones, bringing up her blood pressure, stabilizing her gut, and treating the infections—she only turned the corner once she finally got sleep.

Sleep deprivation is one of the primary reasons that many of my patients remain chronically ill, and it may be holding you back from achieving better health. It is difficult to improve the overall functioning of those with MSIDS until this piece of the medical puzzle is adequately addressed, so don't give up. Get to the bottom of your sleep disorder and work with your doctor to find the right combination of medications and herbs that work for you. Without improving your sleep, you may not be able to resolve your resistant symptoms of Lyme-MSIDS and break the inflammatory cycle.

FOURTEEN

Lyme and Autonomic Nervous System Dysfunction/POTS

atients often come to our practice and complain of fatigue, dizziness, palpitations, anxiety, shortness of breath, exercise intolerance, and brain fog, with difficulty concentrating. Many have seen multiple specialists to evaluate these symptoms, and no cause was found. We have discussed how Lyme disease, associated coinfections, hormonal disorders, environmental toxins, detoxification problems, mitochondrial dysfunction, food allergies, hypoglycemia, sleep disorders, and psychological problems all can cause these same clinical manifestations: Each one of these individually or in combination with the others can be responsible for these symptoms. Yet there is one common disease process that is often missed in the MSIDS patient, which can also mimic these symptoms and explain a poor response to traditional therapies. That is postural orthostatic tachycardia syndrome (POTS), a form of autonomic nervous system (ANS) dysfunction. ANS dysfunction (also known as autonomic dysfunction, or dysautonomia) describes any disease or malfunction of the nerves in the body controlling the blood pressure, heart rate, sweat glands, and bladder and bowel function. It can be due to Lyme disease, but also may occur with other diseases that affect the nervous system, such as diabetes or Shy-Drager syndrome (the degeneration of nerve cells in the brain). Those diagnosed with chronic fatigue syndrome, fibromyalgia, or Lyme disease, who have not adequately responded to treatment may also have ANS dysfunction, and particularly, POTS.

We discussed in Chapter 12 that there were four principal types of neuropathy that can affect the nervous system in the patient with Lyme disease. One of them is autonomic neuropathy. This is a form of polyneuropathy that affects the involuntary nerves of the autonomic nervous system. The ANS involves elements of the central nervous system (brain/hypothalamus and spinal cord), the peripheral nervous system, with its sensory motor branches, and the enteric nervous system, which is made up of nerve fibers that go to the bladder and gastrointestinal tract (including the pancreas and the gallbladder). The ANS also performs its duties by acting through two main branches, known as the orthosympathetic (OS) and parasympathetic (PS) nervous systems. The particular ANS symptoms seen in a Lyme disease patient will depend on which part or parts of the system has been affected: the brain/hypothalamus (causing temperature dysregulation) or peripheral sensory nerves (causing burning, tingling, numbness, and problems with sweating), and whether the parasympathetic or orthosympathetic system has been affected, both of which control heart rate and blood pressure, as well as bladder and bowel function.

The OS and PS nervous systems have opposite effects in the body. The PS regulates automatic body functions, such as breathing, heart rate, and digestion. It does this primarily through the vagus nerve, which when activated secretes a neurotransmitter, acetylcholine, that slows down the heart rate and decreases intestinal function. The orthosympathetic nervous system, on the other hand, secretes the neurotransmitters norepinephrine and epinephrine. Epinephrine (adrenaline) is produced exclusively by the adrenal glands (adrenal medulla), whereas norepinephrine is produced both by the adrenals and the orthosympathetic nervous system. Norepinephrine acts as both a hormone and neurotransmitter and plays an essential role in the functioning of the sympathetic nervous system, helping to control our heart rate and affecting our blood pressure through dilatation of our blood vessels. Epinephrine, on the other hand, is the hormone primarily responsible for the fight-or-flight response to stress, raising the heart rate and blood pressure and causing blood vessels to constrict. When the fight-or-flight response is triggered, the adrenal medulla releases 80 percent epinephrine and 20 percent norepinephrine. These neurotransmitters and hormones also play an important role in increasing muscle tension and sexual arousal. The OS system performs these actions by regulating the contraction and expansion of blood vessels.

Proper regulation of vascular tone is crucial, for we need to be able to remain in an upright position and maintain a normal blood pressure in order to accomplish many of our daily activities. This requires the continuous and rapid responses of the autonomic nervous system. When the ANS fails to function properly, whether through failure of other organ systems (congestive heart failure or renal or hepatic disease), systemic illness (strokes), endocrine abnormalities (hypothyroidism, or a pheochromocytoma, a tumor of the adrenal glands that secretes excessive amounts of catecholamines), or due to other causes of autonomic neuropathy, then blood pressure and cerebral blood flow will be compromised, and POTS can result.

POTS refers to symptoms resulting from the impaired functioning of the autonomic nervous system, when we are unable to maintain our vascular tone. This leads to low blood pressure when standing and/or changing position (postural orthostasis). The heart tries to compensate for the low blood pressure by beating faster, thereby causing palpitations (tachycardia). This acute lowering of the blood pressure causes dizziness, fatigue, exercise intolerance, and difficulty concentrating due to poor cerebral blood flow. These findings were seen in a 2007 Mayo Clinic study, one of the largest clinical studies on this syndrome to date. This study was of particular interest, because many of the participants also had symptoms we commonly see with Lyme disease.

We should be able to maintain a stable blood pressure while standing if our autonomic nervous system is working properly. We can clinically determine the likelihood of POTS in our medical office by checking sitting and standing blood pressures and heart rates. If a patient has a relatively normal resting blood pressure and pulse rate (for example, $^{105}/_{72}$ with a pulse rate of 80 beats per minute), and then stands up and their blood pressure subsequently drops (i.e., to $^{80}/_{55}$ with a pulse rate of 100 or higher) within one or two minutes, this is suggestive of POTS. The diagnosis of POTS would also be suspected if there were associated symptoms of dizziness and palpitations with the change in position, or if the patient had a history of frequent episodes of passing out (syncope) or nearly passing out (presyncope), which are consistent with episodes of low blood pressure.

In order to diagnose POTS definitively, an individual would be sent to the hospital to have a head-up tilt-table test (HUT). This is administered by having the patient lie flat on a special table while the heart rate is monitored (by EKG), and blood pressure is checked. The table then is placed in an upright position, usually at 60 or 80 degrees. If there is orthostatic intolerance (a significant drop in blood pressure, with dizziness/and/or fainting) and an increase in heart rate (an increase of more than 30 beats per minute, or a heart rate greater than 120 beats per minute within ten minutes of the test) while going from the sitting to standing position, that is considered to be a positive head-up tilt-table test.

The pathophysiological changes underlying POTS are complex. There are five reasons why the autonomic nervous system may not work well:

- Abnormal production of hormones and neurotransmitters, such as norepinephrine and epinephrine. Some people secrete abnormally high amounts of plasma norepinephrine on standing (greater than 600 pg/ml), which is responsible in part for their elevated heart rate and palpitations. This increase in sympathetic activation is an early finding of POTS and helps to define the disorder.

- Inability of receptors on blood vessels to properly respond to these hormones.

- Low intravascular fluid volume (hypovolemia), due to leakage of fluid from the small capillaries or from pooling of blood outside the vascular space.

- Autonomic neuropathy, with damage to peripheral nerves, the vagus nerve, autonomic small fibers in the skin, or the nerves connecting the different organs of the body to the central nervous system. This may cause abnormal temperature sensations (feeling too hot or too cold) and sweating, low blood pressure, and symptoms of constipation and bladder dysfunction.

• Autoimmune neuropathy, in which ganglia of the ANS are affected. Ganglia are intermediary connections between different neurological structures in the body, such as the peripheral and central nervous systems, and autonomic ganglia contain the cell bodies of autonomic nerves.

In order to fully understand and properly treat the clinical manifestations of POTS and ANS dysfunction, we must understand how all of these pathological mechanisms work. In the first instance, the symptoms of POTS may be due to neurotransmitters and hormones such as norepinephrine and epinephrine being produced in abnormally high quantities (a hyperadrenergic state). Adrenaline (epinephrine) is the fight-or-flight hormone, and it helps keep us in a state of heightened awareness, ready to respond to danger. If you have been suddenly frightened, your body responds by secreting large amounts of adrenaline into the bloodstream, elevating your heart rate and causing symptoms of anxiety and palpitations. High amounts of norepinephrine are also produced in POTS, and norepinephrine also has many important roles in the fight-or-flight response. It acts as a neurotransmitter released from the sympathetic neurons, increasing heart rate. As a stress hormone, it affects parts of the brain, such as the amygdala and hypothalamus, and increases the brain's oxygen supply, leading to greater wakefulness. It also helps release glucose from energy stores, increases blood flow to skeletal muscles, and increases blood pressure, by increasing vascular tone (the tension of the vascular smooth muscle). It does this through interacting with receptors on the surface of the blood vessels, known as alpha adrenergic receptors, which contract the smooth muscle and increase blood pressure.

We have several different types of receptors on our internal organs, through which the autonomic nervous system controls their function. They are broadly known as alpha and beta receptors. The alpha and beta receptors are found on the vasculature and smooth muscle throughout the body, as well as in the heart and lungs. They help control blood pressure, heart rate, and the contraction or relaxation of smooth muscle. Alpha stimulation of the blood vessels leads to smooth muscle contraction, raising blood pressure. Beta 1 receptors, when stimulated, can raise the heart rate; and beta 2 stimulation relaxes the smooth muscle in the lungs, increasing oxygen supply. However, the receptors on the blood vessels do not work properly for those with POTS. There are several different pathological mechanisms that may be at work (including decreased alpha 1–receptor sensitivity and/or beta 1–receptor supersensitivity).

Other mechanisms contributing to the low blood pressure in POTS that can directly cause dizziness and the sensation of almost passing out (presyncope) or passing out (syncope) is low intravascular fluid volume (hypovolemia). This may be a direct result of small blood vessels (capillaries) leaking fluid upon standing, or from the pooling of the blood in the lower extremities or abdomen. These explain why a certain percentage of patients with POTS feel much better with increased salt and fluids in their diet: Salt helps increase blood pressure, by pulling fluids into the intravascular compartment through osmosis, thereby increasing volume and reversing hypovolemia.

Patients with POTS may also suffer from an autonomic neuropathy. This can affect several different nerves in the body, causing a wide variety of symptoms.

- The autonomic small nerve fibers of the skin impact our sensation of temperature, as well as the functioning of the sweat glands. Patients with POTS therefore may not sweat (anhidrosis) or sweat too much (hyperhidrosis), depending on how these nerve fibers are affected. Small fiber neuropathy would explain the abnormalities seen on sweat testing in patients with ANS dysfunction (the quantitative sudomotor axon reflex test and thermoregulatory sweat testing), in which certain patients with POTS have regional, global, or mixed patterns of sweat loss or hyperhidrosis.

- The peripheral nerves are also affected. This can cause symptoms of burning, tingling, and numbness of the skin (small fiber neuropathy), as well as contributing to the pooling of fluids in the lower extremities, lowering blood pressure.

- The vagus nerve can be affected, and thereby our heart rate. A normal pulse rate is 72 beats per minute, although there are variability's depending on how physically fit we are, and we see a loss of heart rate variability in those with signs of vagal nerve involvement. This would also explain the varied gastrointestinal and urinary complaints in POTS, as the vagus nerve activates and controls the gastrointestinal (GI) and genitourinary (GU) systems. This can interfere with our ability to properly move our bowels and bladder. This was why my patient Larry, who we discussed in Chapter 11, complained that he was in the bathroom for four hours during the day trying to move his bowels due to severe constipation, as well as being up all night trying to relieve his bladder.

• Baroreceptor reflexes can be affected. These are specialized nerve cells present in our arteries (the carotid sinuses and aortic arch) that monitor our blood pressure and feed back the information to the brain (brain stem) and autonomic nervous system. They also help us maintain a stable blood pressure. For example, if the blood pressure starts to decrease too much, it would cause the heart rate to increase, raising the blood pressure. This homeostatic feedback loop does not work well in those with POTS. The result is blood pressure swings without a compensatory increase in heart rate necessary for maintaining blood pressure.

• Nerve fibers of the internal organs can be affected by autonomic neuropathy, further affecting hormonal systems that regulate blood pressure. One of the functions of the kidneys, apart from filtering toxic waste, is the production of hormones such as erythropoietin, which stimulates red blood cell production, increasing the intravascular volume and raising blood pressure. The kidneys also produce the hormone renin, which raises blood pressure through a hormonal feedback loop known as the renin-angiotensin-aldosterone system. If the kidneys are affected by ANS dysfunction, less renin is produced and blood pressure is lowered. Lower renin levels decrease aldosterone, leading to less effective salt retention, which then decreases the production of angiotensin II, another hormone that increases blood pressure through the constriction of blood vessels. Low plasma renin levels are seen with those who have POTS, whereas normally we would expect a high renin level for those with low blood volume (hypovolemia).

• Autoimmune autonomic neuropathy is another mechanism that is occasionally seen with POTS. Autonomic ganglia contain the cell bodies of the autonomic nerves that connect neurological structures such as the peripheral and central nervous systems. In the same study done at the Mayo Clinic, specific autoimmune markers, antiganglioside antibodies, were seen in 10 percent of the 152 patients studied who had POTS. Other studies have similarly described autoantibodies against ganglia in autoimmune neuropathies. We find the same autoimmune markers in many of our Lyme patients who have ANS dysfunction and POTS.

TESTING FOR POTS AND LYME

Many patients in our practice with Lyme disease and MSIDS have autonomic nervous system dysfunction, and oftentimes their previous physicians have missed this diagnosis. The first clue is symptoms of low blood pressure and light-headedness, with weakness upon standing or changing position, for those with generalized profound resistant fatigue and/or episodes of nearly passing out or passing out. If their history also has evidence of autonomic hyperactivity, such as anxiety and palpitations, and they have complaints of hyperhidrosis (too much sweating) or loss of sweating in parts of their body (anhidrosis), then POTS is a likely diagnosis.

According to a 2008 study published in *Current Rheumatology Reports*, POTS has been associated with chronic fatigue syndrome and fibromyalgia, but has not been linked with Lyme disease in the medical literature. I believe, as others do, that POTS may be one of the reasons those with Lyme disease continue to experience chronic symptoms. I see many patients with confirmed POTS and Lyme who have positive tilt-table tests and positive tests for ANS dysfunction by a board-certified neurologist. I have also seen patients come in with early signs of POTS, including high resting heart rates, before they experience any significant drops in blood pressure. Other doctors may mistake this sign for an anxiety or panic disorder if the full clinical picture is not recognized.

On physical examination, patients with POTS often have elevated resting heart rates in the high 80s, 90s, and occasionally over 100 beats per minute. This is consistent with the hyperadrenergic state seen in autonomic nervous system dysfunction. Their resting blood pressure, on the other hand, tends to be in the low normal range, i.e., $^{90}\!/_{60}$, and will drop significantly when they stand up for several minutes. This test of checking a patient's resting and standing pulse and blood pressure can easily be performed in the physician's office, and we do it routinely with our patients to be sure that we have not missed ANS dysfunction as one of the sixteen points on the MSIDS map. The increase in heart rate of more than 30 beats per minute, or a total heart rate greater than 120 beats per minute, is more typically seen on a head-up tilt-table testing (HUT) done in the hospital. Those types of significant responses are not usually elicited in a physician's office, yet a simple screening blood pressure and pulse check with changing position can help lead the medical detective to the right diagnosis.

There are certain common symptoms we see in patients with a positive tilt-table test. In the 2007 Mayo Clinic study, patients with POTS had no evidence of underlying cardiac disease and arrhythmia when they entered the study. Performance of a head-up tilt caused sustained heart rate increases of 30 beats/minute or greater after ten minutes and evoked symptoms of light-headedness, weakness, blurred vision, shortness of breath, nausea, and headache. These symptoms resolved once they were lying down. To meet the strict criteria for POTS, the symptoms have to be present for at least three months in duration.

Apart from the tilt-table, other tests used to evaluate POTS include monitoring the heart rate response to deep breathing and Valsalva maneuvers (pushing on the carotid arteries or increasing intraabdominal pressure by moving the bowels). A second test, quantitative sudomotor axon reflex testing (QSART), which detects abnormal sweating, can also be performed to further evaluate the functioning of the autonomic nervous system.

Neurologists such as Dr. David Younger at NYU have seen many patients with POTS who also suffer with neurological Lyme disease. These patients may present with the classical symptoms of polyradiculoneuritis (inflammation in different nerves coming out of the spine), distal polyneuropathy (neuropathy in the distal nerves), dysautonomia (autonomic nervous system dysfunction), and small-fiber sensory neuropathy. Their complete neurological workup often includes an MRI of the brain, SPECT scans for hypoperfusion, tilt-table testing, quantitative sensory testing

(QST) for heat pain perception thresholds, EMGs, with nerve conduction studies, and epidermal nerve fiber studies of the thigh and calf to screen for small fiber sensory nerve (SFSN) dysfunction. They are also sent for neuropsychological studies, which can show significant deficits in memory and concentration, the slowing of processing speed, and problems with executive functioning.

Along with these tests, I also recommend testing for autoantibodies against nerves (antiganglioside antibodies), one of the manifestations of ANS dysfunction, in order to achieve a comprehensive diagnosis. Lyme disease patients occasionally have positive testing for antibodies against peripheral nerves, which may be caused by an immune reaction against the flagellar proteins of *Borrelia*, leading to the formation of anti-myelin antibodies. We also find antiganglioside antibodies in patients with persistent neurological Lyme disease, which can be a surrogate marker for autonomic nervous system dysfunction and POTS.

Perhaps some of the patients in the Mayo Clinic study who were diagnosed with POTS had Lyme disease. Not only did they have the classic presenting symptoms, but one in seven patients had a positive test for antiganglioside antibodies, which we know to be associated with Lyme disease. When my patients with chronic neurological Lyme disease complain of tingling, numbness, or burning sensations of the extremities (symptoms of peripheral neuropathy), a small percentage will come back positive for antiganglioside antibodies, confirming an autoimmune process is overlapping their bacterial, viral, and parasitic infections. These patients often require IV immunoglobulin therapy to help with their acquired autoimmune peripheral and autonomic neuropathy. In Dr. Younger's published work, sustained subjective and objective neurological improvement was seen in his patients following this type of treatment.

I have seen similar improvements in ANS dysfunction in some Lyme-MSIDS patients following this protocol, but my patients usually require other medical interventions. Those with Lyme and POTS, along with associated severe neuropathy, often require antibiotic therapy for Lyme disease and co-infections such as *Bartonella* until the neuropathy is better, followed by herbal therapies to maintain progress and interventions with nutritional support and LDN to manage the inflammatory cytokines increasing their pain. "Shutting down the faucet of the overproduction of cytokines and opening up the drain to remove toxins" is particularly helpful in some of these patients with POTS and resistant neuropathy.

OTHER TREATMENT OPTIONS FOR ANS AND POTS

There are many treatments available to help relieve the symptoms of ANS dysfunction and POTS. Increasing salt and fluids to help expand the intravascular volume and bring up the blood pressure is the first therapy most commonly tried by health-care providers. You can increase the amount of salt you cook with, or take salt tablets with meals. This is not suggested for those suffering from high blood pressure and certain medical disorders with fluid overload, such as congestive heart failure and cirrhosis of the liver. Even when it is indicated, this protocol does not always work: One study examined thirty-five adolescent patients with POTS who had chronic fatigue and cognitive impairment and found that volume expansion was only effective in relieving symptoms in two of them. Drugs such as Florinef, which directly help to raise the blood pressure, are most commonly used as the next line of therapy, with or without associated beta-blockers to control palpitations. Toprol XL is my preferred beta-blocker, because it has a twenty-four-hour delivery system that prevents breakthroughs. Tenormin, another beta-blocker, can be a reasonable substitute, but it may need to be taken several times a day. Florinef with beta-blockers are a mainstay of treatment in patients who do not respond to more conservative measures of aggressive salt and fluid replacement. This was the case with Michelle that we discussed in Chapter 13, whose fatigue immediately improved after improving her adrenal status and raising her blood pressure.

Another drug that can help raise blood pressure with POTS is ProAmatine, and in my office we use this when Florinef fails a patient or when they cannot tolerate it. Like Florinef, it can also occasionally cause nausea, and rarely cause a rash.

Other therapies that have been shown to be beneficial in POTS are selective serotonin reuptake inhibitors (SSRIs), which are particularly helpful to MSIDS patients, since many also suffer from overlapping anxiety and depression, which SSRIs are usually prescribed for. This classification of drugs, which has been used in clinical trials for POTS, includes

Prozac, Zoloft, and Paxil. They are generally useful in combination with other approaches, such as Florinef, ProAmatine, and beta-blockers, with salt and fluid repletion. Dual reuptake selective serotonin inhibitors such as Cymbalta also have beneficial effects, including decreasing pain with associated fibromyalgia symptoms and neuropathy. Even though Cymbalta is only approved for diabetic neuropathy, we have found it to be useful for those patients with neuropathy associated with POTS and MSIDS. It is also more weight neutral than the other SSRIs and has less sexual side effects. The drug should be avoided in those patients with significant palpitations and anxiety, since Cymbalta can increase levels of both serotonin and norepinephrine, which can produce the same symptoms.

I also treat POTS with Catapres. I first learned to use it almost thirty years ago when I graduated from medical school. At that time it was one of the first-line treatments for hypertension. Catapres is a centrally acting blood pressure drug that acts on alpha receptors in the brain (brain stem), which results in decreased levels of norepinephrine and epinephrine. Since many patients with POTS have high levels of norepinephrine, decreasing this hormone helps to balance out their autonomic nervous system dysfunction. I have had several patients with POTS who only felt better when Catapres was added to their regimen of Florinef.

Other drugs that are occasionally used in the medical literature to treat POTS are Diamox, Mestinon, and IV Procrit therapy. Mestinon is best known for its use in myasthenia gravis, an autoimmune disease that causes fluctuating periods of muscle weakness. Muscles contract when the neurotransmitter acetylcholine binds to receptors on the muscles, but in myasthenia there are anticholinesterase antibodies that block the acetylcholine receptors, preventing the muscles from working properly. Mestinon is an inhibitor of the enzyme that breaks down acetylcholine, raising its concentration at the receptor sites. It can overcome a blockade of acetylcholine by increasing the concentration locally. If a patient with Lyme-MSIDS has tested positively for ganglionic acetylcholine receptor antibodies, they may particularly benefit from use of Mestinon, especially if they have failed to get adequate results with other treatments.

IV Procrit (erythropoietin therapy) works on a different mechanism to help increase the blood pressure in POTS. Some patients have low intravascular fluid volume (hypovolemia) due to leakage of fluid from the blood vessels, or from pooling of the blood outside the vascular space. Increasing salt and water intake is not always enough to increase the amount of fluid circulating in the system. Erythropoietin increases the intravascular volume by working as a hormone at the level of the kidney to produce more red blood cells. This increases the volume circulating in the blood, and erythropoietin also has the ability to constrict blood vessels, thereby raising blood pressure. This is not a commonly used medication in POTS, however, and would only be used as a last resort if the patient has failed all other treatment regimens, since side effects of Procrit include warnings of increased risk of a heart attack (myocardial infarction), stroke, phlebitis (venous thromboembolism), and death.

There are also several natural methods that can help with autonomic nervous system dysfunction, including resistance training (to help with poor muscle tone) and compression stockings to help prevent blood pooling in the lower extremities. Both of these may be used in combination with some of the drug regimens discussed. Biofeedback training with meditation, to help retrain the autonomic nervous system, has also been useful in a select group of my patients with POTS. This is especially useful for those with high levels of circulating catecholamines, such as epinephrine and norepinephrine, which can increase palpitations and cause severe anxiety reactions. Combining the above natural therapies with medications provides a more comprehensive approach to help the resistant MSIDS patient with POTS get better. Oftentimes, when the underlying infections in MSIDS are adequately treated, these symptoms and those associated with POTS also improve.

Nancy Had POTS and Lyme

Nancy was forty-nine-years-old with a past medical history significant for an elevated level of mercury in the blood, allergic rhinitis, irritable bowel syndrome, and Lyme disease. She was first diagnosed with Lyme disease back in 1998 by a Lyme-literate physician. Other co-infection testing was negative except for prior *Mycoplasma* pneumonia exposure and a history of viral infections, including EBV, parvovirus, and HHV-6. Although she felt somewhat better after an initial course of doxycycline, she noticed that her health had taken a precipitous decline several years later after having two children in 2000 and 2003.

When I met Nancy she told me that after each of her children were born, she had severe postpartum depression and anxiety with resistant insomnia. Then, in 2007, she developed increased joint pain in the hips, shoulders, knees, and toes, with debilitating fatigue and dizziness. She went back to her primary care physician, who did another Lyme test that returned positive, and he placed her back on doxycycline, which was continued for several months, since she also suffered from a case of acne. She felt better physically after the course of the antibiotics but still had some resistant fatigue, and the antibiotics did not help the neuropsychiatric symptoms that had developed. She was still depressed despite going for counseling and taking Prozac, and now had developed significant headaches, memory and concentration problems, "vicious" insomnia that no medication helped, and "tremors" in her brain that were unexplained by her doctor or various specialists she had seen. She saw another Lyme-literate doctor in 2009, who felt that her symptoms were consistent with persistent Lyme disease, and tried her on different medication regimens. Unfortunately, when the dose of the doxycycline was increased to get better central nervous system penetration, her stomach couldn't handle the medication. She was tried on minocycline instead, but had a severe Jarisch-Herxheimer reaction. By this time she felt that she could not tolerate any further antibiotics, and went the complementary route. She saw Dr. Zhang, the Chinese medicine doctor who treats Lyme disease with Chinese herbs, and she did a TCM protocol for a year before coming to see us. She had clinically improved on his herbs, as 80 percent of her joint pain and palpitations were better, but she still had resistant fatigue, insomnia, and "brain tremors" as some of her worst symptoms.

We sent out a CBC, comprehensive metabolic profile, vitamin levels for her neuropathy, fatigue, and cognitive issues, co-infection panels to check for associated infections (especially *Babesia* and *Bartonella* to determine the cause of her severe neurological problems), as well as an autoimmune panel, immunoglobulin levels, hormone levels (thyroid, growth hormone, adrenal function, and sex hormones), mineral levels, food allergy testing, and a parasite panel. She came back positive for certain autoimmune markers. Although her ANA, rheumatoid factor, sedimentation rate, and CRP were normal, she was HLA DR4 positive and had a positive antiganglioside antibody, which I've seen in autoimmune peripheral neuropathy with Lyme and POTS. She also had highly elevated liver functions with no associated alcohol use, and no clear toxic exposure to explain the abnormality. Her hormone studies came back positive for a low IgF-1, consistent with possible growth hormone deficiency, and significantly elevated levels of cortisol in the morning and at night. The upper limit of cortisol at 10:00 P.M. is normally 0.5. She was 8.54, more than sixteen times above the normal range. This could have accounted for her resistant insomnia. She also came back positive for antigliadin antibodies with a negative TTG (consistent with gluten sensitivity), with a food allergy panel showing IgG antibodies at high levels against milk, wheat, beef, shrimp, and corn. Her vitamin levels were normal, but she was MTHFR positive with a slightly elevated homocysteine level. Finally, her six-hour urine DMSA challenge showed elevated levels of mercury and lead, and borderline elevated levels of thallium. We discussed rechecking her liver functions and sending out a liver profile for hepatitis A, B, and C, as well as checking for autoantibodies (ANA, AMA), alpha-1 antitrypsin deficiency, and for Wilson's disease (copper overload) and hemochromatosis (iron overload). All of these are diseases that can cause inflammation in the liver. These studies returned negative. We therefore sent her to see a gastroenterologist for a second opinion. Her endoscopy, colonoscopy, and ultrasound of the liver and gallbladder also returned within normal limits, and he could not find a cause for the elevated liver functions.

Nancy was placed on nutritional supplements to support the liver detox pathways (NAC, alpha-lipoic acid, magnesium, milk thistle), and was tried on the herbs Samento and Banderol for her Lyme disease, since she was wary of taking antibiotics. I also wanted to start with the gentlest protocol, because of her elevated liver functions. We placed her on vitamin B_6, methyl B_{12}, and activated folic acid for her positive MTHFR gene status with an elevated homocysteine, as well as Trazodone for sleep with L-theanine and phosphatidylserine to decrease the elevated cortisol levels at night.

Nancy returned one month later. She was flaring on the herbs for her Lyme disease with increased sweats, palpitations, and joint pain, although her headaches, paresthesias, and memory/concentration problems had improved somewhat on this regimen. Her liver functions remained elevated, although slightly decreased from her initial visit. Her sleep was better with the Trazodone, as she went from sleeping two hours to five to six hours a night, but she still did not feel refreshed in the morning, and complained of frequent awakening, fatigue, dizziness, agitation, anxiety, depression, and resistant "brain tremors" that would bother her day and night. We tried her on Sonata for the frequent awakening, with Lunesta at bedtime for sleep, discussed a stricter sugar-free diet to prevent hypoglycemic swings, which could contribute to her fatigue and insomnia, discussed getting off all gluten and allergic foods, and instructed her to check her home for mold: another possible cause for her unusual neurological symptoms. She was also given a trial of oral glutathione for detoxification, since she had resistant neurological symptoms, and her elevated liver functions could represent problems with detoxing chemicals from the environment. Finally, we rotated her to a different herbal regimen for her Lyme disease, since she was flaring with the Samento, and switched her to the Byron White herbal protocol instead.

I received a call from Nancy several weeks later, informing me that they had indeed found mold in her home in New Jersey. Once she moved out, we checked her liver functions several weeks later. They had decreased down to normal. She also found that her muscle and joint pain had improved, and that her fatigue was somewhat better, although still far from normal. Her insomnia was still severe, especially around the second half of her menstrual cycle, and was not responding to the Lunesta, Sonata, Trazodone, and herbs. From days seventeen to twenty-eight of her menstrual cycle she could not fall asleep, and had ongoing complaints of dizziness, increased agitation, anxiety, palpitations, and worsening cognitive difficulties.

On her next office visit I noticed something strange. Her blood pressure had always been in the normal range ($^{110}/_{72}$), but this time it was $^{98}/_{68}$ sitting, with a resting pulse rate of 68, and her standing blood pressure dropped to $^{84}/_{62}$, with a pulse rate in the low 80s. She also felt slightly dizzy upon standing. This was not a severe reaction by any means, but it did make me question whether Nancy was suffering from a mild case of POTS and autonomic nervous system dysfunction, which would account for some of her resistant symptoms.

We discussed going for a head-up tilt-table test at a university center to confirm the diagnosis of POTS, but she was not emotionally ready to subject herself to more tests. We therefore tried adjusting her medication instead. We first discussed changing her Trazodone to Lyrica at bedtime to try and help with the sleep. Next, I wanted her to try the herb crypto-lepis for her resistant sweats. Her *Babesia* testing was negative, but she had normal sex hormone levels, and there was no way to easily explain her resistant sweating. Either she had an infection with *Babesia* (or other piroplasm), which was increasing all of her symptoms, such as the resis-tant fatigue, sweats, joint pain, memory and concentration problems, and sleep disorder, and/or she suffered from autonomic nervous system dys-function. This could also account for the resistant fatigue, dizziness, pal-pitations, anxiety, insomnia, sweats, and cognitive problems she could not seem to get rid of. We therefore suggested a trial of licorice and Flori-nef while increasing her salt and fluid intake (to a minimum of two to three liters per day) and recommended an endocrine consultation to evaluate the low IgF-1 to determine if a growth hormone deficiency was an over-lapping factor contributing to her chronic fatigue.

Nancy returned several months later after following this last protocol. She was elated to report that for the first time in years she was feeling great. Almost all of her symptoms were finally gone, and within one week of starting the Florinef, she started to feel better. Her sleep, fatigue, and dizziness improved, and the resistant "brain tremors" that she com-plained about for years were gone.

She also found that two other suggestions made a big difference. The first was that the hypoglycemic diet stabilized her energy and improved her concentration. The second was that her sweats were now gone after taking the cryptolepis. At the last visit, Nancy told me that she saw a gy-necological endocrinologist who ran all her hormones, and they all came back within normal limits. The resolution of the sweats was probably due to our treating a parasitic infection with *Babesia* or a *Babesia*-type piro-plasm, which was helped by the antimalarial herb. We discussed as the final and last step starting the chelation process to remove her elevated levels of mercury and lead.

Nancy clearly suffered from MSIDS. She had multiple overlapping factors that were responsible for her illness, including infections with Lyme disease, *Babesia*, hormonal imbalances, a severe sleep disorder, food allergies and gluten sensitivity, heavy metals, and mold toxicity. Yet it was the autonomic nervous system dysfunction that was having some of the strongest impact on her resistant symptoms. Until she increased the salt and fluids in her diet and took the licorice and Florinef, we were not seeing the clinical improvements that we were hoping for with her prior rotation of regimens. Her fatigue and dizziness immediately improved after the Florinef, as did her sleep, and this was independent of other changes in her sleep medications. Even the brain tremors that she suffered with for years that were puzzling neurologists went away within one week on the Florinef. It was nothing short of miraculous. Diagnosing and treating autonomic nervous system dysfunction and POTS is one of the essential points on the MSIDS map that is crucial in getting some chronically ill patients with resistant symptoms back on the road to health.

FIFTEEN

Lyme and Allergies

ood allergies and/or sensitivities are extremely common and can be an unrecognized cause for chronic health issues. You may have noticed that many of the patients discussed in the book have been diagnosed with allergic reactions to foods, where these reactions were a contributing factor in their underlying symptomatology. Their symptoms overlap many other disease processes, and they are a common complaint among individuals with low adrenal function and chronic inflammation, as well as in patients with chronic fatigue syndrome, fibromyalgia, EI, and Lyme disease.

There are five main types of antibodies in our bodies that help protect us from foreign invaders. Allergies may present as two different types of hypersensitivity reactions, known as immediate hypersensitivity reactions (due to IgE antibodies) or a delayed hypersensitivity reactions (due to IgG antibodies). IgE-mediated food allergies play a role in acute, severe reactions to foods. These are called type I allergic reactions and cause a range of symptoms, from mild to severe life-threatening anaphylactic reactions, including swelling of the tongue and throat, urticaria/hives, and severe asthmatic reactions with airway closure. IgE-related food allergies can be life-threatening, and affect approximately 1.4 percent of the total population, the most common allergen being peanuts. Unfortunately, IgE testing does not identify all patients with peanut allergies, and there are reports in the scientific literature that some patients can develop adult onset allergies, even if they never suffered from this problem in childhood. Adults with a known history of life-threatening allergies are careful to avoid the offending foods, as food allergies are responsible for up to half of food related deaths in this country.

An allergic reaction takes place because of the interaction between the allergens, IgE antibodies, and mast cells, which are part of our immune system. IgE antibodies are found on mast cells, and mast cells remain inactive until an allergen binds to the IgE receptor sites. An allergic reaction is triggered when an allergen binds to IgE antibodies. When this happens, it causes the release of histamines and cytokines, and causes a dilation of small blood vessels and increases their permeability, which together causes pain, itching, swelling (edema), redness, and warmth, and attract other inflammatory cells to the site of release.

Inside the gastrointestinal tract, an allergic food can come into contact with IgE on the surface of a mast cell and cause an inflammatory reaction that releases histamines as well as inflammatory cytokines. These chemicals can increase intestinal permeability and allow allergens to move into the bloodstream and throughout the body, causing widespread inflammation that leads to anaphylaxis and shock. This entire process can take place within a few minutes of getting a bee sting or ingesting the offending food, although occasionally it can take several hours for a severe reaction to take place.

A second type of food or chemically related reaction is much more common. This is a delayed hypersensitivity reaction (IgG). It is estimated that 80 percent to 85 percent of food allergy/sensitivity reactions are due to IgG antibodies. These cause a delayed reaction, which occurs between twenty-four and forty-eight hours after ingestion of the offending agent, and therefore may not be recognized as a cause of the symptoms. Most individuals would not suspect that their resistant symptoms can be due to food allergies, which is why it is so important to be tested if you have any of the medical problems discussed below.

Scientific studies have shown that symptoms may include:

- Arthritis
- Bed-wetting associated with childhood hyperactivity
- Bladder pain
- Constipation and/or diarrhea

- Eczema and urticaria (hives)
- Fatigue
- Headaches, as well as migraines
- Indigestion and reflux
- Low blood pressure
- Mood swings, with either anxiety and depression
- Respiratory symptoms, with an increase in bronchospasm and asthma
- Stomach upset with abdominal pain

IgG-mediated food and food-chemical sensitivities are complex immune-mediated reactions that cause a cellular activation of other cells of the immune system called "basophils." Basophils are a type of white blood cell that also contains granules, like the mast cells. When basophils are in contact with an allergen, they similarly release histamine and other inflammatory chemical mediators, such as leukotrienes and prostaglandins, but part of their cellular reaction also includes the release of inflammatory cytokines, such as TNF-α, interleukin-1 (IL-1), and interleukin-6 (IL-6). These molecules are released as part of an immune response that causes smooth muscle contraction and swelling, and increases inflammation and pain. This can further exacerbate symptoms for those with Lyme-MSIDS, who already have ongoing inflammatory responses caused by these same cytokines. That is why we place our patients on an anti-inflammatory diet, test them for possible food allergies, and counsel them to avoid these foods so that they can properly heal.

A good starting point for an anti-inflammatory diet is to avoid the most common food allergens: wheat, eggs, dairy, and sugar. We find that the vast majority of our patients are sensitive to dairy, wheat, corn, eggs, nuts, and shellfish. I have found that just by avoiding these allergic foods, many of my patients feel better. Some patients notice that their fatigue, headaches, joint pain, and symptoms of allergic rhinitis, eczema, and asthma improve after eliminating their allergic foods (especially wheat, dairy, and sugar).

Some patients who come to see us are very ill, and have signs and symptoms of significant inflammation, with hot, swollen joints and elevated inflammatory markers in the blood. They also have high levels of inflammatory cytokines, as well as elevated levels of other inflammatory mediators, such as arachidonic acid, and need to be stricter with their diets. Arachidonic acid is produced from consuming foods that are high in omega-6 fatty acids (like red meat) and is a building block for other molecules (thromboxane A2, leukotriene B4, and all two series prostaglandins) that cause further inflammation in the body. (These molecules can be measured by specialized functional medicine laboratories, such as Metametrix.) These patients need to follow a stricter anti-inflammatory diet, decreasing red meats and dairy products while increasing sources of omega-3 fatty acids (especially fatty fish, such as sardines and salmon, which have high levels of DHA), which are anti-inflammatory. Consuming more omega-3 fatty acids helps to decrease production of proinflammatory molecules. This will be discussed in detail in Chapter 19.

Some of my patients also need to avoid the nightshade family of vegetables (potatoes, tomatoes, eggplants, and peppers), because these foods can trigger arthritis symptoms. And for some patients, although they do not have true celiac disease, we have found that they are gluten sensitive and feel better avoiding grains in their diet, such as wheat, kamut, spelt, barley, rye, malts, and triticale. Gluten is also used as a food additive and thickening agent, and can be found in ingredient labels as "dextrin." Many of my patients with gluten sensitivity do not have positive tests for the specific markers for celiac disease (antigliadin antibodies and tissue transglutaminase), while some are antigliadin positive (low, medium, or high levels of antibodies) and are TTG negative (a specific marker for celiac disease). Anyone who has resistant arthritic symptoms and bowel issues should try a diet free of nightshades and gluten for at least two to four weeks to see if symptoms improve.

Some people with gluten sensitivities can also be deficient in secretory IgA (sIgA). This antibody is the first line of defense against gastrointestinal pathogens and forms immune complexes with food allergens to prevent them from being absorbed into the body. If the patient has low levels of secretory IgA (fecal sIgA can be tested, as can salivary levels of it), the GI mucosal barrier may be compromised, which allows allergic foods to enter the body more easily. Celiac disease also involves IgA pathology, due to the presence of antibodies against this particular immunoglobulin, further increasing allergic reactions to foods. This will be discussed in detail in Chapter 16.

Foods that contain artificial food dyes, flavorings, and preservatives can also cause food intolerances. Some integrative doctors specializing in pediatrics believe that eliminating artificial food dyes, flavors, and preservatives that are petroleum-based (BHA, DHT, TBHQ) from the diet can be helpful in sensitive children with enuresis (bed-wetting), frequent earaches, sleep disorders, asthma, and neurological symptoms, including ADHD. This elimination diet is referred to as the Feingold Diet, and has been reported to be helpful in some young children with the above symptoms. Children are usually the most sensitive to these food additives, since food dyes can cross the blood-brain barrier more easily in the younger population.

Some people have been shown to be sensitive to salicylates (the primary ingredient in aspirin), which can cause all of the above symptoms as well as nasal polyp formation and increased asthmatic symptoms. This occurs in up to 10 percent of the population. These people may need to eliminate (at least initially) salicylate-containing foods. This is difficult, as salicylates are found in most plants, as well as in many preservatives and medications.

A diet free of common antigens (an oligoantigenic diet) is more commonly prescribed, and has been used to treat attention deficit disorder, migraines, and arthritis effectively in adults. Once you remove common allergens from the diet, you may find that inflammation significantly decreases, leading to improvement in common chronic health conditions.

There has been a lot of debate about the efficacy of this approach over the last thirty years, and many in the medical establishment and the pharmaceutical and food industries have dismissed its claims. I can certainly attest to the fact that many patients in my practice with chronic resistant symptoms of fatigue, headaches, muscle and joint pain, and allergy symptoms who have failed to find a cause for their symptoms and have failed pharmaceutical drugs have definitely improved with this approach. In those patients who also suffer from chemical sensitivity and environmental illness (EI), eliminating chemicals and preservatives from their diet and periodically detoxifying from other chemicals also helps reverse certain resistant musculoskeletal and neurological symptoms.

TESTING FOR FOOD ALLERGIES

Some allergists will do conventional skin testing with RAST tests to measure IgE-mediated reactions. Although this can be helpful, it cannot identify the delayed, non-IgE-mediated reactions, such as those we see with IgG antibodies. I routinely order both an IgE and IgG food allergy panel to test for immediate and delayed hypersensitivity reactions. Occasionally the patient will have an immediate (IgE) reaction to a food but not have an IgG reaction, or vice versa.

Other tests to consider include a comprehensive digestive stool analysis (CDSA) to look at the digestion and absorption of foods while also looking at the levels of beneficial or harmful bacteria, yeast, and parasites present in the GI tract. This test can be done through functional medicine laboratories such as Metametrix/Genova Diagnostics, and Doctor's Data. An intestinal permeability test can also be used as a means to help diagnose food allergies, along with a salivary or fecal secretory IgA (sIgA) level. Anyone who suffers from inflammation in the GI tract (from *Candida*, for example) may develop leaky gut and have high intestinal permeability, where macromolecules of food in the GI tract are directly absorbed into the body, stimulating allergic reactions and increasing sensitivities to foods. We discussed earlier how secretory IgA is necessary to help form immune complexes with food allergens to prevent them from being absorbed into the body. If testing shows both low sIgA levels and high intestinal permeability, then the likelihood of having leaky gut and multiple food sensitivities is much higher. There is also a molecule in the blood called zonulin that can be measured, and which will indicate current damage to the bowel wall and point to leaky gut. Zonulin acts as "glue" between the cells of the lining of the intestine, and its presence can precede the development of food allergies by nearly three years.

TREATING ALLERGIES AND SENSITIVITIES

The only effective treatment for food allergies and sensitivities is avoidance. The offending allergens must be removed from the diet for at least three months before they can be added back in, via a rotation diet.

Beginning in the first three months, my goal is to correct any imbalances in the microbial flora, heal a damaged intestinal mucosa, and reestablish proper digestion. To maintain bowel health, we usually give high-dose probiotics with *Lactobacillus* and *Bifidobacterium* to replace the beneficial bacteria in the gut, as well as using *Saccharomyces boulardii* to help prevent antibiotic-associated diarrhea. As I've mentioned before, we find high-dose probiotics and occasionally the use of prebiotics with fructooligosaccharides (FOS) to be extremely beneficial in maintaining bowel health when patients are on long-term antibiotics for Lyme-MSIDS. I rarely see antibiotic-associated diarrhea if patients are compliant with this regimen.

I also recommend GI nutritional products that support bowel health. These often contain: combinations of amino acids (glutamine, glycine); vitamins and minerals; anti-inflammatory herbs, such as turmeric and quercetin; NAC and sodium sulfate, for detox support; inulin (from chicory) and arabinogalactans, to help with the production of short-chain fatty acids, which helps decrease intestinal inflammation. I use products containing DGL (D-glycerinated licorice) with aloe vera and glutamine to help heal the stomach and intestines, especially for those with associated leaky gut syndrome. DGL helps to form a mucus barrier in the stomach, aloe vera soothes the stomach, and glutamine helps prevent intestinal mucosal damage and stimulates the repair of the damaged intestinal wall.

I will prescribe enzyme therapies when there is a clear deficiency. Pancreatic enzymes and/or oral betaine hydrochloride will occasionally be needed by those who have associated stomach acid issues, causing poor digestion. A Heidelberg gastric analysis test may be considered if achlorhydria (lack of stomach acid) or hypochlorhydria (decreased stomach acid) is suspected, and a CDSA test may also pick up evidence of pancreatic insufficiency.

After three months of avoiding the allergic foods and allowing the gut to heal, a rotation diet reintroduces foods in a methodical manner. This is done by introducing one previously offending food every three days, keeping a food diary, and recording your health status, so that any adverse reactions can be adequately monitored. Rotation diets can help identify each of the sources of ongoing inflammation that are causing cytokine release and the sickness syndrome in patients with Lyme-MSIDS.

Once we have initially identified and removed all of the allergens from the diet, the next step is to find a healthy nutritional program that can be followed for life. I recommend an anti-inflammatory Mediterranean diet, rich in fresh fruits and vegetables, with smaller portions of red meat, eggs, and dairy (decreased omega-6 fatty acids), healthy fats (increased amounts of omega-3 fatty acids in fish, and increased amounts of omega-9 fatty acids in olive oil), and low in simple carbohydrates.

I have found that this is another dietary modification that helps many of my patients feel better. Increasing the amounts of omega-3 fatty acids in the diet and decreasing the amounts of omega-6 fatty acids is beneficial, since omega-6 fatty acids increase the production of arachidonic acid, increasing inflammation. Lowering the carbohydrate content of meals with a Mediterranean diet also helps, because sugar in carbohydrates drives insulin production and causes metabolic syndrome, whereby elevated blood sugars and associated insulin resistance increase the inflammatory response.

For those who have been diagnosed with hypoglycemia, metabolic syndrome, and/or type II diabetes, I recommend a very low carbohydrate diet, featuring smaller, more frequent meals. Each meal or snack should have a balance of protein (40 percent), complex carbohydrates (30 percent), and healthy fats (30 percent) to avoid swings of blood sugar with high insulin secretion. Reactive hypoglycemia is extremely common in my medical practice and is often a manifestation of metabolic syndrome. Those who suffer from resistant fatigue, headaches, dizziness, palpitations, mood swings, and insomnia might benefit the most. We find that at least half of our patients suffer from reactive hypoglycemia, and its symptoms overlap those of multiple food allergies, as well as those of non-Lyme-MSIDS (especially *Candida*, with adrenal dysfunction) and Lyme-MSIDS. Lyme disease symptoms are also exacerbated during blood sugar swings. A five-hour glucose tolerance test may be necessary to diagnose reactive hypoglycemia for those with resistant symptoms.

Others may need to follow a stricter *Candida* diet, especially if their CDSA test shows elevated levels of yeast in the colon. This type of diet eliminates vinegars, mushrooms, fermented foods, most fruits, and all simple carbohydrates. *Candida* can cause inflammation in the colon and lead to a leaky gut and subsequent food allergies. A course of Diflucan, followed by nystatin and high-dose probiotics, may be necessary in certain resistant groups of patients.

Leigh and Eddie Had Silent Food Allergies

Leigh is a fifty-six-year-old female who came to see me several years ago with a past medical history significant for chronic fatigue, migraines, ADD, with concentration difficulties, some mild neck and shoulder discomfort, dizziness, chronic constipation, gastrointestinal complaints of frequent gas and bloating, and a history of *Candida*. Her constipation was so bad that she frequently had bleeding hemorrhoids, and once required surgery for a rectal fissure. She had been diagnosed with chronic Epstein-Barr for her chronic fatigue and irritable bowel syndrome for her constipation, and she had a history of hypothyroidism and low adrenal function from when she was in her twenties. She was off all medication and glandular supplements by the time she came to see me. Leigh had no recollection of a tick bite but grew up on Long Island and remembers being sick quite often in her childhood. The only thing that was significant in her family history was that one of her parents had colitis.

Her physical exam revealed a normal sitting blood pressure ($^{98}/_{64}$), which went down to $^{84}/_{52}$ after standing for one minute, with an increase in heart rate of twenty beats per minute. This suggested to me that her dizziness was related to POTS, with autonomic nervous system dysfunction. Her skin and hair were particularly dry, and she had decreased Achilles tendon reflexes, which is suggestive of hypothyroidism. We did blood tests to evaluate her fatigue and headaches, which returned positive for a mild anemia, and she had an elevated TSH, confirming the diagnosis of hypothyroidism. Her adrenal testing with a DHEA/cortisol level showed extremely low cortisol levels in the morning, and tick-borne testing returned positive for Lyme disease, babesiosis and *Bartonella*, and she had a positive PCR for *Mycoplasma fermentans*. We also sent off for a food allergy panel and antigliadin antibodies to check for celiac disease and associated food sensitivities, given her GI complaints. It returned positive for antigliadin antibodies with a negative TTG (suggestive of gluten intolerance but not true celiac disease), and her food allergy panel revealed multiple sensitivities, the highest being dairy, wheat, yeast, peanuts, and corn allergies, on an IgG delayed hypersensitivity panel. I told Leigh that her symptoms were caused by MSIDS: She had Lyme disease and associated tick-borne disorders; adrenal dysfunction, with POTS; hypothyroidism; food allergies/sensitivities; and probable *Candida* syndrome with hypoglycemia, all of which were making her sick.

We started Leigh on adrenal support with Adapten-All (which contains B vitamins, pantothenic acid, rhodiola, and ashwagandha), an adrenal glandular extract (she did not want to take low-dose hydrocortisone), Florinef, and Synthroid with Cytomel for her hormonal imbalances. She was given several rotations of antibiotics for the Lyme disease and coinfections. The Plaquenil with Minocin for the Lyme disease and herbs for the babesiosis (artemesinin) was particularly effective in helping her fatigue and cognitive difficulties, as was the Florinef (she tried stopping it on several occasions and felt much worse). Magnesium was also given with extra fluids for her chronic constipation.

When Leigh came back a few weeks later, she reported that one of the greatest improvements in her health took place when she changed her diet. We had instructed Leigh to follow a strict diet for *Candida*, with avoidance of her food allergens. She took powdered nystatin, gradually increasing the dose, while avoiding sugar, yeast, dairy, wheat, and corn. Leigh told me that within one month of starting this regimen, her energy was significantly better, her migraines had disappeared (which she had suffered from since childhood), her neck and shoulder discomfort had decreased, her cognition improved, and for the first time in over twenty years, she no longer had chronic constipation and bowel problems. She felt like a new woman. She also noticed that every time she cheated on her diet and ate sugar, dairy, or wheat, her bowel problems returned, as did her chronic fatigue, muscle pain, and migraines. Food sensitivities were definitely playing a large role in keeping Leigh sick.

Her response to my regimen was so significant that her husband, Eddie, decided to also be checked for food allergies. He had suffered from allergic rhinitis (seasonal allergies) and asthma since childhood and required regular use of antihistamines and asthma medications. He also had a history of midday fatigue like Leigh, with occasional headaches upon awakening. His food allergy profile returned positive for multiple IgG delayed reactions to foods, the most significant ones being to dairy, and he had low-level allergies to wheat, corn, and eggs. We sent him for a five-hour glucose tolerance test to rule out reactive hypoglycemia, and this came back significantly positive. He was then also instructed to avoid all of his allergic foods, especially dairy, and to strictly avoid all simple carbohydrates, eat small frequent meals, with protein, complex carbohydrates, and fats throughout the day.

Eddie returned one month later with Leigh. Although he still required the daily use of over-the-counter antihistamines, such as Allegra or Claritin, his allergy and asthma symptoms were much better. There was less sneezing and dripping on the antihistamines, and he no longer required the use of his asthma spray. Sneezing and wheezing only recurred when he fell off his diet and ate dairy. His energy level was also greatly improved, and his headaches disappeared as long as he avoided sweets and did not miss meals. He and Leigh were amazed by the fact that previously they had had no idea how sensitive they were to their allergic foods, and how strong a role diet played in their health, and in contributing to their chronic physical symptoms.

Food allergies and sensitivities are other hidden sources of inflammation that continue to exacerbate the symptoms of MSIDS patients until they are uncovered. A comprehensive food allergy panel needs to be included in every initial evaluation for those with chronic, unexplained symptoms. We find that a large percentage of our patients finally regain a sense of well-being when they determine which foods are making them feel sick. By eliminating these specific food allergens, gluten, and nightshade vegetables, reducing their intake of simple sugars and foods containing yeast, and eating small frequent meals, they no longer experience many of the symptoms that they had lived with for years.

SIXTEEN

Lyme and Gastrointestinal Health

astrointestinal disorders are a frequent health-related complaint, whether or not they are related to Lyme and associated tick-borne diseases. Digestive disorders have been cited as the second leading cause of absenteeism from the workplace, and irritable bowel syndrome (IBS) alone has been estimated to account for up to 50 percent of all patient visits in ambulatory GI departments. To understand the magnitude of GI disorders affecting the American population, we simply need to look at the numbers reported from NIH studies. In the United States, sixty million to seventy million people have diagnosable digestive disorders; over a quarter of a million people die from GI diseases (including cancer) yearly; and there are over one hundred million outpatient visits every year to gastroenterologists. The most common GI condition is IBS (irritable bowel syndrome), followed by gastroesophageal reflux disease (GERD), gastric and peptic ulcer disease, inflammatory bowel disease (IBD, including Crohn's and ulcerative colitis), and celiac disease (sensitivity to gluten). Yet despite modern advances in medicine—antispasmodics (drugs that decrease spasms in the intestines) for IBS, anti-inflammatory medicines with biological modifiers for IBD (such as Crohn's disease), proton pump inhibitors such as Prilosec (which decrease acid secretion) for GERD, and antibiotic treatment of *H. pylori* for ulcer disease (an infection in the stomach)—many do not find complete relief with these treatments.

Patients with Lyme-MSIDS often present with gastrointestinal problems, including intermittent abdominal pain, nausea, gas, bloating, constipation, diarrhea, or reflux disease, with occasional vomiting. Although these symptoms may be linked to the common GI problems mentioned above or due to other causes, such as food intolerances or gynecological issues (i.e., painful ovarian cysts or endometriosis), these symptoms can also overlap with some of the symptoms of Lyme disease and tick-borne disorders. For example, a review of gastrointestinal and liver problems associated with tick-borne diseases found that in 5 percent to 23 percent of those with early Lyme borreliosis, patients presented with varied gastrointestinal symptoms, such as nausea, vomiting, abdominal pain, anorexia with loss of appetite, and hepatitis, and some even had symptoms of an enlarged liver and spleen. Diarrhea was rare, accounting for only 2 percent of cases.

Just as Lyme disease can be the great imitator, we see that other tick-borne co-infections can also present with varied gastrointestinal manifestations:

• *Borrelia hermsii* can cause nausea, vomiting, abdominal pain, hepatitis, jaundice, and an enlarged spleen. Diarrhea occurred in 19 percent of these infections, and vomiting of blood (hematemesis) or bloody diarrhea rarely occurred.

• Ehrlichiosis occasionally presents with gastrointestinal symptoms of nausea, vomiting, abdominal pain, and jaundice, especially in the early stages of this disease. Diarrhea occurs in up to 10 percent of patients with ehrlichiosis, and can even be one of the primary manifestations.

• Rickettsial diseases (Rocky Mountain spotted fever and Q fever) can cause gastrointestinal symptoms early in the course of the illness, including abdominal pain and tenderness, with vomiting, which when associated with elevations in liver enzymes can be mistaken for other inflammatory diseases of the GI tract, such as hepatitis, appendicitis, peritonitis (inflammation in the abdominal cavity), and cholangitis (inflammation in the gallbladder). Often the classical rash on the hands and soles of the feet with RMSF may follow the abdominal complaints, mistaking these symptoms for gastroenteritis. Gastrointestinal hemorrhage has also been reported for RMSF, due to inflammation in the blood vessels.

• Tularemia can present in several common forms: an ulcero-glandular form (ulcers on the skin with enlarged lymph nodes), an oculo-glandular form (eye symptoms, such as conjunctivitis, with enlarged lymph nodes), as well as the typhoidal form. The last form may cause nausea, vomiting, abdominal pain, and diarrhea, which can be severe in up to 40 percent of cases.

It is therefore the job of the medical detective to determine whether we are dealing with a primary gastrointestinal manifestation of Lyme disease and associated tick-borne infections, or whether there are other overlapping causes for these symptoms. This is where the MSIDS map becomes an extremely useful tool for determining all of the factors impacting gastrointestinal health.

JENA SUFFERED WITH RESISTANT GERD

Jena was forty-nine years old when she came to our medical office for a Lyme consult. She lived in New York and told me that she "pulls ticks off all the time." She had a past medical history significant for: intermittent hypertension; mild hyperlipidemia (elevated cholesterol and triglycerides, and a low HDL cholesterol); metabolic syndrome, with glucose intolerance; recent weight gain; and a history of Lyme and babesiosis, which started about three years before her consultation with me. Lyme and *Babesia* symptoms included drenching day and night sweats, fatigue, especially prominent at 3:00 P.M.; occasional palpitations; eye twitching; migraines several times per month; and an upset stomach. She also had a history of terrible GERD symptoms, with acid reflux that caused her to have a raspy voice, and at night she complained of burning in her esophagus, which interfered with her sleep.

When she started having symptoms of joint pain and increased skin sensitivity, Jena went to her physician, who diagnosed her with Lyme disease despite a negative blood test. He placed her on doxycycline, and within days she had a severe Jarisch-Herxheimer flare with increased fatigue, aching in the lower extremities, and increased brain fog. Then a large rash appeared near her groin. The rash was consistent with an EM rash, and it eventually disappeared, but she still had ongoing fatigue, day and night sweats, joint pain, and mild cognitive deficits. Her family history was significant for her mother having had carotid surgery for carotid stenosis at an early age, a sister who has diabetes and heart disease, as well as having had a cancerous polyp removed from her colon, and a father who suffered with diabetes and had a heart attack with a quadruple bypass.

My physical examination of Jena was unremarkable, although we found a borderline blood pressure reading at $^{142}/_{82}$ and swollen red nasal turbinates (swollen nasal passages) consistent with severe allergic rhinitis. Her laboratory results showed elevated liver functions with signs of mild inflammation (transaminitis), *Borrelia*-specific bands on the Western blot, with a strongly positive *Babesia* WA1 from LabCorp, and elevated inflammatory markers. I believed that Jena suffered from ongoing symptoms of Lyme disease and babesiosis, but we needed to rule out early menopause, since the sweats could have been an indicator of estrogen deficiency (she had just stopped having her period), and her thyroids were normal. We therefore tested her FSH, LH, estradiol, progesterone, and testosterone levels, and she was also sent for a Dual-energy X-ray absorptiometry (DEXA) scan to evaluate her for bone loss, which can be seen in early menopause.

Other tick-borne disorders were considered to explain her elevated liver functions, such as *Ehrlichia* and RMSF, but she had already had a course of doxycycline, which should have been adequate to cover these organisms. Infections such as *Borrelia hermsii* and Q fever were also considered for the elevated liver functions, as well as *Bartonella*. Her prior physician had tested for VEGF (vascular endothelial growth factor), which was elevated, a metabolic marker that suggested a possible associated *Bartonella* infection. For her GI symptoms, we checked her for *H. pylori*, given her history of GERD and stomach problems, sent off a food panel to see if there were allergens that could have been triggering her migraines and eczema, and instructed her to go for a colonoscopy. A DHEA/cortisol test was sent to evaluate her for adrenal fatigue, as she had ongoing symptoms of fatigue and clinical reactive hypoglycemia, with midday energy swings. Finally, a six-hour urine DMSA challenge was sent off to check for heavy metals (she worked with paints and had possible cadmium exposure).

I suggested that Jena begin a comprehensive weight loss program while we waited for the test results, consisting of a significant restriction of simple carbohydrates and small frequent meals to balance her blood sugars and help reduce her high cardiovascular risks (especially considering her strong family history for diabetes, strokes, and heart attacks), and she was instructed to eat organic foods with more cruciferous vegetables (broccoli, cauliflower, brussel spouts, and kale), given her family history of colon cancer.

Laboratory results from her initial consultation confirmed early menopause with elevated FSH and LH and low estradiol and progesterone, and her DEXA scan was positive for osteopenia and bone loss. Lyme disease testing showed a positive Western blot, and tests for co-infections returned positive for *Babesia* WA-1 and exposure to *Mycoplasma pneumonia*, *Chlamydia pneumonia*, and she had a positive West Nile exposure. Screening for hepatitis A, B, and C were negative, and her liver functions returned to normal on antibiotic therapy, implying a tick-borne cause for the elevated liver functions (transaminitis).

H. pylori testing was negative for her upper gastrointestinal symptoms, but her food panel returned positive for multiple allergens. She had a moderate allergy to egg whites, according to the IgE test, and an IgG food panel showed multiple allergens, all in the high range. She had significant delayed hypersensitivity reactions to grains such as barley, oats, corn, rye, and wheat, and allergies to eggs, dairy, soy, peanuts, beef, pork, chicken, fish, and yeast. These allergens were probably a result of leaky gut syndrome. I instructed her to take nutritional supplements to help heal the gut (OptiCleanse GHI, by Xymogen, with flaxseed complex, alpha linoleic acid, betaine, quercetin, potassium D-glucarate, turmeric, NAC, ginger, watercress powder, green tea extract with L-glutamine, and medium chain triglycerides) and told her to strictly avoid her food allergens until her next visit. She was placed on a three-day course of Coartem for the babesiosis, followed by the herb cryptolepis for the day and night sweats, since the sweats could have been due to early menopause and a simultaneous chronic *Babesia* infection.

When Jena returned two months later she had lost five pounds by following our low-carb diet, and she had seen a nutritionist to help her to find other foods to eat, since she had so many food allergies. To Jena's amazement, the GERD symptoms disappeared once she avoided the allergic foods and started taking the supplements, including high-dose probiotics. The burning in her chest from her reflux had completely disappeared, and she no longer felt the urge to regularly clear her throat. She also noticed that her frequent migraines resolved while she was off her allergic foods, her eczema improved, and her energy levels were more stable with a hypoglycemic diet. She even reported having less viral episodes and upper respiratory infections. Her only adverse reaction was a flare of symptoms with her antiparasitic treatment for the *Babesia*, which temporarily caused muscle and joint pain in the hips and knees as well as on the bottom of her feet, along with an increase in her migraines. However, once she went on the cryptolepis for the *Babesia*, all resistant symptoms improved, including her sweats, palpitations, and residual light sensitivity and sleep problems. She felt remarkably better. The MSIDS map uncovered the cause for her resistant symptoms and long-standing GERD.

THE COMPLEX GI SYSTEM

One of the most important functions of the gut is to help with digestion of foods into essential amino acids, fatty acids, and carbohydrates. The gut also plays an important role in immunity. It is the largest organ of immune function in the body. The GI tract houses 80 percent of our immune system, and 70 percent of our lymphocytes, making it the first line of defense against infections. The GI tract also functions as a neuroendocrine organ. Every neurotransmitter from the central nervous system is found in the GI tract. Most of the body's serotonin, which is essential for healthy moods, as well as half of the body's norepinephrine, which is essential for proper functioning of the orthosympathetic nervous system (OS), is found in the gut. At the same time, the gut can hold as many as 100 trillion microbes, referred to as the microbiome. There are ten times more microbial cells than mammalian cells in the body, which means, from a cellular perspective, that our bodies are only 10 percent human—and that they're 90 percent microbial species!

Doctors engage in warfare against bacteria via antibiotics for common infections—urinary tract, sinus, and upper respiratory—without ever giving a thought to replacing the beneficial bacteria that are also destroyed. This indiscriminate killing leads to common problems such as yeast infections, and it may lead to antibiotic-associated diarrhea, including that of *Clostridium difficile*, which is particularly dangerous for immunocompromised individuals.

According to a 2012 *New York Times* report, from 2000 to 2009 the number of patients in the United States hospitalized due to *Clostridium difficile* infections more than doubled, from 139,000 to 336,600. This has a tremendous impact on morbidity and the length of hospital stays, and once *Clostridium difficile* is established, it precludes broad-spectrum antibiotics for other infections that the patient may be suffering from, such as Lyme disease. This is due to the fact that treating one bacterial infection with an antibiotic will potentially worsen the gastrointestinal imbalance with an overgrowth of yeast and the clostridial species responsible for the diarrhea. Yet it is not common practice to instruct patients to take probiotics and beneficial yeast, such as *Saccharomyces boulardii*, during and after antibiotic therapy, even though *Clostridium difficile* can be effectively prevented with just such a therapy.

Bacteria have also been linked to GI cancers, inflammatory bowel disease, and irritable bowel syndrome. Dysbiosis, which is an imbalance of healthy bacteria, yeast, and parasites in the gut, is not a new concept in medicine, but its relationship to many disease processes is now beginning to be understood in new ways. We've known for almost a century that GI flora and increased intestinal permeability were responsible for dermatologic and psychiatric disorders. Then, in the 1980s, it was shown that the GI flora may play a role in the development of arthritis and inflammatory bowel disease. In the late 1990s, a new concept was developed, called "small intestinal bacterial overgrowth" (SIBO), which was found to be one of the causes of irritable bowel syndrome. SIBO was later also found to be associated with chronic fatigue syndrome and fibromyalgia, which, as we have seen, are overlapping syndromes that share similar biochemical and pathological processes to Lyme-MSIDS. Here may be one of the missing links showing how dysbiosis and GI bacteria play an important role in contributing to these seemingly different disease processes that have similar clinical manifestations.

THE CYTOKINE CONNECTION

Gut flora directly impact the production of inflammatory cytokines, and are therefore essential silent contributors to Lyme-MSIDS symptoms. The Human Microbiome Project, the most ambitious survey of the human microbiome yet performed, has shown that the microbiomes of bacteria, viruses, and fungi are constantly interacting with our body, affecting our health.

Bacteria in our gut are now thought to be associated with Crohn's disease, ulcerative colitis, and asthma, as certain bacteria have been found to stimulate chronic low-grade inflammation, an integral part of these diseases. Exciting new research has shown that gut microbes may also shape metabolic and immune network activity, and ultimately influence the development of obesity and diabetes. This may be due to bacterial influences on nutrient absorption: They prolong the time food moves through the intestines, increase the cellular uptake of triglycerides and their subsequent storage into fat (a primary component of obesity and metabolic syndrome, precursors for diabetes) with altered tissue composition of fats in our body. Scientists are now connecting obesity to the gut ecosystem, for when scientists transfer bacteria from obese mice into lean ones, the lean ones put on weight. If the mice are then subjected to a diet that causes weight loss, the fecal flora of the obese mice change, now resembling the flora in the lean mice. Similar changes are seen in the human population. In a 2010 study, eighteen obese men with metabolic syndrome had fecal transplantation (a stool transplant) with bacteria from lean males. The fasting triglycerides of the obese men were reduced and their insulin sensitivity was increased at six weeks posttransplant. We have discussed in prior chapters that abdominal obesity and insulin resistance has been associated with the higher production of cytokines such as IL-6, which is one of the cytokines responsible for the sickness syndrome in Lyme disease.

The roles of bacteria in the gut, and their subsequent effects on cytokine production, even play a role in sleep. At midnight, when cortisol production should be low, bacterial peptides from GI flora stimulate the immune cells of our gastrointestinal tract (intestinal macrophages and T cells) to increase cytokine production and produce IL-1 and TNF-α. These cytokines stimulate non-REM sleep (early deep sleep), and later during the night, as IL-1 beta decreases, this helps to initiate the transformation from non-REM sleep to REM sleep. Some severely ill Lyme patients, who have high cortisol levels at night and can't fall asleep, will not produce the right types and levels of cytokines necessary for the induction of deep sleep, or produce too many cytokines, making them drowsy during the day (hypersomnolent).

The intestinal macrophages and T cells in the gut, and the types of bacteria present in the GI tract, also have an effect on which types of cytokines are produced, affecting sleep and inflammation. Although there are hundreds of different species of bacteria in our GI tracts, there are two major types of intestinal bacteria that are particularly important in cytokine production: *Lactobacilli* and bifidobacteria. Most strains of *Lactobacilli* are robust producers of the cytokines TNF-α, IFN-β, and IL-12, but most strains of bifidobacteria are weak cytokine producers. Bifidobacteria are able to decrease the production of cytokines from *Lactobacilli*, changing their immunological effects. It is therefore possible that by manipulating the types of intestinal bacteria in patients with diverse inflammatory diseases, we can also affect the cytokine production causing the underlying inflammation that is responsible for making them so ill. This would apply to those with non-Lyme and Lyme-MSIDS with overstimulated immune systems, as well as those with metabolic syndrome, obesity, diabetes, asthma, and diseases in which diarrhea is a primary component, such as irritable bowel syndrome and inflammatory bowel disease.

Diarrhea is known to be caused by several different cytokines: TNF-α and IL-6 directly correlate with both fever and the number of diarrheal episodes, and cytokines in general are directly involved in intestinal injury and the severity of the diarrhea. TNF-α is a central mediator of intestinal inflammation, and it is elevated in inflammatory bowel disease (IBD) as well as in Lyme.

Cytokines play a role in the infectious and noninfectious causes of diarrhea. This is seen in many community-based diarrheal outbreaks that are viral in origin, such as in rotavirus infections in children and adults and common bacterial food-borne infections due to *E. coli* 0:157, Salmonella, Shigella, Yersinia, and Campylobacter. These organisms can cause serious medical complications in immune-compromised individuals. They may present with sudden episodes of severe diarrhea, fever, nausea, vomiting, and blood in the stools, and may require prompt intervention with aggressive hydration and electrolyte replacement and appropriate antimicrobial therapy to prevent serious complications.

Since inflammatory cytokines have been associated with GI diseases, do Lyme flares worsen the bowel inflammation in IBD by further increasing systemic levels of cytokines? Does IBD with elevated cytokine production conversely worsen the symptomatology of Lyme disease? Down-regulation of cytokines is one of the primary treatments used in the management of Crohn's disease, and LDN (low-dose naltrexone) has now been recognized in the medical literature as being effective in helping to control the intestinal inflammation in Crohn's disease. We also find that LDN is extremely beneficial in controlling the symptoms of fibromyalgia in Lyme-MSIDS patients. It can be dangerous to try and decrease inflammation by giving a TNF-α blocker like Enbrel to a Crohn's disease patient with active Lyme disease, as these drugs may significantly worsen Lyme disease symptoms. However, LDN can help balance the immune response, as can the right types of probiotics, and these have the potential to decrease inflammation in patients who suffer simultaneously from both diseases.

GASTROINTESTINAL BACTERIA AND NEUROTOXINS

Gut bacteria can also secrete neurotoxins, and the most commonly known is ammonia, often found to be elevated in cirrhosis. Those patients with cirrhosis of the liver require a low-protein diet, since the enzyme urease induced in colonic bacteria, such as *Klebsiella*, *Proteus* and *Bacteroides*, break down urea to form ammonia, which is increased with a high-protein diet. The ammonia also raises stool pH, which has been associated with a higher risk for colon cancer. We occasionally see elevated levels of ammonia in Lyme-MSIDS patients, even without evidence of cirrhosis.

Other neurotoxins found in gut bacteria include D-lactic acid and octopamine, chemicals that are generated by the action of colonic bacteria on undigested protein. In patients with cirrhosis of the liver, these compounds enter the blood and contribute to the confusion and encephalopathy seen in liver failure. Some people with MSIDS also suffer from detoxification problems, and these chemicals may play a role in increasing cognitive difficulties in those with Lyme disease. We have already discussed the possible role of neurotoxins such as quinolinic acid, chloral hydrate, and mold neurotoxins in adversely affecting cognitive function-ing in the MSIDS population. Other biotoxins may include chemicals produced by living organisms (such as staph, strep, and certain blue-green algae), those from food (preservatives), and xenobiotics (chemicals such as dioxins and PCBs). Richie Shoemaker, MD, and others have found that these biotoxins affect the HPA axis and hypothalamus, lowering levels of hormones such as Leptin, MSH (melanocyte stimulating hormone), ADH (vasopressin/antidiuretic hormone), and VIP (vasointestinal peptide), re-sulting in increased pain, fatigue, and poor sleep, and that correcting these abnormalities (using drugs such as Questran, DDAVP Nasal Spray, VIP Nasal Spray) have provided clinical improvement. Further studies are required to determine the efficacy of this approach in varied patient groups, and if ammonia, D-lactic acid, and octopamine are also of signifi-cance in causing CNS symptoms for those with MSIDS.

Patients with MSIDS also occasionally suffer from systemic candidia-sis, and have been found to have elevated levels of alcohol in their blood even when they did not consume any. The sugar and yeast fermentation in the gut produced acetaldehyde, which was then converted into etha-nol, causing them to feel constantly drunk. This was first discovered in Japan and labeled "drunk disease." We need to include the gastrointesti-nal tract as a possible source of neurotoxins potentially affecting the cognitive symptoms in MSIDS.

MAINTAINING NORMAL GUT MICROFLORA

The *Lactobacilli* and bifidobacteria provide colonization resistance against other harmful organisms, stimulate GI immunity, produce vitamins and short-chain fatty acids, and aid in digestion and absorption. These short-chain fatty acids (SCFA) are important for colon health, as they play a role in sustaining the activity of normal colonic epithelial cells and help de-crease inflammation. We can increase the healthy bacteria in our gut by not only taking probiotics, but also by taking prebiotics with FOS (fruc-tooligosaccharides) and using fermented vegetables. This can be benefi-cial in patients suffering from inflammatory bowel disease with colitis or in patients who do not manage to maintain adequate levels of beneficial bacteria in the gut with the use of antibiotics and probiotics.

There are four major mechanisms responsible for keeping the proper balance of good bacteria in our GI tract. These include: gastric acid secretion; pancreatic enzyme secretion; small intestinal motility; and maintaining the proper structural integrity of the GI tract. When any or all of these four mechanisms are out of balance, we may develop GI-related diseases. For example, SIBO is an overgrowth of bacteria in the small intestine, yet bacteria should not normally be found there in any significant quantity. A deficiency of stomach acid permits harmful bacteria to pass through the stomach into the small intestine, contributing to dysbiosis and SIBO, and leads to chronic infection with *Helicobacter pylori*. Low acid secretion from the stomach (hypochlorhydria) results when the specialized cells of the stomach that make hydrochloric acid do not function efficiently enough, particularly when we get older: 50 percent of people over sixty years old may have hypochlorhydria. This is clinically important, as *H. pylori* was discovered as the cause for ulcer disease, and has also been found to be one of the contributing factors in gastric cancer and lymphoma.

Lowered stomach acid not only contributes to chronic infection with *H. pylori.*, we also need hydrochloric acid to help kill off other harmful bacteria. That would explain why patients on proton pump inhibitors for GERD have higher rates of diarrheal episodes with Salmonella and *Clostridium difficile*, and may contract hospital-acquired aspiration pneumonia. These harmful bacteria are no longer killed off effectively by adequate stomach acid. In fact, hypochlorhydria has been hypothesized to be related to many disease processes, from osteoporosis to iron deficiency anemia (due to poor absorption of minerals), and the medical literature has shown that proton pump inhibitors (PPIs) also contribute to hypomagnesemia (low magnesium levels). This can be dangerous in those with detoxification problems requiring magnesium, as well as in those with coronary artery disease and a history of cardiac arrhythmias who are already taking diuretics (water pills), which can further increase both potassium and magnesium loss. Magnesium loss with low potassium can contribute to arrhythmias, and low levels of magnesium can cause muscle spasms, bronchospasm (bronchoconstriction in asthma), and Raynaud's phenomenon (constriction of the peripheral circulation in cold weather). So although low stomach acid is not usually considered a problem by most physicians, we see that it can be linked to multiple disease processes, including SIBO.

The signs and symptoms of SIBO and dysbiosis include:

- Bloating and flatulence after meals
- Constipation
- Diarrhea
- Fatigue
- Indigestion
- Iron deficiency, with weak or cracked finger nails (poor absorption of minerals)
- Nausea
- Rectal itching
- Systemic reactions after eating with food intolerances
- Undigested food in the stool or greasy stools (suggestive of pancreatic enzyme deficiency)

The clinical workup would include: a CBC, a CMP, and hormone testing; checking for food allergies (IgG and IgE) and antigliadin antibodies, with a TTG (tissue transglutaminase, a specific test for celiac disease and gluten sensitivity); checking pancreatic enzyme levels (amylase and lipase); antibody testing against common parasites (blood and stool); a stool CDSA (comprehensive digestive stool analysis); H. pylori antibody and breath tests; and a breath test for SIBO. An upper endoscopy and colonoscopy should be considered in patients with chronic resistant symptoms when no clear etiology is found. However, overlapping causes for bloating and indigestion with SIBO could also include lactose intolerance, fructose intolerance, or Candida overgrowth.

Many patients with MSIDS and SIBO have positive tests for food allergies and sensitivities that are related to an imbalance in gut microflora. These multiple food allergies may be responsible for increased cytokine production and imply that the patient may also suffer from dysbiosis and leaky gut. As we discussed in the prior chapter on food allergies, leaky gut is a term used to describe a loss of the integrity of the GI lining of the gut, where macromolecules of food pass through the intestinal barrier and antibodies against them are formed, as they are seen to be foreign invaders. This loss of integrity of the tight junction system in the gut can also take place when patients have cancer and are exposed to radiation or chemotherapy; have chronic bacterial and/or parasitic infections or significant yeast overgrowth; have taken antibiotics long term, leading to an overgrowth of *Candida* and other fungi, or in the case of certain autoimmune diseases.

Scientific reports are now emerging that new mechanisms for food allergies have appeared in hundreds of adults across the United States that are not related to leaky gut, but instead to the bite of the lone star tick. Dr. Scott Commins, assistant professor of medicine at the University of Virginia, recently reported on a group of four hundred cases in which patients who ate beef had a delayed allergic reaction, ranging from hives to full-blown anaphylaxis. Ninety percent of the patients reported a history of tick bites. The hypothesis is that the saliva from the tick enters the site of the bite and subsequently causes the severe allergic reaction. Studies are presently being carried out to confirm the theory, by researching the effect of tick saliva on the human body's antibodies to alpha-gal, which is contained in red meat, lamb, and pork. This is a new and potentially fatal problem that can be acquired from a tick bite.

Those who suffer from both food allergies and SIBO can be treated with Betaine hydrochloric acid before meals to increase gastric acidity, digestive enzymes with meals, and fiber (soluble and nonsoluble, including ground flaxseeds), as well as L-glutamine before, during, and after meals. These patients also need to decrease their intake of carbohydrates and sugars, avoid hydrogenated oils, alcohol, nicotine, caffeine, artificial sweeteners, allergic foods, and, when possible, stop antibiotics that can contribute to a *Candida* overgrowth. Dietary interventions to increase healthy prebiotics include increasing fermented foods in the diet, such as sauerkraut, kimchee, pickles, pickled ginger, olives, and kefir (as long as you are not diagnosed with systemic candidiasis). Healthy probiotic supplementation should include a minimum of at least 10 billion organisms with a good quality probiotic daily, but higher doses of probiotics are preferable for those with severe dysbiosis, as seen on a CDSA test.

Phase I of treatment for SIBO and IBS uses the antibiotic Xifaxan, followed by a breath test to confirm if there has been eradication of the small intestinal bacterial overgrowth. Occasionally, phase II treatment for SIBO will be needed, and it will require a low-dose antibiotic, such as erythromycin, to continue to eradicate the bacterial overgrowth if Xifaxan has been unsuccessful.

For treatment of leaky gut, we suggest glutamine; OptiCleanse GHI, by Xymogen, and phosphatidylcholine, to help heal the gut lining; high-dose probiotics; digestive enzymes; gamma-linoleic acid (as borage seed oil); and avoidance of allergic foods, followed by a rotation diet.

When patients are on antibiotics for Lyme disease, we use probiotics with acidophilus (over 200 billion colony forming units/CFUs) and *Saccharomyces boulardii*, the beneficial yeast that has been proven to decrease the incidence of *Clostridium difficile* diarrhea. According to a metaanalyses that appeared in a 2011 article in the *Journal of Clinical Gastroenterology*, three types of probiotics (*Lactobacillus rhamnosus GG*, probiotic mixtures, and *Saccharomyces boulardii*) have all been shown to significantly decrease the incidence of antibiotic-associated diarrhea, but only *S. boulardii* is effective for the prevention of *Clostridium difficile* diarrhea. Some patients will develop *C. difficile* diarrhea, however, despite taking probiotics, and will need to be treated with a course of antibiotics, such as Flagyl, oral Vancocin, or Dificid. In resistant cases, fecal transplantation may be used to restore a diverse, healthy microbiome in the intestine.

Probiotics have multiple mechanisms of action that allow them to be especially beneficial for health, as they balance intestinal microflora. They help reduce gut permeability, preventing leaky gut and multiple food allergies. They promote the production of mucin, which helps protect the gut's lining, and produce antimicrobial compounds. They need, however, to be of human origin, resistant to destruction by gastric acid and bile, and be able to adhere to the intestinal epithelial tissue in order to effectively colonize the GI tract. They also have an effect on our immunity: They decrease inflammatory cytokine production, while also affecting the gut-associated lymphoid tissue (GALT), part of the immune system found in the GI tract. This is especially important when we consider the causes of infectious diarrhea.

While the most common causes of infectious diarrhea are the bacterial and viral infections we've discussed, certain parasites can also cause inflammation and disrupt microflora, leading to diarrhea. Common parasitic infections include giardiasis, amebiasis, cryptosporidium, hookworm, pinworm, roundworm (including filariasis), and strongyloides. We have found that certain patients with resistant symptoms of MSIDS improved once intestinal parasites were discovered and treated. These infections are all treated differently and, unfortunately, testing for many of these parasites may be unreliable, as is the case with testing for Lyme disease and associated co-infections. It is therefore important that we understand the limitations of standard GI testing and examine other methods for determining the parameters of gastrointestinal health.

EVALUATING GI HEALTH USING THE COMPREHENSIVE DIGESTIVE STOOL ANALYSIS (CDSA)

One excellent method for evaluating gastrointestinal health is the comprehensive digestive stool analysis (CDSA) that is available through many functional medicine laboratories such as Metametrix, Doctor's Data, or Diagnos-Techs. The gastrointestinal function profile from Metametrix is the one that we most often employ. It evaluates many of the markers of intestinal health, and although the CDSA is generally not taught to physicians in medical school, I have found it to be invaluable in expanding the GI workup for patients with gastrointestinal disorders that could not be explained by routine testing. It includes testing for:

• Bacteria: The CDSA identifies the predominant bacteria in the gut, including obligate anaerobes (bacteria that will not grow in an oxygen-rich environment) such as *Bacteroides spp.*, *Clostridial spp.*, *Fusobacterium*, and others; facultative anaerobes, such as *Lactobacillus* and *Bifidobacterium spp.*, and obligate aerobes (bacteria that need an oxygen-rich environment to flourish) such as *E. coli*. They also evaluate the gut for the presence of opportunistic bacteria, pathogenic bacteria such as *H. pylori*, *E. coli* 0157:H7, *Campylobacter spp.*, and *Clostridium difficile*. Knowing if there are opportunistic bacteria is important, as they can affect digestion, absorption of nutrients, pH, and immune status.

• Yeast: An abnormally high overgrowth of yeast on the CDSA can point to possible candidiasis in the right clinical setting, requiring treatment with antifungal agents.

• Parasites: We need to check MSIDS patients for intestinal parasites if they suffer from resistant symptoms despite standard treatment protocols. These parasites can increase the symptoms of Lyme-MSIDS, and often go undetected. The majority of our patients are now co-infected with *Babesia*, a blood-borne parasite, and *Babesia* can suppress the immune system, allowing other parasitic infections to emerge. Parasites can also cause GI symptoms similar to yeast overgrowth, such as gas and bloating, confusing the clinical picture. They can be difficult to pick up on standard ova and parasite testing, and we have found the presence of hidden parasites on CDSA testing from specialized laboratories when local laboratory evaluations were negative.

• Inflammation: The CDSA also looks for signs of inflammation in the colon, checking for white cells and mucus that are found in elevated levels in inflammation and/or infection. It also evaluates the level of lactoferrin, an iron-binding glycoprotein that is released in inflammatory bowel disorders such as Crohn's disease and ulcerative colitis, but not in irritable bowel syndrome. This marker is one way to differentiate between IBS and IBD, apart from doing a colonoscopy.

Finally, measuring the levels of short-chain fatty acids (SCFA) in the stool helps to determine the risk of colon inflammation (colitis). SCFAs are produced by the fermentation of foods in our diet (dietary polysaccharides and fiber), and one of their products, N-butyrate, has been shown to lower the risk of colitis and colorectal cancer.

• Fecal sIgA (secretory IgA) and antigliadin sIgA: The CDSA can determine if there are immune system reactions to antigens from bacteria, yeast, or other microbes, and help evaluate for the presence of gluten sensitivity.

• Intestinal pH: The CDSA evaluates the intestinal pH related to pH-lowering organic acids and pH-raising ammonia levels from certain bacteria.

• Essential markers of digestion and absorption: The CDSA evaluates pancreatic enzyme secretion for malabsorption due to pancreatic or biliary insufficiency.

We have been finding that many patients with resistant symptoms of Lyme-MSIDS who have not adequately responded to standard antibiotic protocols do, in fact, test positive for multiple abnormalities on the CDSA. Using that information and treating associated yeast overgrowth, dysbiosis, enzyme deficiencies, and/or parasitic infections can be a turning point in getting patients to the next level of wellness.

FOR ELIZABETH, LYME DISEASE WAS HALF THE PROBLEM

Elizabeth was forty when I met her. She had been inexplicably sick for the previous ten years; she was finally diagnosed with Lyme disease and babesiosis (positive IgM Western blot, positive *Babesia* IFA). Although she had some of the classical symptoms of Lyme-MSIDS, with severe fatigue, day and night sweats, myalgias, neuropathic symptoms in the lower extremities, and cognitive difficulties, some of her worst symptoms were gastrointestinal: She suffered from gastroparesis, a particularly severe form of delayed gastric emptying with nausea, gas, and abdominal pain. Elizabeth could also go for days without moving her bowels. The only thing that used to help her was intermittent colonics to clean out the colon. In Lyme disease patients, we occasionally see problems with abnormal gastrointestinal motility, but gastroparesis is a particularly rare and severe manifestation, related to ANS dysfunction. Clinical manifestations include patients complaining of fullness after eating, abdominal pain, nausea and vomiting, and an inability to eat. It is a challenging condition to treat, since available pharmaceutical drugs, such as Reglan, may have short-term benefits in stimulating gastric contractions, but it is not an option for long-term use, due to significant side effects. Interestingly, Elizabeth told me that whenever she would take antibiotics, such as Augmentin, for a sinus infection, many of her chronic health problems would improve, including her severe chronic constipation.

During our medical workup she was checked for hypothyroidism, adrenal dysfunction, food allergies, gluten sensitivity, and magnesium deficiency. We also sent off a CDSA to check for enzyme deficiencies, imbalances of healthy bacteria and yeast, and parasites. Her tests showed magnesium deficiency (low red blood cell magnesium levels) and multiple food allergies (especially grains, tomatoes, some nuts and fruits), and her CDSA test revealed the presence of two parasites—strongyloides and another that was unidentifiable. Her laboratory tests were otherwise unremarkable, except for adrenal dysfunction, with some elevated cortisol levels in the morning.

We placed Elizabeth on a strict avoidance diet for her food allergens, gave her high doses of magnesium to help stimulate GI bowel activity while increasing her fluids, and prescribed probiotics as well as medications for her Lyme, babesiosis, and intestinal parasites. We discussed giving her a broad spectrum antiparasitic regimen for one week, consisting of several doses of Biltricide, one dose of ivermectin, and one dose of Pin-X, followed by three days of Alinia (nitazoxanide), since we could not identify all the parasites present.

Elizabeth returned one month later. She had a big smile on her face as she reported to me that her gastrointestinal symptoms and gastroparesis had cleared up for the first time in years. It no longer took her days to have a bowel movement, and her nausea and abdominal discomfort were gone. She also had more energy, and her sweats and muscle and nerve pain were significantly better. We had found an answer for issues that had plagued her for years and eluded some of the best subspecialists she had seen. Treating her Lyme disease, co-infections, food allergies, magnesium deficiency, and parasites was the answer to her chronic health complaints and gastrointestinal problems.

The health of the gastrointestinal tract is important for everyone, especially those who suffer with chronic illness. Poor digestion can lead to poor nutritional absorption, impairing normal cellular functioning. An improper balance of healthy bacteria and yeast play a role in contributing to irritable bowel syndrome with SIBO, inflammatory bowel disease, systemic candidiasis, food allergies, and GERD. The GI tract also plays a pivotal role in coordinating metabolic activities, affects our sleep, weight, and moods, and is also a key player in the production of inflammatory cytokines. It houses our first line of immune defense and plays an important role in controlling and balancing the inflammatory response, which we have repeatedly shown is the underlying common denominator for most chronic disease.

SEVENTEEN

Lyme and Liver Dysfunction

nother gastrointestinal issue that frequently arises in MSIDS patients is elevated liver functions. This phrase refers to abnormalities that appear in specific blood chemistry tests that measure inflammation in the liver (tests: AST, ALT, GGT) or obstruction/congestion in the liver (tests: Alkaline phosphatase +/− bilirubin). Unfortunately, these liver chemistry abnormalities are not always accompanied by symptoms, at least early in the course of the illness, and are only diagnosed by going to your doctor and getting these blood tests. For example, some liver diseases, such as hepatitis, can be present without symptoms for years, all the while leading to significant damage.

Some diseases can cause inflammation in the liver, while others cause a blockage (obstruction) both in and leading from the liver to the pancreas or the gallbladder. A third issue occurs when there is congestion in the liver, as in the case of congestive heart failure. For example, hepatitis is an inflammation of the liver that occurs without significant congestion. It can cause elevations in AST, ALT, and GGT as well as nonspecific symptoms, including fatigue, poor appetite, weight loss, nausea, and muscle and joint pain. Other diseases, such as cirrhosis of the liver, have a significant congestive/obstructive component. The obstruction causes jaundice and fluid accumulation in the abdomen, an enlarged spleen, and enlarged blood vessels in the esophagus. Diseases such as pancreatic cancer can cause a bile duct obstruction with minimal inflammation (primarily raising levels of alkaline phosphatase and total bilirubin). Pancreatic cancer often does not cause symptoms early in its course, but symptoms later in the disease can include painless jaundice, pale colored stools, itching, poor appetite, weight loss, and upper abdominal pain. It is therefore vital to identify which liver functions are elevated so we can create a proper differential diagnosis and order appropriate follow-up testing. It is also important to differentiate whether these elevated liver functions are directly affected by tick-borne diseases, or are medication side effects due to other diseases that are not only affecting the liver but mimicking the symptoms of Lyme-MSIDS.

Some of the diseases that cause elevated liver functions can be fatal, and there may be no clinical signs of an illness until the abnormalities become severe. When symptoms do occur, they can include:

- Breast development (gynecomastia) in men
- Confusion or difficulty thinking (encephalopathy)
- Fatigue
- Impotence
- Joint pain
- Loss of appetite
- Nausea and vomiting (with occasional vomiting of blood)
- Nosebleeds, bleeding gums, gastrointestinal bleeding (secondary to esophageal varices, i.e., dilated veins which often bleed in cirrhosis, and coagulation defects)
- Pale or clay-colored stools
- Redness of the palms of the hands (palmar erythema)
- Small, red spiderlike blood vessels on the skin (spider angiomas)
- Swelling or fluid buildup in the legs (edema) and in the abdomen (ascites)
- Weight loss
- Yellow color in the skin, mucus membranes, or eyes (jaundice)

LIVER DISEASE AND LYME

Elevated liver functions are frequently seen in those with Lyme disease, as well as in patients with other tick-borne disorders. Patients who present with localized EM rashes have been found to have elevated liver function assays 37 percent of the time. In patients who have disseminated Lyme disease, in which the disease has spread throughout the body, the incidence is even higher. In one study, published in the journal *Hepatology*, 115 patients with EM rashes were evaluated; other causes for abnormal liver functions were excluded (they were not yet on antibiotics), and they found that 66 percent of the patients had elevated liver functions in disseminated Lyme disease, compared to 34 percent with localized disease. These improved or resolved three weeks after the onset of antibiotic therapy in most patients. Cytokines causing inflammation or direct *Borrelia* invasion of the liver were the postulated mechanisms responsible for the elevation in liver functions.

We see the same elevated liver functions accompanying other tick-borne diseases. Blood testing of those with confirmed ehrlichiosis or anaplasmosis will often reveal elevated liver functions. These will generally promptly resolve with tetracycline treatment (although, rarely, antibiotics will temporarily raise liver functions; changing the medication or lowering the dose resolves the problem). In the case of babesiosis, mild elevations of serum bilirubin, alkaline phosphatase, and AST are common. Relapsing fever with *Borrelia hermsii*, as well as rickettsial diseases, such as Rocky Mountain spotted fever (RMSF) and Q fever, are also associated with elevations in liver functions. Q fever may lead to chronic symptoms such as Q fever endocarditis, an enlarged liver, hepatitis with liver enzyme elevations, and rare cases of jaundice.

OTHER CAUSES OF LIVER INJURY

Apart from a fatty liver (steatosis of the liver) described below, there are many systemic diseases that can affect liver functions. Often we pick up elevated liver functions on routine blood testing when a patient comes in for an initial consultation, or the liver problem may develop and/or appear during their treatment course, as in the case of a toxic chemical exposure, viral infection, or new medication.

- Acute and chronic pulmonary diseases: This includes both acute lung diseases caused by the infectious agents responsible for pneumonia, as well as chronic lung diseases such as cystic fibrosis. Infections causing pneumonia, such as *Legionella pneumophila*, *Mycoplasma pneumonia*, or *Pneumococcus*, may all raise serum ALT concentration and total bilirubin, and patients with chronic pulmonary diseases may also have elevations in GGT, ALT, and alkaline phosphatase.

• Alpha-1 antitrypsin deficiency: This is a genetic disorder responsible for decreased production of the enzyme alpha-1 antitrypsin. It can cause both liver disease and emphysema. Specific treatment involves IV alpha-1 antitrypsin augmentation therapy, although there have been no randomized controlled trials to prove the efficacy of this therapy in improving the decline in pulmonary function seen in this disorder.

• Autoimmune hepatitis: Autoimmune hepatitis is a chronic disorder in which there is progressive liver damage from a cell-mediated immunologic attack against liver cells, leading to inflammation, liver necrosis (cell death), and fibrosis, and eventually to cirrhosis and liver failure. Symptoms include fatigue, poor appetite (anorexia), joint pain (arthralgias), and jaundice. The mainstay of treatment is steroid therapy, followed by immunosuppressive therapies such as azathioprine or 6-MP, which have been proven effective in controlled clinical trials.

• Cancer: Patients with chronic hepatitis B and C are at risk for developing cirrhosis of the liver as well as primary liver cancers, i.e., hepatomas. These patients should be screened regularly with blood tests (LFTs and alpha-fetoprotein) and imaging studies (ultrasound/MRI) for early detection of liver cancer. Elevated liver functions can also be seen with secondary metastatic tumors (i.e., breast cancer), as well as with pancreatic cancer.

• Chemical exposures: Certain toxic chemicals, such as carbon tetrachloride, have been implicated in cases of acute liver failure. These chemicals can cause a rapid decline in liver function, leading to changes in mental status function (hepatic encephalopathy) with associated bleeding defects (coagulopathy). Dialysis and liver transplantation may be necessary in severe cases.

- Connective tissue diseases: Lupus (SLE), juvenile idiopathic arthritis (JIA), rheumatoid arthritis, Sjögren's syndrome, scleroderma, and polymyalgia rheumatica (PMR) may all present with liver abnormalities. Elevations in liver enzymes have been observed in up to 21 percent of patients with autoimmune diseases such as SLE, and there have been reports of patients with overlapping lupus and autoimmune hepatitis. It is important to differentiate between true lupus, autoimmune hepatitis, and a patient with MSIDS who has an overstimulated immune system producing elevated levels of antinuclear antibodies (ANA), since the treatments for these diseases are completely different. A patient with Lyme disease will rapidly relapse on high-dose steroids, due to suppression of their immune system, but patients with SLE and autoimmune hepatitis (AIH) require steroids to prevent disease progression. It is also important to differentiate between a lupus-related chronic hepatitis and an autoimmune hepatitis, since patients with AIH require adequate doses of steroids, or they may rapidly progress to liver cirrhosis.

- Drug-induced liver injury: The most common over-the-counter drug to cause liver injury is Tylenol. People who take 3,000 mg to 4,000 mg per day on a regular basis may experience a rise in liver functions with hepatotoxicity, and therefore the dose should be lowered if it is needed for long-term pain control. The total daily dose should be even lower in the elderly or in those with associated liver disease, and should not exceed 2,000 mg per day. Any elevation of liver functions while on Tylenol requires stopping the medication and taking high doses of cysteine (orally or IV, in severe cases), which helps detoxify the Tylenol through the glutathione pathway, preventing liver failure, which can be fatal. We routinely suggest 600 mg twice a day of NAC (N-Acetylcysteine) to those who require acetaminophen for pain.

- Endocrine diseases: Hyperthyroidism, hypothyroidism, hypercortisolism (Cushing's syndrome), hypocortisolism (Addison's disease), as well as diabetes may also cause elevations in liver chemistries. These abnormalities may include liver injury, with either liver congestion or inflammation, with nonalcoholic fatty liver disease being a complication in 32 percent to 78 percent of those with type II diabetes. This may lead to liver cirrhosis and hepatocellular carcinomas. The difficulty in evaluating patients with MSIDS who have overlapping systemic diseases such as hypothyroidism and diabetes (which are not uncommon in this population) is that antibiotics may cause transient elevations in liver chemistries, and these same biochemical abnormalities can be seen with the underlying endocrine disorder. Getting the hormones and blood sugars back into the normal range will help to eliminate any overlapping pathologies.

• Fatty liver with/without alcoholism (NASH, nonalcoholic steatohepatitis): Many people associate liver disease with alcoholism. However, liver disease can also occur without an alcohol component, as in the case of nonalcoholic fatty liver disease (NASH), where excess fat deposition in the liver causes inflammation. Extreme alcoholic consumption is linked to liver disease, and telltale signs include spider angiomas (red dots on the chest and face that blanch with palpation), gynecomastia (abnormal breast enlargement in men), and palmar erythema (unusually red palms). Blood tests will often reveal abnormal elevations in uric acid levels, with a macrocytic anemia (increase in the size of the red cells). These are classic manifestations of excessive alcohol intake and reflect high estrogen levels, with early signs of cirrhosis. A nonalcoholic fatty liver (steatosis) causing elevated liver functions can also be seen in overweight individuals. If no apparent cause of elevated liver functions is found in an individual with obesity, an ultrasound of the liver and gallbladder can be performed to check for fatty infiltration.

• Gallstones: Gallstones are produced in the gallbladder and may be asymptomatic or symptomatic, depending on their size and quantity and whether they pass into other parts of the biliary tree, causing inflammation and obstruction. Mild gallbladder dysfunction may cause symptoms of nausea, bloating, and abdominal pain after eating a fat-laden meal, but if they obstruct the bile ducts, symptoms may include severe stomach pain (in the right upper quadrant of the abdomen) with nausea, vomiting, fever, and jaundice (as in the case of acute cholecystitis, ascending cholangitis, and pancreatitis). These conditions can be diagnosed with a proper history and physical examination, an imaging study of the liver, gallbladder, and pancreas (ultrasound, CAT scan, MRI), and by a combination of blood tests that look at the CBC, liver functions, and pancreatic enzymes. Abnormalities would include elevated white cell counts (consistent with infection), elevated liver enzymes (especially alkaline phosphatase and total bilirubin, consistent with obstruction), and elevated pancreatic enzymes, such as amylase and lipase, reflecting inflammation in the pancreas. Asymptomatic gallstones may not require therapy, but gallstones obstructing the bile ducts or ampulla of Vater (connecting the bile and pancreatic ducts) may require surgery and antibiotics.

• Hematological diseases: These include sickle cell anemia, thalassemia, Hodgkin's disease, non-Hodgkin's lymphoma, acute myelogenous leukemia (AML), acute lymphocytic leukemia (ALL), chronic lymphoid leukemia (CLL), chronic myeloid leukemia (CML), hairy cell leukemia, multiple myeloma, and myelodysplasias. These may all cause elevated liver functions either through infiltration of malignant cells or through iron overload in the liver.

• Hemochromatosis: This disease is due to iron overload in the liver, which can lead to cirrhosis of the liver, darkening of the skin with diabetes (brown diabetes), testicular failure, arthritis, and congestive heart failure (cardiomyopathy). There are also generalized symptoms including weakness and nonspecific neurological symptoms. The genes for this disease may be carried by 8 percent to 13 percent of the population, and it is one of the most common genetic disorders seen in a medical office. Treatment for hemochromatosis includes avoiding foods rich in iron and periodic bloodletting: removing one or two units of blood (250 ml to 500 ml) weekly in symptomatic patients and those with a serum ferritin level of at least 1,000 mcg per ml, until the iron levels have been depleted and returned to the normal range. Then phlebotomies are continued every two to four months to maintain serum ferritin levels between 50 mcg and 100 mcg per L.

• Infectious diseases: Other infectious diseases, apart from Lyme and its co-infections, may cause liver damage with inflammation. Viral illnesses such as chronic hepatitis B and C (including all forms of hepatitis: A–E) and other infectious diseases, such as GI infections (Salmonella, *Clostridium*, and *Campylobacter*), fungal infections, mycobacteria (tuberculosis), syphilis, HIV, parasitic infections (amoeba, liver fluke), and fungal infections can all cause abnormalities in liver functions.

• Inflammatory bowel disease: Ulcerative colitis and Crohn's disease often have abnormal liver functions, especially if their disease is severe enough to require surgery. These diseases can cause hepatobiliary disorders, including primary sclerosing cholangitis (PSC), fatty livers, granuloma formation, amyloidosis (which can be seen in many chronic inflammatory diseases), and hepatic abscess formation, and be associated with gallstones and an autoimmune hepatitis (AIH).

• Right-sided heart failure: This is manifested by an enlarged liver found on physical examination (hepatomegaly), an enlarged spleen (splenomegaly), ascites (fluid in the abdominal cavity), with peripheral edema and fluid in the cavity surrounding the lungs (pleural effusions), as well as occasional jaundice.

• Wilson's disease: This is a rare disease caused by a defect in the excretion of copper that affects the liver and brain, where a copper overload leads to neuropsychiatric symptoms and liver disease, with associated hepatitis and cirrhosis and occasional esophageal bleeding. Neurological manifestations of Wilson's disease include tremors, problems with speech, and personality changes with severe mood swings.

Testing for Elevated Liver Functions

Since many liver diseases can be silent with long-term health consequences, it is important to have your liver functions checked once a year, and understand the strengths and weaknesses of the currently available testing. Many of these tests are not specific for the liver yet give us clues that there may be disease processes at work.

• Aspartate transaminase, AST (GOT): This is a liver enzyme that is considered to measure inflammation in the liver. Normal values are usually less than 35 U/L but will depend on the individual laboratory's reference range. In diseases such as chronic hepatitis, values of AST can be greater than twice the normal range, and in some cases are more than ten times the upper limit of normal, which may reflect severe liver and/or biliary disease. This enzyme may be slightly elevated due to certain drug reactions (such as antibiotics), moderately elevated in those who drink too much alcohol (alcoholic hepatitis, with enzymes in the 200 IU to 300 UL range), and very elevated, as in the case of acute viral hepatitis (above 1,000 UL). We can suspect which disease is present based on the patient's history and level of elevation of AST. However, in the case of a massive hepatic necrosis and severe destruction of the liver from hepatitis, the levels of these enzymes may fall: The liver is so severely damaged that there is very little enzyme activity. This clearly hampers the effectiveness of this test.

Another difficulty in interpreting the AST test is that some of these enzymes are not completely disease- and liver-specific. For example, even though AST is considered to be a liver enzyme, AST levels can be elevated during a heart attack and in diseases causing inflammation of the skeletal muscle (myositis). And while AST is generally considered to be a marker of inflammation, and is not commonly associated with bile duct obstruction, sudden increases of AST above fifteen times normal may be seen in acute cholangitis, which is due to acute obstruction of the gallbladder, and can be accompanied by a sudden increase in abdominal pain in the right upper quadrant (biliary colic) with jaundice, fever, and chills. This combination of symptoms is known as Charcot's triad.

• Alanine transaminase, ALT (GPT): This is a more specific enzyme test for liver disease with associated bile duct and gallbladder dysfunction (hepatobiliary dysfunction) and will generally not be affected by other disease processes. This is a better marker to determine if we are primarily dealing with a process unique to the liver and not due to an inflammatory process from another source. Normal values are usually less than 40 U/L.

• Alkaline phosphatase: This test identifies an enzyme that is associated with congestion and obstruction in the liver. Normal values are between 33 U/L and 115 U/L (Quest Diagnostics). Elevated levels of alkaline phosphatase may be seen with gallstones; if pancreatic cancer is obstructing the bile duct; with bile duct strictures; with congestive heart failure; with cirrhosis of the liver; and with liver cancer. The highest levels of alkaline phosphatase are usually seen in severe liver disease, with bile duct obstruction that is usually associated with elevated levels of bilirubin. Bilirubin is formed when old or damaged red blood cells are broken down in the spleen, forming the compound unconjugated bilirubin, which is then shuttled to the liver via transporter proteins (albumin). An elevated alkaline phosphatase level together with an elevated total bilirubin level is indicative of liver congestion and obstruction, and can cause jaundice (yellowing of the skin, mucous membranes, and the eyes).

As with AST, isolated alkaline phosphatase levels are not specific for the liver. These enzymes are also present in the bone, intestine, placenta, and white blood cells. An elevated alkaline phosphatase level might therefore suggest a bone disease (such as Paget's, a bone disorder in which there is an abnormal turnover of the bone, leading to skeletal deformities and musculoskeletal pain), or breast cancer, with metastases to the bone. Elevations in alkaline phosphatase levels can also occur during pregnancy and in children during a growth spurt (without an increase in bilirubin). Therefore, if the source of the elevation is not obvious, other tests need to be run in order to determine the origin of the abnormality. One such test, called the serum 5'-nucleotidase, parallels the activity of the enzyme in the liver, but not the bone. There are also ways of breaking down the alkaline phosphatase into different isoenzymes to determine the source of the elevation, i.e., whether it is coming from the liver, bone, uterus, or white cells.

• Total bilirubin: This test can help determine if there is an obstruction in the liver, especially with an associated elevation of alkaline phosphatase. However, isolated levels of total bilirubin without an elevation of alkaline phosphatase are not necessarily indicative of an obstruction. This is usually due to Gilbert's syndrome, a hereditary disorder in which there is impaired bilirubin uptake and storage, due to a decrease in the enzyme that conjugates bilirubin. Although this can produce jaundice, it is completely benign. It affects roughly 7 percent of the total population, and we see Gilbert's disease frequently in our patients. Normal values of total bilirubin range between 0.2 mg/dL and 1.2 mg/dL (Quest Diagnostics).

• Gamma-glutamyl transpeptidase (GGT): GGT is a very sensitive marker for inflammation, but it is not specific for any one disease process. An elevated GGT does not indicate the cause of an inflammation but may be useful in helping to determine whether an alcohol problem may exist; i.e., if the levels are greater than 30 U/L, with an associated increase in the size of the red blood cells (macrocytosis).

• Supplemental tests to evaluate liver function—albumin levels, prothrombin time, alpha-fetoprotein levels: I run these additional tests if the blood work listed above shows that there are abnormalities in liver function, or when a patient tells me that they are taking anticoagulants such as Coumadin, or that they have a history of liver cancer. Serum albumin is a protein produced in the liver that enters the bloodstream (plasma) and helps bind water (increasing the osmotic pressure and decreasing edema); it also transports fats (fatty acids), hormones, bilirubin, and medications in the blood. Low albumin levels can be seen with chronic disease states and liver damage. The prothrombin time is a measure of coagulation in the blood, and the normal reference range is ten to fourteen seconds. Elevated prothrombin times are seen in some cases of jaundice (obstructive and hepatocellular jaundice) and may lead to increased bleeding, as the liver is unable to produce the proper proteins necessary for coagulation. Elevated prothrombin times are not specific for liver disease, and can also be seen in cases of vitamin K deficiency, malabsorption, and use of an anticoagulant medication (Coumadin). Alpha-fetoprotein is a serum protein like albumin that transports bilirubin and fatty acids in the blood. Levels can be elevated in pregnancy and indicate developmental disorders in the fetus; they can also be elevated in those with germ cell tumors, a primary cancer of the liver (hepatoma), and metastatic disease to the liver. Alpha-fetoprotein levels can be monitored in these circumstances to evaluate treatment and tumor progression.

SCREENING FOR SPECIFIC LIVER DISEASES

Apart from testing for tick-borne disorders, which is a common cause of abnormal liver functions, I also perform the following blood tests to rule out other causes of liver disease. The majority of them are genetically determined, and some can be fatal. I recommend that everyone be tested for hepatitis B and C at some point in their adult life, and be screened for hemochromatosis. When cross-referenced with symptoms and a complete patient history and physical, these tests will usually help to differentiate the cause for any liver abnormalities:

- Alpha-1 antitrypsin level: A decreased level is seen in cases of a genetic enzyme deficiency, and can cause liver disease and emphysema.

- Antinuclear antibody (ANA): Elevated levels are seen in autoimmune diseases of the liver, such as lupus.

- Anti–smooth muscle antibodies: Elevated levels are seen in autoimmune hepatitis.

- Iron-TIBC and ferritin level: Elevated levels are seen in hemochromatosis (iron overload); however, elevated iron and ferritin levels are not specific for hemochromatosis. This can also be seen with iron replacement therapy, red blood cell disorders, and significant alcohol consumption, as well as during inflammatory states, including the inflammation seen in severe Lyme arthritis, hepatitis, other liver diseases, and cancer.

• Ceruloplasmin levels: Ceruloplasmin is the major copper-carrying protein in the blood produced in the liver. Low levels of ceruloplasmin are seen in malabsorption (Menkes disease), with high levels of vitamin C consumption, and in Wilson's disease.

• Antimitochondrial antibody (AMA): Elevated levels are seen in primary biliary cirrhosis, a disease in which there is destruction of the small bile ducts that can cause cirrhosis.

• Hepatitis screen for hepatitis A, B, and C: This would include antibody levels, level of antigens, and measuring the amount of DNA or RNA of the virus in the blood. Acute hepatitis may present with significantly elevated levels of liver enzymes (AST, ALT), yet chronic hepatitis (B and C) may present with only minimally elevated levels of liver enzymes (transaminases) and be silent causes of liver disease decades later. Hepatitis A usually resolves spontaneously (although rare cases of acute liver failure do exist), but chronic hepatitis B and C can lead to cirrhosis of the liver and liver cancer, and be fatal. Hepatitis sufferers may complain of chronic fatigue, arthralgias, and joint pains, the same symptoms seen in Lyme-MSIDS. These symptoms stem from the virus causing deposition of immune complexes in the joints, as well as viral deposition of immune complexes in the arteries and kidneys, leading to an inflammation in the blood vessels (vasculitis) and in the kidneys (glomerulonephritis). Many chronic hepatitis patients are asymptomatic, and the disease can remain silent for many years, until the liver is severely affected. Many young Americans may have chronic hepatitis C, while Americans of all ages, as well as those of Asian, Indian, and Tibetan descent, often also suffer from chronic hepatitis B. Sexual transmission, maternal-neonatal transmission, IV drug use, body piercing, tattoos, and hemodialysis are associated risk factors. Regular screening of liver functions, viral loads, alpha-fetal-protein levels (an early marker for hepatocellular carcinoma), and imaging studies of the liver are essential in following patients with known hepatitis. Fortunately, some of the newer antiviral combinations for hepatitis B and C are proving to be more effective than prior regimens, and may put the disease into remission.

JIM'S SILENT LIVER DISEASE CONTRIBUTED TO HIS SYMPTOMS

Jim was twenty-one years old and had a past medical history significant for severe depression, anxiety, and mood swings. When he came to see me he also complained of fatigue, migratory joint and muscle pains, headaches, tingling and numbness in the extremities, tremors and neurocognitive deficits, and pronounced difficulties with speech. He told me that he dropped out of college because of the severity of his symptoms. He had a history of several tick bites over the years, and one EM rash. At that time he had received twenty-one days of doxycycline, was pronounced "cured" by his physician, and was told that his ongoing symptoms were due to chronic fatigue syndrome, depression, and fibromyalgia.

His physical examination was essentially unremarkable, except for the tremors and his marked anxiety. His vital signs were stable, heart and lung examinations were normal, there was no evidence of swollen joints, and there was no hepatosplenomegaly (increased size of the liver or spleen). His laboratory tests revealed a CDC positive Lyme IgM Western blot and prior exposure to *Mycoplasma pneumoniae* and *Chlamydia pneumonia*; his tests for other tick-borne diseases, including *Ehrlichia/Anaplasma*, babesiosis, *Bartonella*, Rocky Mountain spotted fever, Q fever, typhus, tularemia, and brucellosis, were all negative. He was slightly anemic, and his comprehensive metabolic profile (CMP) was completely normal, including his liver functions. Hormone testing showed normal thyroid functions, and we sent off a salivary DHEA/cortisol test, which returned with a borderline low cortisol in the morning, which may have been responsible in part for his chronic fatigue. We performed a six-hour urine DMSA challenge, which showed an elevated level of mercury (28, normal is less than 3) and an elevated level of lead (36, normal is less than 2). We initially hypothesized that Jim's depression, anxiety, mood swings, tremors, fatigue, and musculoskeletal symptoms were due to his Lyme disease and associated heavy metal burden and borderline adrenal function.

During the first month of treatment, Jim was taking Omnicef, Plaquenil, and Zithromax, as well as nystatin tablets. He had a severe Jarisch-Herxheimer reaction within the first two weeks, and we stopped the antibiotics. We retried the same antibiotics one week later with a flare protocol, including having him increase his intake of lemons and limes in order to alkalize his system, and using high-dose oral glutathione. Unfortunately, he had the same reaction, and the antibiotics were discontinued. Jim was then switched to doxycycline and Plaquenil with meals, but again, within the first two weeks of treatment, we had to stop the antibiotics due to a significant increase in his fatigue and joint pain.

We then performed a new set of routine laboratory tests: His blood counts were normal, but his liver functions had dramatically increased. Although they were normal on his initial screening test, his AST was now 510 and his ALT was 682. These levels were over ten times normal, and although we occasionally see mild elevations in liver functions with antibiotic therapy, this was an extremely unusual elevation. We therefore sent off blood work for ANA, AMA, ceruloplasmin, ferritin, alpha-1 antitrypsin levels, and screens for hepatitis A, B, and C. These screening tests all came back normal except for the ceruloplasmin. It was low, at 16 mg/dL; normal values are between 20 mg/dL and 40 mg/dL. This suggested Wilson's disease, as the symptoms associated with it were exactly what Jim was experiencing. They were also the same symptoms that we frequently see with Lyme disease and mercury exposure, yet there was one essential difference in this case: Jim's tremors and mood swings were extremely severe. I often see patients with tremors, and I am used to seeing depressed patients with anxiety and mood swings. But there was an extreme nature to Jim's symptoms, and based on his low ceruloplasmin level, I had wondered if he had a copper overload, and if Wilson's disease was responsible for the severity of his complaints, on top of neurological Lyme disease with exposure to mercury. The last test confirmed my suspicion.

We sent Jim for an eye exam to rule out Kayser-Fleisher rings, an abnormal eye finding found in Wilson's disease, in which copper deposits at the margins of the cornea lead to a golden brown or green discoloration that can be observed during an eye examination. It can also present in rare cases of biliary cirrhosis and liver congestion (intrahepatic cholestasis). His eye exam was inconclusive. The ophthalmologist reported changes in the eyes but was unclear as to whether they were classic Kayser-Fleisher rings. We therefore sent him to a university center that specializes in liver diseases, and referred him to a physician who had extensive experience with Wilson's disease.

The gastroenterologist agreed with our findings that Jim's case was certainly suggestive of Wilson's disease, and he performed a liver biopsy. The hepatic copper levels were elevated. Jim's Lyme disease and elevated levels of mercury were contributing to his tremors and mood swings, but his elevated levels of copper were responsible for making these symptoms more severe. If he hadn't shown an unusual increase in his liver functions with antibiotic therapy, we wouldn't have screened him for Wilson's disease. We might have assumed that his symptoms were due to Lyme and mercury, since we already had several probable causes that could adequately explain his symptoms.

TREATMENT OPTIONS

The treatment of elevated liver functions depends on the cause of the elevation. In the case of viral hepatitis, there are newer drug regimens (pegylated interferon and Ribasphere, Baraclude, Viread, Epivir, Hepsera, and Tyzeka) that have helped decrease viral loads and put patients in remission. For hepatitis C, the new standard is a peglyated interferon plus ribavirin, and a protease inhibitor such as Incivek and Victrelis. For iron and copper overload disorders (hemochromatosis and Wilson's disease), the treatment is to remove the iron (through giving blood regularly, i.e., phlebotomy) and by chelating out the copper (with drugs like Cuprimine). In lupus and autoimmune diseases, as with an autoimmune hepatitis, steroids and immunosuppressive drugs may be needed (such as Imuran) to decrease signs and symptoms of inflammation. In endocrine disorders, balancing out the hormone abnormalities will normalize liver functions, and in tick-borne diseases, antibiotic therapy will reduce elevated liver enzymes.

One newer treatment that shows promise for patients with inflammatory bowel disorders with associated Lyme disease and elevated liver functions is low-dose naltrexone. Drugs like LDN may be a better choice for patients with elevated liver functions caused by inflammatory bowel disease with overlapping co-infections, since LDN does not suppress the immune system and worsen associated infections. We have used LDN effectively (4.5 mg at bedtime) to treat pain disorders and inflammation in patients with Lyme-MSIDS. A complete explanation of its use in chronic disease states and pain will be discussed in Chapter 18.

When the cause of the liver dysfunction has been established and properly treated, other integrative therapies may be useful in decreasing inflammation and supporting liver function. These include antioxidant therapies and supplements that support detoxification reactions. The supplements NAC and alpha-lipoic acid help with the production and regeneration of glutathione, aid in detoxification, and protect the liver from free radical damage. NAC will also help protect the liver if the patient is taking large amounts of Tylenol, since cysteine is used in acetaminophen toxicity, and alpha-lipoic acid has been shown to have liver-protective effects, as is the case with mushroom poisoning. Milk thistle (silymarin) is also a useful supplement; extensive scientific research has been done on its liver-protective effects. Finally, there are traditional Chinese herbal formulas, such as Hepa #2, by Dr. Zhang, that have been found to be useful in treating inflammation in the liver. Dr. Zhang treats many patients with chronic hepatitis. The formulation he calls Hepa #2 is useful in lowering liver functions for those with chronic liver disease, and we have confirmed the utility of this herbal formulation for our patients with elevated liver functions.

Liver abnormalities are commonly seen with Lyme-MSIDS, and patients may be asymptomatic for them early on in the course of the illness. Liver diseases such as hepatitis, and genetic disorders such as hemochromatosis, can be life-threatening, are very prevalent in the general population, and can only be identified in the earliest stages through proper blood work. By using the above differential diagnostic categories and testing protocols, it is possible to move through the complicated maze of options, improve your health, and discover one more clue to your symptoms.

EIGHTEEN

Lyme and Pain

One of the most disabling symptoms for the patient with MSIDS is chronic pain. For those suffering from Lyme-MSIDS, over-the-counter medications such as acetaminophen (Tylenol), ibuprofen (Advil), or naproxen sodium (Naprosyn/Aleve) only provide minimal relief. By the time they see me, some of the patients are on high-dose narcotics to control their pain. These patients frequently have seen rheumatologists and, depending on their clinical presentation, they may have been told that they suffer from seronegative rheumatoid arthritis or from a nonspecific autoimmune disease. They are then placed on steroids such as prednisone, or disease-modifying anti-rheumatic drug regimens, such as methotrexate, arava, or TNF-α blockers, such as Enbrel. These agents might give temporary relief but can have significant side effects.

Pain can be so debilitating that some people lose their ability to function in a meaningful and productive way. Many turn to pain management specialists, who then often prescribe multiple drug regimens of neuroleptic drugs and narcotics, combined with nerve blocks to provide pain relief. Despite these physicians' best attempts, the patients may still have pain, and as the narcotics wear off, higher and higher doses are required to control their discomfort. Often the end result is that pain sufferers end up on disability, and are unable to work or go to school.

PAIN AND LYME DISEASE

Lyme disease can cause pain in every part of the body. Although this pain may be limited to one or two areas, and be more or less constant, one particular hallmark of tick-borne disease, and particularly *Borrelia burgdorferi*, is that pain comes and goes and migrates. This includes arthritis pain, myalgias (muscle pain), and neuropathic pain (nerve pain), all of which normally do not tend to migrate. In women the pain is also influenced by hormonal cycles, since women usually flare for several days right before, during, and after their menses. We can also suspect a tick-borne disorder when antibiotic use increases pain (from a Jarisch-Herxheimer reaction) or decreases pain. This will occasionally happen in patients treated for an unrelated bacterial infection, such as a sinusitis or urinary tract infection, who are unaware that they have Lyme disease.

If pain is associated with multiple systemic symptoms, especially the ones listed in the Horowitz Lyme-MSIDS questionnaire, then it is quite likely that it is caused by Lyme-MSIDS. A patient who just presents with neck pain or an isolated pain in a joint might simply have a herniated disc with neuropathy, or osteoarthritis. If a patient circles many of the symptoms on this sheet, one should suspect a tick-borne disorder and order the appropriate tests. This includes testing for co-infections such as *Babesia*, which increases all of the underlying symptoms of Lyme disease; *Bartonella*, a frequent cofactor in neuropathy; as well as *Mycoplasma* and *Chlamydia*, which can increase arthritis pain. Similarly, viruses and yeast may impact pain syndromes, and should be tested for and treated if patients do not improve with treatments for bacterial and associated parasitic infections.

Establishing a proper pain etiology can be difficult, because as we have seen in numerous other chapters in this book, Lyme-MSIDS can mimic most common pain syndromes. For example, MSIDS can cause chronic fatigue syndrome and fibromyalgia, with widespread pain. It can cause symptoms of common autoimmune diseases such as rheumatoid arthritis, lupus, and multiple sclerosis with associated inflammation. It can present with a varied list of neurological syndromes that cause pain, including headaches and migraines, peripheral neuropathy, neuropathy of the face, dental pain syndromes, trigeminal neuralgia, radiculopathy, associated cranial nerve palsies, and carpal tunnel with ulnar neuropathy. It may present with painful gastrointestinal and genitourinary syndromes, with irritable bowel syndrome, associated inflammatory bowel disease, or interstitial cystitis. We have seen patients with painful gynecological syndromes, including vaginal neuralgia and dysparaneuria (painful intercourse), and painful cardiac presentations, such as resistant chest pain (due to costochondritis, with inflammation in the nerves and cartilage of the chest wall) and pericarditis (inflammation of the sac surrounding the heart). Patients also may present with painful eye syndromes, such as conjunctivitis, uveitis, retinitis, or optic neuritis (inflammation in different parts of the eye) and psychiatric symptoms such as depression and anxiety that result from tick-borne diseases may further increase their perception of pain.

You may remember that there are both strains and species of *Borrelia*. Pain syndromes depend on the particular strains and species. Some cause significant pain, and others do not. There are approximately one hundred different strains of *Borrelia* in the United States, and three hundred strains worldwide, and they can cause different clinical syndromes. In Europe, a different species of *Borrelia*, *Borrelia afzelii*, is responsible for the classic purplish skin rash of acrodermatitis chronicum atrophicans (ACA), but another species, *Borrelia garinii*, is responsible for symptoms of Lyme neuroborreliosis with associated neuropathic pain syndromes, like Bannwarth's syndrome. *Borrelia burgdorferi sensu stricto* is the primary form of *Borrelia* found in the United States, and the B 31 strain will have different clinical manifestations than the European species, and cause especially severe pain syndromes, depending on the length of the infection, and the patient's co-infection status and genetic makeup (HLA status). All of these spirochetes have proteins on their outer surface, called lipoproteins, and are known to be proinflammatory, but more than 8 percent of the genetic coding sequence of strain B 31 found in the United States is devoted to these lipoprotein sequences. Researchers reported in the journal *Infection and Immunity* that *Borrelia* lipoproteins attract immune cells (neutrophils) to the site of infection and are fifty- to five-hundred-fold more active inducers of inflammatory cytokines than lipoproteins of other common bacterial organisms, such as *E. coli*. These cytokines, such as TNF-alpha, IL-1, and IL-6, increase pain in the muscles, joints, and nerves by having a direct effect on nerve fibers. In the peripheral nervous system, cytokines such as interleukin-1beta also can cause the release of other inflammatory molecules from the nitric oxide pathway, as well as increase the production of pain-inducing molecules such as bradykinin and/or prostaglandins. Another possible source of pain arises from the body's production of *Borrelia*-specific antibodies. These may target the 41 kDa flagella and other outer surface proteins (especially Osp A) in an attempt to disable the bacteria, then cross react with antigens on the surface of our own nerves and organs, which are structurally similar. This process is called "molecular mimicry," and immune reactions against such shared antigens could play a role in the chronic manifestations of Lyme borreliosis, including pain.

Simultaneously treating the three I's of Lyme disease—infection, inflammation, and immune dysfunction—may be the key to alleviating chronic pain. Blebs secreted from the surface of *Borrelia burgdorferi* can cause a nonspecific stimulation of the immune system (apart from the role of co-infections such as *Babesia*, *Bartonella*, and *Mycoplasma fermentans* previously discussed). Blebs are shed particles containing partial DNA, from *Borrelia burgdorferi*. These blebs are highly stimulatory to the immune system, and intracellular blebs convert host cells into targets for the immune system. We also discussed the role of the nitric oxide (NO) pathway and its ability to increase oxidative stress and increase cytokines in Lyme disease, fibromyalgia, environmental illness, and chronic fatigue syndrome. Diverse stressors, whether viral, bacterial, physical, emotional, or exposure to volatile organic solvents or pesticides can all increase nitric oxide and its oxidant product peroxynitrite, leading to an increase in cytokines and pain syndromes. This would be one of the common mechanisms linking these different diseases, which all have similar clinical presentations. Finally, inadequate phase I and phase II liver detoxification, with inadequate production or overutilization of glutathione, and the subsequent inability to remove neurotoxins and cytokines often seen with Lyme-MSIDS, will also result in pain.

OTHER CAUSES OF PAIN

Many different medical problems that are listed on the MSIDS map can cause pain, and may be contributing overlapping factors. Each of these different factors can increase free radical production and increase cytokines, and may need to be simultaneously addressed to achieve adequate pain control in both Lyme-MSIDS and non-Lyme-MSIDS. These would include:

- Detoxification problems
- Endocrine abnormalities
- Food allergies
- Heavy metals and environmental toxins
- Nutritional and enzyme deficiencies
- Other infections, including bacteria, parasites, viruses, and opportunistic infections (*Candida*)
- Sleep disorders

Psychological disorders may also increase discomfort, as the amygdala is the part of the brain that deals with emotions and pain sensation. When patients suffer from depression and anxiety, their pain thresholds can be lowered, leading to increased perception of pain.

BRETT'S PAIN WOULDN'T GO AWAY

Brett was twenty-seven years old from Boston with a past medical history significant for kidney stones, hypokalemia (low potassium), low vitamin D, and hyperlipidemia, but his biggest complaint when he came to see me was his chronic pain. He complained of severe joint and neuropathic pain and was taking MS Contin (morphine sulfate) and Dilaudid: These are high-dose narcotics that were barely addressing his pain. He also had spinal disc problems (located at L5-S1), which he was told were causing his chronic back pain, and it was keeping him up at night, causing insomnia and depression. He had been diagnosed with a nonspecific autoimmune disease as well as seronegative rheumatoid arthritis. He had seen over one hundred doctors in the previous several years (you read that number correctly), including eight rheumatologists. He had been on multiple immunosuppressive and biological agents, including prednisone, methotrexate, Enbrel, and Humira. His history included multiple tick bites (five to ten), and he complained of drenching night sweats every night for over a year, severe fatigue, decreased libido, chronic constipation, chest pain, migratory joint pain in the wrists, hands, elbows, shoulders, hips, and ankles, and a slight swelling of the joints. Other symptoms included sore muscles, headaches, facial pain with intermittent Bell's palsy, tingling, numbness and burning sensations in his arms and legs, floaters in his eyes, and tremors.

His physical examination was unremarkable except for low blood pressure while standing (BP 86/54) with associated dizziness and palpitations (pulse rate: 112 beats per minute), swollen nasal turbinates, and decreased sensation in his hands. Laboratory testing showed a low potassium, low serum zinc, low serum iodine, low RBC magnesium, normal B_{12} and folic acid levels, normal thyroid functions, borderline hypercortisolism, multiple food allergies (IgG positive for milk, soy, wheat, beef, peanuts), and increased levels of lead and mercury. We determined that his autoimmune reaction was connected to antiganglioside antibodies against his nerves. A previous physician had ordered Lyme testing, which revealed a borderline Lyme IgG Western blot and a decreased CD 57 count (an alternative blood test used to help support the clinical diagnosis of Lyme disease and to follow the disease's progression). We then ordered more blood work, which revealed positive titers for *Mycoplasma pneumoniae*, as well as a low-level EBV and HHV-6 titers. All other co-infection testing was negative.

In my clinical judgment, Brett suffered from Lyme disease with co-infections, particularly babesiosis, and autonomic nervous system dysfunction. I started him on Coartem, followed by Omnicef, Plaquenil, Mepron, Zithromax, nystatin, and Serrapeptase. This regimen would address the cell wall forms, cystic forms, and intracellular location of *Borrelia* as well as treat biofilms and associated parasitic infections. An anti-inflammatory protocol was given, including alpha-lipoic acid, resveratrol, curcumin, and glutathione. He was advised to avoid his allergic foods, and use EDTA suppositories with DMSA to remove his heavy metals; his mineral deficiencies were addressed by replacing them with a high-potency multimineral supplement that contained calcium, potassium, magnesium, zinc, iodine, and other trace minerals.

Once he started this protocol, his pain and depression initially worsened, but his drenching night sweats became less frequent. After several weeks his incessant joint pain finally decreased to a point where it was tolerable. Cymbalta was added for the depression, fibromyalgia symptoms, and neuropathy, as well as Lyrica for sleep and ongoing neuropathic pain. Florinef was then added for his low blood pressure and autonomic nervous system dysfunction, and Omnicef was rotated to IM Bicillin LA for ongoing severe symptoms.

One month later there was a slight improvement in his pain, and he felt increased energy with the Bicillin injections, but he had a significant relapse of day sweats off the Mepron. Due to the severe pain and neuropathy, I suspected *Bartonella*, and Factive was prescribed with cryptolepis for the clinical symptoms of babesiosis. Once the *Bartonella* and *Babesia* were treated, Brett was able to start lowering the doses of the MS Contin and Dilaudid for the first time in years. He reported that he was doing "really well," with a significant decrease in pain while on Factive, but he noticed significant relapses of his pain whenever he was off of it. He was on his sixth cycle of pulsed therapy with a quinolone, implying an intracellular organism such as *Bartonella*, and/or *Mycoplasma* as one of the primary causes of the pain. Since he relapsed when he was off intracellular meds, minocycline was added to the regimen, as double intracellular antibiotics are often more effective against intracellular infections. Once the minocycline was added, his energy showed further improvement, and the sweats were no longer drenching. We were able to decrease the MS Contin over a two-month period, and he was eventually able to get off all his narcotics for the first time in years. Once his Lyme disease and associated tick-borne infections were properly treated, the pain was much more manageable.

TREATING PAIN RELATED TO MSIDS AND LYME

The pain in Lyme disease and MSIDS is often resistant to standard treatment modalities such as NSAIDS, SSRIs, and neuroleptic medications such as Neurontin, and is incompletely controlled with narcotics. Some MSIDS patients given oral and IV glutathione will have dramatic decreases in musculoskeletal and arthritic pain, as well as improvements in their headaches, fatigue, and neurocognitive difficulties within minutes to hours of receiving treatment. In a study I performed in 2004, patients reported improvement in fatigue, joint pain, muscle pain, mood swings, headaches, balance, dizziness, speech problems, and cognitive difficulties within thirty minutes of the administration of glutathione. Glutathione may be acting to metabolize toxins in the short term, and may have an effect on cytokines, prostaglandins, interleukins, oxidative stress, and immune modulation in the long term. We have found detoxification to be crucial in helping patients deal with their chronic resistant pain.

Aside from glutathione, I divide pain treatments into two basic categories. The first would be a pharmaceutical approach, in which we simply treat the symptoms, and the second would be an integrative approach, in which we treat the whole person. This would include a body/mind/spiritual approach, while addressing biochemical/immunological imbalances. We always attempt to get to the "source" of the pain.

Using the Horowitz sixteen-point differential diagnostic map we have found that a multifaceted approach works best in treating patients with overlapping CFS and FMS. Those who complain of severe headaches, neuralgia, myalgias, and arthritis find that a combination of antibiotics and/or nutraceuticals and herbs for Lyme disease and co-infections can effectively treat pain. Usually the sickest patients will require a combined approach, using pharmaceuticals and nutraceuticals along with classical pain medications to help relieve their suffering.

CLASSIC PAIN MEDICATION TREATMENTS

Multiple treatments from each of the following six categories are often necessary to achieve adequate pain relief:

1. NSAIDS (nonsteroidal anti-inflammatory drugs): effective analgesics for muscle pain; includes medications such as Motrin, Aleve, Naprosyn, Voltaren, and Zipsor. Contraindications include a history of ulcer disease, bleeding disorders, liver abnormalities, and uncontrolled blood pressure.

2. Antidepressants: Some antidepressants are effective in helping to relieve pain. Among the class of SSRIs, which includes Prozac, there are several medications that not only block serotonin uptake in the brain, but also block the uptake of another neurotransmitter, norepinephrine. We first learned about norepinephrine in the chapter on autonomic nervous system dysfunction, where we saw that norepinephrine acts as both a hormone and neurotransmitter, and has an effect on blood pressure and heart rate. Norepinephrine also has an effect on decreasing pain. Those SSRIs (like Cymbalta) that increase serotonin and norepinephrine simultaneously have been proven to be helpful in decreasing both muscular

pain and neuropathic pain. Elavil is another antidepressant in a different class of medication (tricyclic antidepressants), which also has been shown to have an effect on neuropathic pain.

3. Single-dose Decadron and Neurontin: Occasionally Lyme patients have to go for surgery from an unrelated illness. Steroids are generally contraindicated in Lyme disease, because of their immune suppressive effects, but a single dose of the steroid Decadron administered with Neurontin has been shown to improve postoperative pain and may be useful. Antibiotics should always be used pre- and postsurgery to prevent a worsening of symptoms.

4. Combination drug regimens: Lyme-MSIDS patients may have resistant pain that is not controlled with one medication, and combination regimens may improve pain control at lower doses than single analgesics alone. Examples of effective combination drug therapy include using tricyclic antidepressants (Elavil, Pamelor) and Neurontin with or without opioids. This regimen is particularly effective in patients with overlapping migraines and neuropathic pain (burning sensations of the extremities).

5. IVIG: This is the treatment of choice for pain secondary to small fiber neuropathy and chronic inflammatory demyelinating polyneuropathy (CIDP), which is an immune-mediated inflammatory disorder of the peripheral nervous system seen with Lyme disease. We use IVIG for patients with significant immunoglobulin deficiencies, as well as for neuropathic pain that has persisted in patients with Lyme-MSIDS. IVIG is used for patients with resistant neuropathy despite treating *Borrelia* and co-infections such as *Bartonella* and despite detoxing heavy metals such as mercury and lead that can both affect nerve function and cause neuropathy.

6. Nondestructive, minimally invasive techniques for refractory pain: This would include electronic stimulators, pulsed radiofrequency, and Botox injections. Some Lyme disease patients do not adequately respond to pharmaceutical regimens for pain, as in the case of severe back pain unresponsive to standard therapies. Electronic stimulators (peripheral, spinal, and motor cortex) can improve difficult to manage chronic pain syndromes, pulsed radiofrequency can decrease pain without tissue damage, and Botox may be able to decrease targeted neuropathic pain.

INTEGRATIVE TREATMENTS

1. Low-dose naltrexone (LDN): We have found LDN to be an extremely useful and effective medication in patients with resistant pain, and it should be routinely considered in patients with Lyme-MSIDS with overlapping pain syndromes. LDN has been studied for treating multiple sclerosis and fibromyalgia. A study published in 2010 in *Online Annals of Neurology* showed that LDN was well tolerated, and it significantly improved mental health quality-of-life indicators, with a 1.6 point improvement on the pain effects scale (P = .04). This confirmed a prior study published in 2008 in *Multiple Sclerosis* on the use of LDN for MS: It was studied for its effects on pain, fatigue, depression, quality of life, safety, and tolerability. Protein concentrations of beta-endorphins increased during this trial, which is significant, because endorphins are one of the mechanisms the body has for helping to decrease pain. Similar results were found with drugs such as naltrexone and naloxone, which were able to reduce inflammatory reactions in microglial brain cells in animal studies. These studies have important implications for those with MSIDS, because the same cytokines seen in Lyme disease, FM, and CFS that increase inflammation and pain are also found in those with inflammation from Crohn's disease and MS. LDN helped decrease pain and inflammation in each of these diverse groups.

I performed a study of LDN with my patients. It started in 2009 and is continuing to date. Patients with CFS- and fibromyalgia-type symptoms, who had been diagnosed with Lyme disease and co-infections, are given LDN at gradually increasing doses. Patients are started at 2 mg at bedtime for one month, and then increased to 3 mg at bedtime for a second month, until reaching a final dose of 4.5 mg at bedtime. Over seven hundred patients have participated in this clinical trial to date. The results have shown that approximately 75 percent of patients with Lyme-MSIDS improved their FM and CFS symptoms, including fatigue, myalgias, and arthralgias. LDN was well tolerated without any significant side effects, although a small percentage (10 percent to 20 percent) had to decrease the dosage or stop the drug due to insomnia. Those who cannot tolerate LDN at bedtime can take it upon awakening in the morning.

2. Antioxidant therapies: These would include pharmaceuticals such as glutathione, and nutraceuticals such as alpha-lipoic acid, NAC, glycine, sulforaphane, resveratrol, and curcumin. NAC, glycine, and alpha-lipoic acid all help augment the production of glutathione, which has been shown to be clinically beneficial in decreasing pain, fatigue, and brain fog in the resistant Lyme patient. Antioxidant therapies may be helpful, especially in patients with overstimulated immune systems producing large numbers of inflammatory cytokines. These supplements lower oxidative stress, which subsequently decreases the stimulation of NFKappaB, thereby turning off the switch which is responsible for the production of inflammatory cytokines.

In our medical practice, we combine the antioxidants mentioned above to achieve a synergistic effect, especially if lipid peroxide levels are elevated (a biomarker of oxidative stress) or if patients have resistant pain. In our study on LDN, we often combined LDN with antioxidants such as alpha-lipoic acid, glutathione, resveratrol, and curcumin to reduce free radicals and inflammation, which increase pain, as well as using supplements to support detoxification and removal of the inflammatory cytokines from the body. These combinations can be particularly effective in the Lyme-MSIDS patient with chronic pain.

3. Angiotensin receptor blockers (ARBs): Angiotensin II is a hormone that regulates vascular tone, stimulates the release of proinflammatory cytokines, activates NFKappaB, and increases oxidative stress, thus functioning as an inflammatory molecule. ARBs are known to decrease levels of TNF-alpha. ARBs such as Benicar may be useful in certain cases of persistent inflammation, especially when associated with uncontrolled hypertension. These medications are often associated with the Marshall protocol for treating Lyme disease, which incorporates ARBs and lowering vitamin D levels as a means of controlling inflammation. It is occasionally useful for those with ongoing, severe Jarisch-Herxheimer reactions who cannot tolerate intracellular antibiotics such as tetracyclines and macrolides.

Several of our patients have had a positive response to ARBs, but I have been hesitant to use the high doses recommended in the Marshall protocol because of concerns about lowering blood pressure significantly. I prefer to use other methods, such as LDN and antioxidants, to decrease inflammatory cytokines. Similarly, a very small percentage of my patients describe flare reactions after sun exposure, possibly due to increased vitamin D levels increasing inflammation. However, the great majority of patients in our practice (close to 90 percent) are vitamin D deficient and do not have any difficulty tolerating vitamin D supplementation. Based on recent scientific evidence that vitamin D can help to decrease morbidity and mortality in certain patient groups, I believe that the benefit outweighs the risk of using it in the MSIDS population. Using ARBs and lowering vitamin D would only be a reasonable intervention for those with inflammation who are unresponsive to other treatment protocols.

4. Following an anti-inflammatory diet: Anti-inflammatory diets consist of increasing the amounts of omega-3 fatty acids and decreasing omega-6 fatty acids. The goal is to achieve the proper balance of fatty acids, because when the ratio of omega-3 to omega-6 fatty acids is out of balance, this contributes to inflammation, thus increasing pain. Levels of fatty acids can be tested through functional medicine laboratories such as Metametrix. If the ratios are too high toward the omega-6 side, and there is evidence of inflammation, we recommend a diet change and add nutritional supplements, such as high doses of omega-3 fatty acids in the form of mercury-free fish oils that are also high in DHA.

Anti-inflammatory diets consist of Mediterranean-style menus that incorporate the use of increased fresh fruits and vegetables, decreased consumption of red meat, eggs, and dairy, and eating more fish (omega-3 fatty acids). This is typically combined with the occasional consumption of red wine (for increasing resveratrol) and avoiding simple sugars, although I do not recommend drinking alcohol to my MSIDS patients while they are being treated with antibiotics, since most patients with tick-borne diseases tend to feel worse after drinking (especially if they are on Flagyl or Tindamax). Due to the high levels of mercury often found in seafood, I recommend wild organic salmon and limiting consumption of farm-raised fish unless you know how they are raised, as well as avoiding eating raw fish or sushi, due to the possibility of parasites. Eating smaller fish is also advisable, since larger fish, such as tuna, tilefish, and swordfish, accumulate more mercury, as they are higher up in the food chain.

A newer diet plan, the Paleo diet, has had some provocative results with chronically ill patients. The diet consists of eating lean meat, fish, low-carb fruits such as berries, vegetables, nuts, and healthy fats, while avoiding high-carb foods, grains, dairy, and salt. This type of diet may be warranted in those with resistant fatigue, headaches, dizziness, palpitations, mood swings, and insomnia that have failed other treatment and dietary interventions. These symptoms overlap those of Lyme-MSIDS, and patients report that their Lyme disease symptoms are exacerbated when their blood sugars swing toward the low side. The Paleo diet helps stabilize hypoglycemia, and can also be beneficial for those patients with overlapping food allergies and food sensitivities to gluten and grains, which may account for its clinical effect. An avoidance of gluten in foods may be indicated in patients who continue to complain of resistant fatigue, myalgias, arthralgias, headaches, and gastrointestinal complaints. There are those who do not have true celiac disease but are still sensitive to grains and report that they feel much better avoiding these foods on this diet.

5. Stress reduction techniques: Meditation, yoga, and Tai chi can be helpful, since repeated episodes of acute or chronic psychological stress can induce an acute phase response and subsequently a chronic inflammatory process. Through the relationship of mind-body medicine, and the intermediary of psychoneuroimmunology, if we can integrate the practice of mindfulness meditation (Kabat-Zinn), calm abiding meditation, or other stress-reduction techniques into our daily routines, we will not only be providing a way to better cope with our illness, but also will be helping to decrease stress as another factor driving the inflammatory response. These are discussed in more detail in Chapter 20.

6. Treatments for Jarisch-Herxheimer reactions: This would include alkalizing the body, and using methods described above to decrease the levels of cytokines. Herxheimer reactions increase pain cycles due to production of cytokines, especially TNF-alpha, IL-1, and IL-6. The key to controlling Jarish-Herxheimer reactions is to "shut down the faucet and open the drain," i.e., decrease the production of cytokines and flush them out of the body, as well as remove any associated neurotoxins causing illness. I have found a five-step approach to be effective in up to 70 percent of my Lyme disease patients.

a. Alkalize: During Jarish-Herxheimer reactions, as well as in severe illness in general, the body can get acidic. This is detrimental to health, as the enzymatic processes of the body function best at a neutral pH of around 7.4. We therefore want to shift the acid/base balance, and balance the pH if we become acidic. This involves the use of Alka-Seltzer Gold during a Jarisch-Herxheimer flare, or using an equivalent medication, such as sodium bicarbonate tablets. Other effective methods include buffered vitamin C and lemon-lime water.

I presented a paper at the International Lyme and Associated Diseases Conference in 2003 on the use of "lemon-lime" therapy for the treatment of Herxheimer reactions. We know that alkaline reserves act as buffers to maintain a pH balance in the blood, which is essential to proper metabolic functioning. During periods of inflammatory responses, acid by-products are produced that may deplete alkaline reserves with a corresponding increase in free radical production damaging tissues. Lakesmaa and colleagues published in the *Journal of Infectious Diseases* that the effects of these tissue and circulating cytokines can explain many of the symptoms and inflammatory reactions seen with Jarisch-Herxheimer reactions. The study we performed was designed to observe whether antioxidant supplementation and increasing the alkaline reserves during the Jarisch-Herxheimer flare would have an appreciable effect on symptoms in a cohort of Lyme patients during antibiotic therapy. The methodology involved patients squeezing one to two fresh lemons or limes in a glass of water and drinking it over several minutes at the onset of a Jarisch-Herxheimer flare. Among thirty patients surveyed, 70 percent reported mild to moderate improvements in symptoms within several hours. Symptoms that improved included fatigue, muscle and joint pain, fever, sweats, hot flashes, muscle spasms, and paresthesias, with several patients reporting an improvement in overall wellness within minutes.

We know that fruits and vegetables are generally alkaline-containing foods. Lemon and lime juice, although tasting acidic, are converted to alkaline ash in the body, thereby temporarily raising alkaline reserves. These will buffer acid by-products of infection and provide an increase in water-soluble antioxidants that are available to counter increased free radical production. Alkalinization can also augment the effect of certain antibiotics in killing intracellular bacteria. These results imply that in certain Lyme disease patients depleted alkaline reserves and increased free radical damage with oxidative stress may be temporarily responsible for increased symptoms during Jarisch-Herxheimer reactions, apart from intermediary cytokines and their overall metabolic effects on the body.

Another study, published in the *American Journal of Epidemiology*, reported on data from the thirty-thousand-subject Iowa

Women's Health Study. Results indicated that beta-cryptoxanthin, a substance present in citrus fruit, helped decrease the incidence and risk of developing rheumatoid arthritis. It is therefore possible that other substances in citrus fruits were playing a beneficial role apart from increasing the alkaline reserves in our patients with J-H flares.

b. Support the elimination of toxins: Glutathione has already been discussed in this book in terms of its effectiveness in patients with severe Jarisch-Herxheimer flares. Other supplements that support liver detoxification (milk thistle, dandelion, phosphatidyl-choline), or different methods of intestinal detoxification, such as using charcoal, bentonite clay, zeolite, or occasionally using enemas in the very sick patient can be beneficial.

c. Shut down the production of cytokines: This involves the use of LDN and antioxidants to decrease the stimulation of NFKappaB (alpha-lipoic acid, resveratrol, curcumin, DIM, and sulforaphane).

d. Supplement with minerals used in the detoxification reactions. These include magnesium (used in more than three hundred detox enzymes), zinc (needed in phase I liver detoxification and alcohol dehydrogenase), and copper (used in SOD), which can be found in a good multimineral supplement.

e. "Open up the drain." There are different nutraceutical drainage remedies available, such as ones that work on lymphatic drainage (i.e., Itires, Pekana drainage remedies) or general drainage formulas, such as SyDetox (Syntrion) or those in the Cowden protocol, such as Parsley and Burbur (NutraMedix), that are helpful in a percentage of patients. Taking in extra fluids and getting adequate sleep, combined with a mild exercise program and infrared saunas for further elimination of toxins, can also be helpful.

7. Transdermal pain medications: Some patients have pain localized over one or two areas and do not require oral medications. The benefits of topical treatments include delivering higher drug concentrations at the site than can be achieved through oral delivery, while significantly reducing or eliminating GI, hepatic, and systemic side effects. One readily available example is Voltaren gel, which is mainly used for osteoarthritis and is usually applied up to four times a day to the affected site.

8. Herbal therapies: As discussed earlier, the herbs most commonly used in our practice for those with Lyme disease and pain are andrographis, *Polygonum* (a form of resveratrol), Stephania root, *Smilax*, redroot, and boneset. These all have strong scientific support and can be useful for those with ongoing symptoms and inflammation. These herbs can be added to any regimen to help decrease inflammation and pain, and one herbal protocol made by Greenwood Herbals in Maine combines three herbs: *Smilax*, redroot, and boneset for Herxheimer reactions. Patients have reported that this combination has been effective in decreasing pain associated with Jarisch-Herxheimer flares.

MARTHA HAD TO GET RID OF LYME AND OTHER TOXINS BEFORE HER PAIN WENT AWAY

Martha had a history of Lyme disease, depression, and anxiety, as well as Hashimoto's thyroiditis (an autoimmune disease) and high levels of ANA antibodies. She also was diagnosed with chronic inflammatory demyelinating polyneuropathy (CIDP), which is a very painful nerve disorder seen occasionally in those with Lyme disease. Her severe neuropathy was present for three years, and she had been on IVIG for six months when I first saw her, without any significant response to therapy.

Martha was forty-eight years old when we first saw her, and her symptoms included fatigue, deep muscle pain in the lower back and legs, severe burning pains in her arms and legs, and occasional night sweats. She had failed antibiotic therapy with amoxicillin prescribed by a prior treating physician, and she had been placed on IV Rocephin, which was somewhat helpful for her pain. Other antibiotics caused severe Jarisch-Herxheimer flares, and her neuropathy flared so badly that all treatments needed to be stopped. Her co-infection testing was positive for *Babesia*, but treatment with Mepron and Zithromax also caused severe flares of pain and neuropathy, and could not be continued.

Her physical examination was essentially unremarkable. Other medications used for pain had included Neurontin, with Mobic (an NSAID) and IVIG, but these medications were ineffective at controlling the pain. Her sleep was also significantly disturbed, and she had been using Klonopin to fall asleep, but she still awoke frequently from her discomfort.

Further lab testing revealed a positive *Babesia* titer and FISH assay, elevated viral titers of CMV, EBV, and HHV-6, an elevated sedimentation rate consistent with inflammation, and positive Raji cell immune complexes. She also had decreased B cell levels on immunological testing (*Borrelia* kills B cells), with elevated titers of antinuclear antibodies (ANA), and the HLA DR4 marker was positive. Heavy metal testing was performed with a six-hour urine DMSA challenge, and it revealed elevated levels of mercury and lead. She also had low folic acid levels and elevated liver functions, but the workup for the liver abnormalities was negative. There was a normal level of alpha-1 antitrypsin, no signs of hepatitis B or C, and normal levels of iron and copper, ruling out hemochromatosis and Wilson's disease. An MRI of the lower back revealed a dorsal nerve root compression that, apart from the CIDP, was contributing to her neuropathic pain.

We started her on a new treatment course that included adding Septra (Bactrim double strength) to the Mepron and Zithromax to treat the *Babesia* and possible *Bartonella* infection. She had never tried Septra, and *Bartonella* is known to be a frequent associated cause of neuropathy. *Bartonella* testing is known to be highly unreliable, as it is an intracellular co-infection, and both *Babesia* and *Bartonella* can respond favorably to sulfa drugs like Septra. Within days of adding the Septra, her severe pain started to decrease. Re-treatment with IV Rocephin was tried, and also decreased the pain, but she kept relapsing off medications and was failing IVIG almost one year into the therapy. We then used LDN combined with resveratrol, alpha-lipoic acid, glutathione, curcumin, DIM, and sulforaphane. DIM assists in balancing phase I liver detoxification, and sulforaphane is the most potent nutritional stimulator of phase II liver detoxification pathways, as well as being a potent antioxidant. Herbs to fight the Lyme disease, such as Samento and Banderol, were added slowly and in low doses as we started to taper her off of the antibiotics for the first time in over a year.

After following this new course of treatment for one month, Martha came back to my office elated. There was significant improvement in her pain for the first time in years! She noticed it almost immediately after the LDN was added to her regimen. She was able to come off her antibiotics and IVIG, which previously was unthinkable. She was then chelated with low-dose DMSA to remove the mercury and lead (which is a cofactor in neuropathy) and was sent for physical therapy for mild ongoing low back pain (due to the compression that showed up on her MRI). Over time, the resistant neuropathy completely cleared, and she remained on

Samento, Cumunda, and Plaquenil for two more years without a significant relapse in any of her symptoms.

Martha's case illustrates that proper treatment of co-infections and
heavy metals with antioxidant therapies and LDN may be effective in
those with Lyme-MSIDS who have failed traditional pain therapies alone.
Relieving a patient's suffering by decreasing their pain or helping them
become pain free, is one of the most rewarding aspects of treating Lyme
disease and associated tick-borne illnesses. If we can decrease the total
load of the organisms, balance an overstimulated immune system, and
decrease inflammatory cytokines (treating the three I's), we can significantly improve resistant pain syndromes.

NINETEEN

Lyme and Exercise

The most basic component of our overall health lies in our genetic code: our DNA. Just as we know that we inherit certain physical characteristics and social/emotional traits from our parents, we also inherit their health profile. This is why doctors have been taught to take a comprehensive family history during an initial consultation. However, we now know that these genes do not equal our destiny. In many instances, environment and lifestyle choices can affect the way genes are expressed. Instead of resigning yourself to the fact that you will have a chronic disease because one or both of your parents experienced the same illness, we have come to understand that you can prevent this scenario by taking better care of your overall health before symptoms present. This involves changing your diet and getting enough exercise. These simple steps not only make you feel better, but actually change the structure and function of your DNA. The science that backs up this theory is known as epigenetics.

The two most important lifestyle changes that influence health are diet and exercise. The scientific literature is beginning to show that there are exercise-induced changes in gene expression in specific organ systems that may result from inactivity. For example, the capacity of skeletal muscle to oxidize fuels is directly dependent upon the duration and intensity of exercise. Cytochrome c protein is a marker of mitochondrial density and capacity to oxidize fuels, and it will increase or decrease depending on the level of exercise or inactivity. More exercise translates into increased mitochondrial production and increased energy. Patients with Lyme disease, fibromyalgia, and chronic fatigue syndrome (myalgic encephalomyelitis) find that their fatigue and pain syndromes improve with increased exercise, independently of other changes in their medical regimens.

We need a certain amount of nitric oxide (NO) in the vascular system, produced by the vascular endothelium, to support cardiac health. Physical inactivity can lower NO expression in vessel walls, which may prevent dilatation of the coronary arteries leading to angina and a worsening of heart disease. Insulin resistance and elevated blood sugars are also higher in patients who are sedentary, since contracting muscles not only increase glucose uptake, but also lead to gene expression of AMP-activated protein kinase (AMPK). This in turn affects stimulation of gene expression for glucose transporter 4 (GLUT4) and hexokinase, which are both enzymes important in glucose regulation. GLUT4 transcription is decreased with physical inactivity, and diabetes prevalence has been found to be much higher in developed countries versus the levels in physically active agricultural societies, implying a strong role for exercise and regular physical activity in preventing diabetes.

Vigorous walking for at least twenty minutes per day may positively influence many chronic health conditions, ranging from diabetes to cancer. Studies have shown that those who are able to adhere to the American Heart Association's seven ideal cardiovascular health components not only reduced the incidence of cardiovascular disease but even lowered the incidence of several major types of cancer as well. These include:

1. Maintaining a body mass index (BMI) below 25 (visit http://nhlbisupport.com/bmi/ for more information and to access a BMI scale)
2. Refraining from smoking
3. Maintaining an untreated total cholesterol below 200 mg/dl
4. Maintaining an untreated blood pressure below 120/80 mm Hg
5. Maintaining an untreated fasting blood glucose below 100 mg/dl
6. Performing at least 150 minutes per week of moderate exercise, or 75 minutes per week of vigorous physical activity. Moderate exercise would include fast walking, a slow jog, and slow

bicycling (an activity where you can still carry on a conversation), and vigorous physical activity would include high-intensity aerobics (running, cycling, swimming, elliptical training, Stair-Master, kickboxing, Zumba, team sports) where the level of activity would preclude talking because of the increased intensity

7. Following a healthy diet, as outlined in this book

There is an inverse relationship between compliance with diet and exercise recommendations and the incidence of cardiovascular disease (the higher the compliance, the lower the incidence of disease). This was confirmed in a similar analysis of data by investigators at the American Cancer Society, where a high level of adherence to cancer prevention recommendations regarding obesity, diet, alcohol consumption, and increased physical activity not only decreased cancer rates, but also decreased cardiovascular mortality. In that study there was a 48 percent reduction of cardiovascular mortality in men, and a 58 percent reduction in cardiovascular mortality in women, as well as being associated with a 30 percent and 24 percent reduction in cancer mortality in men and women respectively. By losing weight and exercising, we are helping to decrease inflammation and increase detoxification, which are of paramount importance in MSIDS. Patients feel much better, both physically and mentally, once they have adopted a healthy lifestyle program.

MSIDS AND EXERCISE

The medical literature has abundant examples of the use of exercise, and behavioral, nutritional, and physiological interventions to treat fatigue in both autoimmune diseases and multiple sclerosis. Applying the MSIDS model, it may be reasonable to assume that some of these same patients may also have Lyme and associated co-infections. I have seen patients significantly improve their symptoms and recover their health using these same exercise and nutritional interventions.

Aerobic exercise has been shown to be effective in reducing fatigue among adults with chronic autoimmune conditions, as well as those with depression, cancer, multiple sclerosis, and chronic fatigue syndrome. Lack of exercise contributes to obesity and presents a significant health challenge to those with arthritis. Researchers from the CDC reviewed data from

432,607 adults aged eighteen years and older who responded to telephone surveys as part of the Behavioral Risk Factor Surveillance System. The interviewers found that adults with arthritis accounted for at least 20 percent of those with no leisure-time physical activity. Another study showed that patients with fibromyalgia have diminished levels of physical fitness, which may lead to functional disability and exacerbate complaints. Once exercise training was combined with cognitive-behavioral therapy, these patients achieved clinically relevant changes in their health and fitness.

The majority of patients who come to my medical office have been ill for an extended period of time. Some are bedbound or are forced to use wheelchairs, and have lost a significant amount of muscle tone. Others continue to suffer from chronic fatigue, dizziness, muscle pains, joint pains, and weakness of the lower extremities that make starting an exercise program difficult. While we can address and treat their symptoms based on the differential diagnoses on the MSIDS map, none of these measures will address the severe deconditioning that can take place. This is why physical therapy and progressive reconditioning with stretching are often essential to get Lyme sufferers back to an optimal level of functioning.

In a case report that was published in the journal *Physical Therapy*, Myriam M. C. Moser, PT, DPT, profiled a typical scenario that we see in our medical office. She presents the case of a fourteen-year-old girl who had been infected with Lyme disease one year before receiving appropriate treatment. The patient could not participate in any sports due to her fatigue, pain, total body tremors, and a significant decrease in strength and endurance. Therapeutic exercises and gait training were used for treatment, and after four and a half months of therapy, she was able to return to playing sports with an increase in muscle strength and a decrease in tremors. This young girl had received antibiotic therapy for Lyme disease but still had impaired functional mobility in the activities of daily living. It wasn't until she participated in a combination of therapeutic exercise and a home exercise program that her energy, strength, and range of motion deficits improved.

CREATING A LASTING EXERCISE PROGRAM

The ideal exercise program for those with Lyme disease is one that can be built up slowly, gradually increasing levels of exertion. This will ensure that you can stick with the program, and that you won't overdo it early on in therapy and subsequently feel worse. There is a view among exercise physiologists known as the "energy envelope theory." Simply stated, each individual has an amount of energy perceived to be available to him/her at any point in time, and if the individual expends only as much energy as they perceive they have available, they will remain in their energy envelope. If they expend more energy than they perceive they have available, then overexertion can lead to worsening symptoms. The physical and psychological functioning of individuals who are able to remain in their energy envelope is significantly better than those individuals who ignore their body's basic signals. Those with Lyme and non-Lyme-MSIDS often tell me that as they begin to feel better and have good days, they tend to overdo it, and then crash, and they may be in bed for days. They ignored the signals that they were pushing too hard without having adequate physical stamina and ended up paying the price. This is why I believe that a graded exercise program that improves your stamina and keeps you within your energy envelope offers the best results for relieving symptoms and improving health.

Set a scheduled time each day for exercise. Scheduling it as a part of your everyday routine will ensure that it becomes an integral part of your health plan. Before you begin, you'll need to discuss your goals with your doctor and make sure you are physically able to exercise. If you are severely deconditioned, a trained physical therapist may be needed to evaluate your current health.

An exercise program typically includes stretching, aerobic or cardiovascular exercise, as well as strength training. Some of these exercises can be home-based, but supervised training is advised if you have been ill for a long time and are deconditioned. If you haven't exercised in a long time due to your illness, especially if you are new to exercise in general, I strongly recommend that you begin with a gentle whole body stretching and conditioning program. The goal of this is to restore range of motion and regain flexibility. Working with a trained yoga professional is preferable; however, you can also follow along with yoga instructional books or DVDs. This program should include gentle yoga stretches and postures for ten to fifteen minutes every morning, which will help with range of motion and flexibility. Never push beyond your body's level of comfort. Slow and gentle is always preferable. Be present and in your body as you breathe deeply, stretch, and hold the position. As you improve over time, you can lengthen your practice and increase the range of postures, especially those that help with balance.

The second component is aerobic exercise. If you have been severely ill and deconditioned, you may only be able to do five minutes of a slow, gentle walk each day. Each week, try and gradually increase the level of exercise, but do it in a systematic fashion, keeping a diary of your progress and always staying in the energy envelope, not pushing beyond your limits. Try and work up to at least twenty-five minutes a day, as this will ensure that you get all of the cardiovascular health benefits. Water-based exercise is also a good choice for those with chronic illness, as patients can exercise longer in water than on land without increased effort or joint or muscle pain, and with all of the cardiovascular benefits.

As you become stronger over time, endurance training, resistance and weight training, and combined training may then be used. Strength training with weights has been shown to be beneficial in relieving fatigue, increasing muscle strength and endurance, and improving mood in patients with chronic illness. If you are new to working with weights, I strongly recommend that you work with a personal trainer to make sure that you are performing the exercises correctly, and therefore averting injury.

NUTRITIONAL SUPPORT CAN FACILITATE EXERCISE

There are many nutritional supplements that are useful to help with fatigue and deconditioning, and research has shown that they are the same ones we frequently use with our MSIDS patients. For example, a statistically significant reduction in fatigue of deconditioned patients was achieved with the use acetyl-L-carnitine, which I commonly prescribe to support mitochondrial function. L-carnitine helps to shuttle fatty acids into the mitochondria as an energy source, and they may be useful in deconditioned patients who are too weak to exercise. In a randomized, double-blind, crossover trial published in the *Journal of the Neurological Sciences*, researchers compared the effects of acetyl-L-carnitine and prescription amantadine for the treatment of fatigue in multiple sclerosis. They found that acetyl-L-carnitine was superior to, and better tolerated, than amantadine, which is usually used as a first-line pharmacological treatment for MS fatigue. The use of mitochondrial support with L-carnitine should therefore routinely be considered for those with Lyme and MSIDS who are fatigued and don't have adequate energy to participate in a reconditioning program.

Fish oil has long been shown to help decrease inflammation, primarily through decreasing the production of inflammatory prostaglandins. In a study of patients with rheumatoid arthritis, those consuming fish oil were able to exercise over two hours longer before fatigue onset compared to a placebo group. Similarly, antioxidants such as vitamins C and E, combined with exercise, have been shown to be superior to exercise alone in patients with fibromyalgia. In this study, lipid peroxide levels (a marker for oxidative stress) were lower, and reduced glutathione levels were higher in the vitamin-supplemented group who exercised. As we have previously discussed, glutathione can help detoxify chemicals and modulate prostaglandins and cytokines, which subsequently may have an effect on decreasing fatigue and pain. This explains why glutathione is often helpful in patients in a medically supervised exercise program, in which pain and fatigue limit their ability to fully participate in physical therapy.

THE BENEFITS OF MASSAGE

Medical massage and whole body vibration (using electric vibrators over the major muscle groups) should also be considered for those whose pain interferes with their ability to participate in graded exercise therapy. In a 2008 study published in the *Journal of Alternative and Complementary Medicine* researchers recorded the effectiveness of a six-week traditional exercise program, with or without supplementary whole-body vibration therapy (WBV). They found that pain and fatigue scores were significantly reduced from the baseline of those in the exercise and vibration group, but not of those in the control group or in the group with exercise alone. Whole-body vibration therapy should therefore be considered for those with resistant symptoms who suffer with chronic fatigue syndrome, fibromyalgia, and MSIDS.

Medical massage therapy is another option to improve outcomes during physical therapy and rehabilitation, especially for those whose pain and stiffness interferes with their participation in a physical therapy program. In a widely reported 2012 study that evaluated the effects of massage therapy, researchers found that massage had several important effects on cellular function, mitochondrial biogenesis, and cytokine production. Massage was shown to improve energy by increasing the production of new mitochondria through its effects on PGC-1α (the switch which regulates mitochondrial development and metabolism) and decreased pain, by decreasing levels of NFKappaB, thereby lowering the production of the inflammatory cytokines TNF-α and IL-6. Massage was shown to decrease inflammation and promote mitochondrial biogenesis, two of the most important factors necessary for reducing fatigue and pain for those with Lyme-MSIDS.

Although we may address all of the other fifteen points on the MSIDS map and improve our health, without putting a proper exercise and progressive reconditioning program in place, those who have been chronically ill will have a much more difficult time maintaining their gains. Meditation and stress reduction techniques are another way to improve our physical and mental health, and optimally would be used in conjunction with a focused diet and exercise plan. We will discuss this in detail in Chapter 20. If you are suffering from chronic fatigue, depression, and/ or muscle and joint pain, speak to your health-care provider about the next steps you should take to integrate a customized healthy diet, exercise, and stress reduction program into your life.

TWENTY

Meditation, Mind Training, and Medicine

Over the years I have found that the pain and suffering associated with Lyme disease and MSIDS not only manifests as physical symptoms but has a strong emotional component. The vast majority of my patients share their emotional life with me, and their experiences range from mild sadness to severe depression, with elements of anxiety, shame, anger, guilt, fear, and grief.

Sometimes these emotions are directly related to their physical symptoms and coping with their ongoing illness. However, some experience posttraumatic stress disorder that comes from issues completely unrelated to their Lyme disease. This can often include emotional, physical, and sexual abuse. These are the patients who are the most challenging to treat. There is evidence that early trauma can damage the immune system, and it makes these individuals, once infected, more vulnerable to the worst ravages of the disease. However, I know that once they have gathered up the courage to go into their own pain and suffering and transform it, they will have an easier time healing. I have seen this happen over and over again.

When patients tell me about their migraines, irritable bowel syndrome, and asthma, I know it is possible that some underlying emotional wound might be contributing to the illness. This phenomenon has been described in detail in the scientific literature. I'm not saying that migraines can't be triggered by food allergies, lack of sleep, stress, hypoglycemia, nutritional deficiencies, and Lyme disease with co-infections. Yet my clinical experience has convinced me that we are carrying around our emotions within our bodies, and that they have a profound effect on our health. Books such as Bruce H. Lipton's *The Biology of Belief* and Candace Pert's *Molecules of Emotion* discuss studies on psychoneuroimmunology, the complex interaction between psychosocial factors such as stress and trauma and the nervous, cardiovascular, endocrine, and immune systems. We know that the immune system can be influenced by the outside world. For example, high levels of the stress hormone cortisol can trigger cell death of white blood cells and other changes in inflammatory processes during traumatic experiences. In this way the mind and body work as one. Psychiatric medications can be helpful with symptom relief, but they do not address deeper emotional wounds and the way they affect our immune system. There are some doctors trained in integrative medicine who have devoted their lives to understanding mind-body interactions at an even deeper level to help their patients with emotional trauma. They have combined Western and Eastern traditions to help find new solutions for their patients. Working within the framework of the Chinese, Tibetan, and Ayurvedic systems of medicine, these doctors work to balance and strengthen the subtle energy channels in the body (known as the energy meridians in Chinese medicine), which, when out of balance, lead to diseases of the body and mind. I have worked with Dr. Yeshe Donden, the Dalai Lama's personal physician, as well as with other highly talented physicians who practice Chinese, Tibetan, and Ayurvedic medicine, and I have seen results when Western approaches might not have been successful.

While there is no one right way to resolve an illness, a multidisciplinary approach while working with the mind to clear emotional issues and past trauma is often helpful. Talk therapy and cognitive-behavioral therapy can be beneficial, and techniques such as EMDR (eye movement desensitization and reprocessing), neurofeedback (EEG biofeedback), and hands-on bodywork (for example, Rosen Method Bodywork) can also help in those cases of deep trauma associated with grief. Working with the mind and learning to find peace in the midst of pain and suffering is essential when dealing with significant illness. This is where the practice of meditation can be of immense benefit.

MEDITATIONS TO CALM THE MIND
AND HEAL THE BODY

Those who practice meditation know that it is accessible to all of us. I have been blessed by having the opportunity to study for more than thirty years with meditation masters of the Kagyu school of Tibetan Buddhism. They have passed down an unbroken lineage of teachings from twenty-five hundred years ago that is still accessible and fresh today. These teachings allow us to develop greater loving-kindness and compassion that can help deepen a person's faith and devotion irrespective of their own spiritual path. That is because these teachings transcend religious beliefs, as they deal with the direct experience of the mind itself, and allow one to experience a deep peace and joy that may not have been previously known to the individual. As you learn to calm your mind and listen to the body, the body will speak its truth, allowing our hidden innate potential to surface, ultimately having a healing effect.

Meditation has been proven to have scientific health benefits that can assist us in our healing and in maintaining our well-being. We are all living in a fast-paced world, challenged by circumstances that are potentially stressful. Stress management techniques that include relaxation demonstrate the most consistent benefits. Meditation may be one way to mute the impact of stressful events on our lives and give us a chance to experience this deep relaxation. It is like taking a minivacation in the midst of a busy working life.

The health benefits of meditation were first studied by Dr. Herbert Benson at Harvard, when he studied the relaxation response. He found that there were numerous beneficial effects of meditation on our physiology, including decreased sympathetic nervous system activity with a decrease in our heart rate, respiratory rate, and cortisol levels, as well as decreased oxygen consumption and decreased blood lactate levels, implying better metabolic activity, with an increase in alpha and theta waves on the EEG (deeper, calmer states of consciousness), with hemispheric symmetry (symmetric brain-wave patterns in both the right and left brain). As we have seen, patients with Lyme-MSIDS often have problems with their autonomic and endocrine systems, with abnormal levels of norepinephrine and cortisol secretion. These patients are often anxious about their illnesses, with associated significant neurocognitive difficulties. By meditating we can help balance these abnormalities and teach the mind to be clear and rest in a relaxed state.

Since Benson's introduction of the relaxation response in 1975, other researchers have demonstrated the benefits of meditation on health and healing. For example, one 2008 study, which was published in the *Journal of Personality and Social Psychology*, found that the practice of loving kindness meditation produced increases over time in daily experiences of positive emotions, which produced increases in a wide range of personal resources (e.g., increased mindfulness, purpose in life, social support). In turn, these increments in personal resources predicted increased life satisfaction and reduced depressive symptoms, as well as decreasing symptoms of the patient's illness. Similar studies verified earlier work, in which mindfulness-based stress meditation has been found to have health benefits, enabling patients to better cope with their illness. A recent study published at the University of Wisconsin in 2013 also showed that meditation lowers inflammatory cytokine levels, an important effect for those suffering from the "sickness syndrome" in MSIDS.

A simple meditation practice that I often share with my patients has three parts. The first part is the motivation behind meditation, the second part is the meditation practice itself, and the third part involves a dedication of merit after completing the practice. The motivation behind the meditation is important. We are certainly meditating because we want to find peace and happiness and relieve our own suffering. But others are also suffering, and if we develop a broader motivation of loving-kindness and compassion for others, then, according to my teachers, the meditation practice will bear the greatest fruit. Love is wanting others to be happy and compassion is wanting others to be free from suffering. Loving-kindness and compassion are the highest level of motivation, and they prepare the ground for a successful practice.

Next we have the meditation practice itself, which is also divided into three parts. The first part is calm abiding meditation, the second part is insight meditation, and the third part is Mahamudra meditation, which integrates calm abiding and insight meditation.

Last, when we are done with the meditation practice, we dedicate the merit for the sake of all beings limitlessly throughout time and space. Whatever qualities you may develop from this meditation, use them to benefit yourself and others, which is the essence of virtue. By following this three-step process, you will learn to access the deeper states of meditation by calming the mind and then examining the nature of what arises in that state.

Before You Begin

You can start to practice meditation in short, five-minute sessions, and eventually expand this to a half hour per day. All you need is a space where you can be quiet and alone during your practice.

Your physical posture is important when meditating. This allows the proper flow of energy to take place during the practice, so that we do not fall asleep or become too agitated. Be free and easy and deeply relaxed with the posture! Do not force it, and do not hold the body too tightly or too loosely. Simply be mindful of your body and gently try and keep the following seven essential points in mind while performing the different meditation exercises.

1. Sit cross-legged on a cushion (sattva posture), or if you are an experienced meditator and have experience doing yoga, you can sit in a full lotus posture (vajra posture). Never force the position. If either of those are too difficult, simply sit in a chair.
2. Position your arms and hands so that the hands are folded on the lap with the right hand resting in the left hand ("gesture of equanimity"), or the hands are placed on the knees, the fingers extended toward the ground ("the gesture of ease").
3. Sit with the back straight and upright in either a chair or cushion. This allows the energies in the subtle channels to flow more freely and straight, allowing the mind and attention to remain at ease.
4. Extend the shoulders and elbows until they are straight.
5. Slightly tilt the neck, and tuck the chin in slightly toward the chest.
6. Connect the tip of the tongue to the palate. This helps stop the flow of excessive saliva.
7. Keep your eyes open, gazing toward the tip of the nose (forty-five degrees downward).

The First Meditation: Calm Abiding Meditation

In the seated posture described above, you will perform the following meditation for five minutes, three times a day. Over time, you can combine these sessions into one longer session, working your way to a total length of one thirty-minute session once a day. If you are new to a meditation practice, work with this exercise until you are not distracted by your own thoughts and feelings. When this occurs, you will know that you are ready to move to insight meditation.

There are two different techniques that can be used: calm abiding meditation with a support and calm abiding meditation without a support. The first is practiced by choosing a physical object as a mental support, such as a small pebble, flower, picture, statue, or staying focused on your breath. The technique is simply to gently place your awareness on the object. Don't examine the object and mentally discuss its qualities, just use the object as a way of anchoring your attention. Don't follow thoughts of the past (the past is gone), don't follow thoughts of the future (where fear lies), and don't follow thoughts of the present (which are gone the moment you notice them). Just place enough attention on the object to anchor the mind and not be distracted. Constant mindfulness and awareness are necessary. If you lose your mindfulness and your attention wanders off of the object of meditation, as it is likely to do, once you notice that you have been distracted, bring your attention back to the object.

One simple way to practice calm abiding meditation is to focus on your breath. Watch your breath go in through the nostrils, and watch it go out. Breathe naturally, and try and follow the breath nondistractedly for several minutes while the mind is in an open and relaxed state. Another variation of this practice is to count your breath twenty-one times, where an in breath and an out breath are counted as one. If you make it to twenty-one without being distracted, start over again. If you notice that you have forgotten what number you are on, or are no longer watching the breath, start counting again. This method allows us to track our progress, and see how far we can get before we are distracted.

Once you have attained some level of stability with the meditation practice, and your mind is no longer frequently distracted while observing the object, you can practice calm abiding meditation without a support. This means that you simply fix your attention on the mind, without the support of the breath or a physical object. If you get distracted by thoughts, bring your attention back to the mind. Again, do not follow thoughts of the past, thoughts of the present, or thoughts of the future. Do not block thoughts and do not analyze them in a conceptual manner. Be natural and simply rest, nondistractedly looking at your mind, resting in the nature of whatever arises. You can alternate doing calm abiding on an object and calm abiding meditation without an object during the same meditation session. You can also keep it fresh by occasionally changing the objects of meditation during the same session, or in different sessions.

Obstacles to Overcome

There are two main obstacles that frequently arise in meditation, both of which cause distraction: drowsiness and agitation. If you become drowsy, straighten your posture and raise your gaze. If this does not work, imagine a white lotus at the level of your heart with a small bright sphere the size of the pea that sits in the center of the lotus. This pea is white on the outside and red on the inside and represents your mind and awareness. It is the nature of light and should not to be visualized as a solid object. With a forceful exhale, imagine shooting this small sphere up through the top of your head into space. Continue to visualize this bright white sphere in space above your head until the drowsiness resolves.

The second obstacle to meditation is agitation: When you try to settle your mind, it gets caught up in thoughts. Remedies for this include cutting thoughts at their root: take the attitude from the beginning that you are not going to get involved in any thoughts whatsoever during the meditation, no matter how interesting. If you become too agitated, relax your posture and lower your gaze, and if this is ineffective, imagine a four-petal black lotus upside down at the level of the heart (also of the nature of light) with a dark pea-sized sphere of light in its center. Imagine this sphere slowly traveling down through the body into the earth. Continue to visualize this heavy and dark sphere nondistractedly until the agitation resolves.

Insight Meditation

Each of us can become confused as to who we really are when we are in the midst of chronic illness. We can't find the happiness we once experienced, because we are drowning in the pain or confusion of dealing with our symptoms. This is particularly true for my MSIDS patients. Even when we are feeling well, human nature has us experience the world in terms of opposites: good/bad, happy/sad, man/woman, life/death. Insight meditation allows us to realize that the ultimate nature of consciousness is a more unified state of perception instead of a dualistic one. This helps us to break the connection between pain and suffering.

During this meditation you will be looking directly at the mind to see the nature of thoughts and emotions, and the nature of mind itself. You will not focus on the content of thoughts, whether they are good or bad, virtuous or not. Instead, you will simply ask yourself the following questions and look at the mind to directly see the answers, rather than taking an intellectual or conceptual approach to them. This process is creating a direct experience of the answer not an intellectual approach to answering it. Don't worry if this seems complicated: You have to sit down and do it to see what your direct experience is.

These instructions are particularly helpful for those who suffer with strong emotions, especially great anxiety and fear regarding their illnesses. Instead of running from the fear, we learn to relax our minds and turn toward it, looking at its essential nature. This was eloquently stated by the meditation master, Mingyur Rinpoche: "At any given moment you can choose to follow the chain of thoughts, emotions, and sensations that reinforce the perception of yourself as vulnerable and limited. Or you can remember that your true nature is pure, unconditioned, and incapable of being harmed." We can then use meditation as a way to help us transform our illness and fear about our illness. Once we are able to relax and see the deeper truth of our experience, it cannot harm us in the same way.

Focus on one question for each session during insight meditation. You can break up each one into several parts and focus on each individually for several minutes, until you are ready to move on to the next. Once you have practiced calm abiding meditation for several minutes, and your mind is calm and not distracted, ask yourself the following questions during the practice of insight meditation:

- Where does the mind come from, where does it reside, and where does it go?
- Where do thoughts come from, reside, and go?
- Where do emotions come from, reside, and go?
- Look at the mind when it is still, and look at the mind when it is in motion. Is there a difference?
- Look at the essence of the one who is meditating. Who is meditating?

- Does the "I" that is experiencing suffering have a color or form? Does the mind experiencing suffering have a color or form?
- Where does fear come from, reside, or go? Does it have a color or form?

After you have asked these questions, and directly looked and seen whatever you have seen, rest naturally and at ease in the essence of the mind (clarity and emptiness) nondistractedly, without effort, and without grasping on to concepts. This is the final stage of Mahamudra meditation.

Working with the Mind in Postmeditation

When we arise from the meditation cushion, we should try and maintain the mindfulness and awareness that was developed during meditation. Being able to rest the mind is not enough. We need to enhance our meditation practice in order for it to develop. In postmeditation we try and maintain the state of "nondistractedness" more or less continuously, so that progress can occur. To enhance the mind that has been stabilized, we also need to apply "watchfulness," which is being aware of what the mind is doing, similar to the activity of a spy. Throughout the day, recognize what thoughts are present. If virtuous thoughts arise, recognize them as virtuous. If nonvirtuous thoughts arise, recognize them as being negative. By doing this we are sure to progress on the path, and we will not find ourselves easily distracted by the sounds and activities around us that can tend to disturb our minds.

In practical terms, this means that you must be grounded in your body and aware of what you are experiencing. You must be conscious of what you are seeing, hearing, and so on. This does not mean that you attempt to interfere or block what you see or what you hear. You are simply trying to maintain awareness of your experiences. You must know what you are seeing, know what you are hearing. Also, you do not stop thoughts, but don't allow yourself to drift in following them. Throughout the day we are usually distracted by the forms and sounds themselves, and everything becomes vague; the mind is allowed to drift aimlessly, and we are unaware of the details of the forms and sounds. By using watchfulness, with mindfulness and awareness in postmeditation, we are aware of the details of our outer experience and also aware and recognizing what is happening in our minds. This absence of distraction helps bring progress to our meditation practice. When we learn to rest in the fresh, direct experience of the present moment, not judging or grasping thoughts, then we can help ourselves to attain greater levels of healing. There is the possibility of resting in our basic nature of peace, joy, love, and wisdom that is one of nature's greatest healers.

At the end of your practice, take a few moments to dedicate the merit of the practice for the sake of all sentient beings limitlessly through time and space. Such a motivation will seal the merit of the practice and be like a seed planted in the ground that will grow and bear fruit. All the wisdom masters of all the different spiritual traditions have invoked this motivation in order to reach their full potential and benefit others.

Finish the meditation by reciting a four-line prayer that encapsulates the essential meaning of this meditation, known as the Four Immeasurables. Repeat this calmly at the end of each session:

May all beings have happiness and the causes of happiness.
May all beings be free from suffering and the causes of suffering.
May all beings know the great bliss which is free from all suffering.
May all beings know the great equanimity which is free from
   attachment and aversion.

I wish you peace, joy, love, and healing as you proceed on your journey.

TWENTY ONE

Solving the Mystery of Lyme and Chronic Disease

N ow that you have read this book, you have become a medical detective. You have followed my journey and have investigated the many ways that MSIDS can be causing and/or exacerbating your symptoms. As you've learned, there are up to sixteen possible reasons that you may not be feeling well, and the three I's–infection, immunity, and inflammation, with associated cytokines—are likely to be responsible for many of the clinical manifestations of your illness. More important, there is not one cause for one disease: There can be multiple causes for your symptoms, and each needs to be fully addressed before you will begin to feel better.

It's time to put the lessons of this book to the test. The first step is to fill out the Horowitz-MSIDS thirty-eight-item questionnaire and discuss your findings with your physician. If you have a score of 46 or higher, there is a strong likelihood that you are suffering from Lyme disease, other tick-borne diseases, and overlapping factors on the MSIDS map that are making you ill. In that case, ask your physician to send off an IgM and IgG Lyme Western blot test through a reliable specialty lab, and to check for other tick-borne diseases, especially *Babesia*, *Bartonella*, *Ehrlichia/Anaplasma*, *Mycoplasma*, *Chlamydia*, Rocky Mountain spotted fever, and Q fever. If any *Borrelia*-specific bands return positive (23, 31, 34, 39, 83–93), and you have good and bad days during which the symptoms come and go and pain migrates around your body, then there is a high likelihood that Lyme disease and associated co-infections are responsible for your illness. This is especially true if you have been diagnosed with chronic fatigue syndrome, fibromyalgia, an autoimmune disorder (such as MS or seronegative rheumatoid arthritis), or have unexplained neuro-psychiatric symptoms, and if you have had tick bites with symptoms improving or worsening with antibiotic treatment. Even if you have not been diagnosed with any of these conditions, if you suffer from resistant symptoms of fatigue, headaches, joint and muscle pain, tingling, numbness or burning sensations, memory and concentration problems, sleep problems, and psychiatric symptoms that are unresponsive or poorly responsive to standard medical therapies, it is possible that Lyme-MSIDS, or non-Lyme MSIDS underlie your illness.

As you've learned, Lyme disease is a clinical diagnosis: Your doctor will need to assess the signs of your disease, your symptoms, and your laboratory findings in order to arrive at a proper diagnosis. Introduce your doctor to the comprehensive table that lays out the differential diagnostic map in Chapter 1 to sort through and prioritize testing in order to get to the root cause(s) of your symptoms. Remember, the tests involved can be inconsistent or inconclusive, and your response to treatment will be determined by how other aspects of your health are currently affected by Lyme, or by previous illnesses. Lyme disease is spreading worldwide in epidemic proportions, and it is the modern day's Great Imitator: It imitates many chronic illnesses, and at the same time it can exacerbate the symptoms of all of them. Using the Horowitz sixteen-point differential diagnostic map will help provide you with answers as to why you are not getting better.

If you bring this information to your health-care provider and find that he or she is not responsive to the philosophy or the treatment plans outlined in this book, it may be due to the fact that they are not fully informed. Science and medicine are ever changing, and the MSIDS model gives both patients and doctors a different way to connect symptoms and chronic disease. This is not a model taught in medical school. Bringing this information to your doctor may put you in a position of being perceived as "pushy" or "misguided," but this is a risk you might want to take: It is your health that is most important. The potential for patient–physician conflict is high, and if the situation becomes too combative, you might feel devastated. Or you might feel empowered and decide that it's time to seek new opinions for your medical care.

There is an ongoing debate among physicians as to how to properly diagnose and treat tick-borne disorders, and your doctor, especially if he or she is a primary care physician outside of the northeastern United States, may not have a full understanding of the complexities of Lyme disease. In fact, they may not have even heard of MSIDS. You can share with your doctor what you've learned about the new treatments that are available. Have your physician read the book and review the extensive scientific references on these newer diagnostic and treatment regimens, so that you can work together in a healing partnership. You may find that doctors trained in integrative medicine are more familiar with these concepts, and can be part of your medical team, in order to implement the testing and treatment protocols that I've described.

The biggest difference between the MSIDS model and the standard medical approach to illness is a new emphasis on several distinct aspects of treatment: detoxification, improving functional medicine pathways, and resolving chronic infections with associated immune dysfunction and inflammation. Perhaps you have undiagnosed food allergies, vitamin and mineral deficiencies, environmental toxicity, mitochondrial dysfunction, or undiagnosed hormonal abnormalities, while having been exposed to multiple infections. Using this protocol ensures that you receive a comprehensive diagnostic and treatment plan for your symptoms. It has the potential to change the way we look at and treat chronic illness, both for Lyme disease and all of the other conditions on the MSIDS map.

By using these tools you may find out that you have Lyme disease, or Lyme disease and other co-infections. You may also learn that you have an autoimmune disorder, or CFS/FM without having been exposed to Lyme, but still may reap significant benefit from using this approach, because it deals with the underlying biochemical abnormalities driving symptoms. You have learned that cytokines can cause the same symptoms in all of these diseases, and once the cytokines and inflammation are properly addressed, you will feel better. In treating over twelve thousand patients during the last twenty-six years, 90 percent to 95 percent of my chronically ill patients have improved by applying the MSIDS model as a map to get to the multifactorial causes of their illness. Some get slightly better, some moderately better, and some significantly better, while some become symptom-free.

You are now empowered to take control of your health. As you work through the differential diagnostic map with your doctor, implementing the strategies discussed in this book, you'll notice that your overall health will improve as well as your specific symptoms. You may notice that your energy improves, your joint and muscle pain is better, that your brain fog has lifted, and that you no longer have difficulty concentrating. Your sleep may improve, and at the same time, you might find that your mood is better. People may start telling you that you look well.

My greatest wish is that you will grant yourself the gifts of time and patience while you are on the road to healing. Restoring health takes work, and perseverance, but you have already taken the first important step. You can now continue on your journey with the confidence of knowing that you can, and will, feel better.

Appendix A

Treatment Protocols for Lyme Disease–MSIDS
for Health-Care Providers

Treatment of Lyme disease

Treatment of Lyme disease can be divided into two major categories: acute Lyme disease and persistent Lyme disease. In both cases, the most important thing to keep in mind is that *Borrelia burgdorferi* has several forms: the cell wall form, cystic forms, and organisms in the intracellular compartment and biofilms. We also must take into account aspects of the biology of the organism, such as its long replication time, and that certain antibiotics that are bactericidal, such as penicillins and cephalosporins, will only work when the organism is actively dividing and reproducing. This implies that several rounds of antibiotics may be necessary to cover the cycles of the organism. Other antibiotics, such as the tetracyclines, are bacteriostatic, so we must have a healthy immune system to fight the infection. Unfortunately, *Borrelia* and multiple co-infections can suppress the immune system, so we must take this into account when simultaneous infections need to be cleared.

ACUTE LYME DISEASE:
In the case of an uncomplicated EM rash with no systemic symptoms

According to the scientific literature, approximately 75 percent of patients are cured with a three-week course of doxycycline (100 mg PO BID) or cefuroxime axetil (500 mg PO BID). However, if patients have multiple EM rashes, or a stiff neck, headache (central nervous system symptoms), or tingling/numbness in the extremities (peripheral nervous system symptoms), then the organism has disseminated, and one month of antibiotics is insufficient, since such patients often go on to develop persistent symptoms. Another explanation as to why a three-week course of doxycycline alone may be inadequate is that doxycycline does not address cystic forms and allows spirochetes to survive.

Although three weeks of doxycycline 100 mg PO BID, or Ceftin 500 mg PO BID, cures a significant percentage of all uncomplicated EM rashes, the biology of *Borrelia burgdorferi* suggests that it may be worthwhile to offer patients the following regimen with their consent for an uncomplicated EM rash:

Month one: Plaquenil 200 mg, one PO BID, doxycycline 100 mg, two PO BID, nystatin tablets 500,000 units, two PO BID, with pulse Flagyl or Tindamax three days a week, based on body weight (body weight less than 120 pounds: 750 mg per day; between 121 and 150 pounds: 1,000 mg per day; greater than 150 pounds: 1,500 mg per day). The addition of the Flagyl or Tindamax eradicates some of the cystic forms that may arise during initial treatment. Serrapeptase, one PO BID (or similar enzymes that affect biofilms) may be used concurrently.

Month two: Plaquenil 200 mg PO BID, Omnicef 300 mg PO BID, Zithromax 250 mg PO BID (pulsed four days in a row per week), with Flagyl or Tindamax three days a week (the days off the Zithromax), with Serrapeptase one PO BID, and nystatin tablets, 500,000 units one PO BID. In the second month, we have now added a cell wall drug (Omnicef, or a different cephalosporin, such as Suprax, Cedax, or Ceftin; or a penicillin, such as amoxicillin), since cell wall forms may have persisted during the initial month of treatment with a tetracycline. Rotating the regimens in this fashion attempts to address all of the different forms of *Borrelia,* and prevent the establishment of a persistent infection.

Once the patient becomes asymptomatic for two months on treatment, stop the antibiotics and consider moving them over to an herbal protocol, as described in Chapter 9. They should remain on that for several months to ensure that there are no new symptoms.

Each situation is unique, and general guidelines may not be applicable to a specific patient. For example, a patient presenting with early neuropathy, or with a history of severe *Candida,* may not be an ideal candidate for Flagyl or Tindamax, as these drugs have the potential to increase those symptoms. However, these medications play an important role in clearing complicated infections and may help prevent patients from going on to the chronic form of Lyme disease, with the inherent suffering and disability that often ensues. Choosing a treatment regimen for a specific patient requires an open and informed dialogue. The discussion should cover the potential side effects and likely benefits of the different treatment options, as well as the patient's goals and preferences.

For an EM rash with systemic symptoms, or multiple EM rashes

Complicated EM rashes (multiple EM rashes, with or without peripheral and/or nervous system involvement) imply dissemination of the organism, and since a single tick bite may transmit multiple co-infections, it is inherent upon the practitioner to choose drugs with good CNS penetration (e.g., doxycycline, minocycline, high-dose amoxicillin, IV Rocephin), to treat all forms of *Borrelia burgdorferi,* and to expand the regimen so as to simultaneously treat associated co-infections.

If the patient presents with an EM rash and has associated day sweats, night sweats, chills, an unexplained cough, and air hunger, these symptoms are suggestive of babesiosis, and adjuvant treatment with Mepron or Malarone may be indicated early on in the treatment course. Babesiosis can go on to develop into a chronic carrier state, like Lyme disease, and keep the MSIDS patient chronically ill, so early and aggressive treatment is indicated. Testing for *Babesia* often requires a panel approach to pick up the organism (Giemsa stain, IFA for *Babesia microti* and *duncani, Babesia* FISH test, and/or PCR), so one negative test does not rule out the disease. An inadequate response to a Lyme regimen, and a positive clinical response to antimalarial therapy, most likely indicates the presence of the organism.

When a patient presents with unusual stretch marks, new severe neurological symptoms (neuropathy, severe encephalopathy, and a new onset of a seizure disorder), or new ophthalmological symptoms, with or without enlarged lymph nodes, consider a diagnosis of *Bartonella.* In that case the patient may require rotations of double intracellular drug combinations such as doxycycline and rifampin, doxycycline and a macrolide, or doxycycline and a quinolone drug.

Lyme Disease: Diagnosis and Treatment Regimens		
SYMPTOMS	**TESTING**	**TREATMENT**

• EM rash
• Flulike symptoms
• Migratory joint &
  muscle pain
• Fatigue
• HA
• Paresthesias c&g
• Cognitive difficulties
• Psych abnormalities
• Sleep disorders
• Neck stiffness
• Photophobia &
  photophobia
• Sx generally c&g
	• ELISA/C6 peptide
	• Western blot IgM, IgG
	  (combining multiple
	  strains yields better
	  results. Look for *Borrelia*
	  specific bands, i.e., 23, 31,
	  34, 39, 83–93 kDa)
	• PCR urine and blood
	• Lyme dot blot/RWB
	• Lyme serum antigen
	• Lymphocyte
	  transformation test
	• Test for co-infections
	• Rarely, biopsy & culture
	• Silver staining
		• Cell wall:
		  penicillins,
		  cephalosporins,
		  carbapenems,
		  vancomycin
		• Cystic:
		  Plaquenil, GSE
		  Flagyl, Tindamax
		• Intracellular:
		  macrolides,
		  tetracyclines,
		  quinolones,
		  rifampin

LYME DISEASE AND ASSOCIATED INFECTIONS

Bacterial Infections

Lyme disease (*Borrelia burgdorferi*): Combine antibiotics to address all bacterial forms of *Borrelia* so as to overcome its ability to shift between different forms or go dormant and evade immune surveillance. Use natural enzymes to address biofilms, and continue treatment until the patient is symptom-free for two months.

Cell wall forms: Use cell wall agents (primarily penicillins and cephalosporins). Oral options include amoxicillin, Augmentin, Ceftin, Cedax, Omnicef, or Suprax, and intramuscular (IM) Bicillin is an extremely effective choice in persistent Lyme disease/MSIDS. IV medications such as Rocephin and Claforan are especially useful in patients with significant CNS disease, or who have failed oral and IM regimens. Although Rocephin has been better studied, Claforan can be used in patients with gallstones, where IV Rocephin is relatively contraindicated. Other useful cell wall agents include IV vancomycin. IV vancomycin can be a particularly effective choice in the patient whose other drug regimens have failed. The initial dosage is based on the patient's body weight and may be adjusted subsequently based on trough levels. Most patients have required dosages in the range of 1,000 to 1,250 mg Q twelve hours to get a trough level in the proper range (check with your laboratory for trough ranges).

The following are examples of dosages of oral cell wall medications in adults: amoxicillin 500 mg, and 875 mg capsules or tablets are frequently used in several different combinations. Typical dosages of antibiotic regimens described in the medical literature to treat Lyme disease have often been found to be ineffective in clinical practice. Higher dosages may be necessary, and in my clinical experience, I have found them to be safe and well tolerated. Examples: amoxicillin 875 mg, two to three PO BID with probenecid 500 mg, one PO BID with meals. Beginning dosages will depend on the patient's body weight. Check an amoxicillin peak and a trough level and adjust the dose. The peak should be between 12 and 15. If the peak is suboptimal, or the patient has an inadequate response, increase the dose. Effective dosages are typically 875 mg, three PO BID or 500 mg, six PO BID in adults. Some physicians increase dosages to 7,000 mg to 8,000 mg/per day if CNS disease is present or the response to treatment is inadequate. Probenecid is used to increase the levels of the cell wall drugs in the blood, but probenecid should be avoided if there is a sulfa sensitivity, and used with caution if there is a history of kidney stones.

Other cell wall drugs/penicillins include: Augmentin, 875 mg to 1,000 mg, one to two PO BID or Q 12. This may be used alone or added to amoxicillin if the patient has done well with longer-acting drugs in the past (such as Bicillin) but has clinical breakthroughs due to inadequate trough levels when solely on amoxicillin. For severely ill patients, and patients who cannot easily tolerate oral medications (GI intolerance, *Candida*), IM Bicillin 1.2 million units IM, two to four times per week versus 2.4 million units two times per week should be considered. This is one of the most effective treatment regimens we have found to treat Lyme disease, especially in patients who have failed with other oral medications. The higher the dose of Bicillin, often the better the clinical efficacy. Use Emla or lidocaine cream one hour prior to the injection and warm the Bicillin to body temperature just prior to use to decrease pain over the injection site. An ice pack may also be applied one or two minutes before the injection to minimize discomfort. Massage the area well right after the injection for two to three minutes, and repeat several times per day, to both prevent localized inflammation, and ensure deep tissue penetration of the drug.

Other cell wall drugs: Oral and IV cephalosporins. These are also particularly effective in the patient with Lyme-MSIDS.

Simply because a patient has not responded to one cell wall drug (penicillin or cephalosporin) does not mean that they won't have a positive clinical response to different drugs in the same class. Frequently used medications and dosages that have been found to be effective include:

Oral cephalosporins: Ceftin, 500 mg, one to two PO BID; Omnicef, 300 mg one to two PO BID; Cedax, 400 mg one QD to BID; Suprax, 400 mg one QD to BID. Second- and third-generation cephalosporins are preferable to first-generation drugs (Keflex is ineffective and should not be used).

IV cephalosporins: IV Rocephin or similar agents should be considered for patients with resistant neurological syndromes or manifestations of Lyme disease that could lead to significant disability (optic neuritis, Bell's palsy, severe meningitis/encephalitis) and in those who did not respond to oral or intramuscular therapies. Informed consent as to the potential side effects of the drugs and IV lines must be discussed with patients, including allergic reactions, line infections, phlebitis, and gallbladder complications.

Rocephin: 2 g IV QD, five to seven days per week, up to 2 g IV Q 12 pulsed four to five days per week. Use Actigall, 300 mg one PO BID, to help prevent sludge and gallstones. The utility of Actigall has not been demonstrated in a published clinical trial, but we have found it to be effective in our clinical practice in helping to prevent gallbladder complications. A gallbladder ultrasound prior to the start of treatment may be appropriate in patients with risk factors for cholecystitis. We also regularly use a baby aspirin and fish oils to try and prevent the occurrence of phlebitis. While on Rocephin, check a CBC and CMP with liver functions every two weeks, and use liver support (e.g., NAC, alpha-lipoic acid, Hepa #2, milk thistle) as necessary if there is any evidence of a transaminitis (elevated liver functions). Liver functions often return to normal quickly after the drug is stopped.

Other common IV medications: Claforan, 2 g IV Q8–12. May be used as a substitute for Rocephin if there are gallbladder problems. Precautions: agranulocytosis (leukopenia/neutropenia, thrombocytopenia, with or without anemia). Check a CBC and CMP every two weeks, or more frequently if any significant hematological abnormalities appear.

IV vancomycin: 1 to 1.25 gms/Q 12 hours is the typical dose for most patients (check peak and trough levels—acceptable trough levels vary by laboratory, but the usual range should be between 10 and 15). "Red man syndrome," which is not a true allergic reaction but a common side effect of the drug, can often be prevented or minimized by administering Benadryl 25 mg to 50 mg PO or IV before each dose. Using a nonsedating antihistamine (Zyrtec, Allegra, Claritin) to block H1 histamine receptors with Zantac or Pepcid to block H2 histamine receptors can be helpful if there are breakthrough symptoms. IV vancomycin can be useful in patients if other IV regimens have failed, and with those patients who are allergic to penicillins and cephalosporins.

IV Primaxin: 500 mg IV Q6. It is a less commonly used drug regimen, due to the inconvenience of the frequent dosing regimen.

IV Cleocin: This is the last of the common IV regimens to consider. It may be useful for Lyme patients with overlapping babesiosis for whom other oral *Babesia* regimens have failed and with patients who are intolerant of other medications. The dosage is typically 600 mg IV Q8, or 900 mg IV Q12.

Cystic forms (L-forms, S-forms, spheroplasts, cell wall deficient forms): Use Plaquenil, +/− grapefruit seed extract (GSE), Flagyl, or Tindamax. GSE can be used when there is a contraindication to using Plaquenil (such as in the case of psoriasis) and also when Flagyl and Tindamax need to be avoided because of a history of associated *Candida* or a significant neuropathy (although they also can decrease neuropathy in certain Lyme patients). Flagyl and Tindamax can also cause an Antabuse-type effect (alcohol should be avoided while using them) and have the potential to cause severe Jarisch-Herxheimer reactions. Therefore, they may need to be pulsed (i.e., several days in a row per week, or two weeks on, two weeks off), and we routinely use high doses of B vitamins (B_6, B_{12}) and nystatin to decrease potential side effects. If any new neuropathic symptoms appear, or older neuropathic symptoms increase in severity and/or duration (i.e., increased tingling, numbness and/or burning), the drug should be stopped, and the patient reevaluated.

Intracellular location: Use tetracyclines (doxycycline, minocycline, tetracycline), macrolides (Zithromax, Biaxin), quinolones (Cipro, Levaquin, Avelox, Factive), and rifampin. Since many intracellular co-infections can persist in the Lyme-MSIDS patient with single-drug therapy, combination regimens are often more successful.

Macrolides: Zithromax: 250 mg one PO BID with meals versus 500 mg to 600 mg QD or, rarely, 2 g one to two times per week. Biaxin or Biaxin XL: 250 mg one PO BID, children; 500 mg one PO BID, adults. Biaxin XL is generally tolerated better and may be more effective with its longer half-life. Biaxin has more potential interactions with other medications than Zithromax, and both must be used carefully in patients, especially if they are on other drugs that can affect QT intervals on the electrocardiogram.

Other options: roxithromycin (Europe), ketolides such as Ketek. I have used roxithromycin effectively in treating European patients. Ketek is no longer commonly used due to black box warnings in the United States (increased LFTs).

Tetracyclines: doxycycline 100 mg, 2 PO BID with meals. Use 100 mg one PO BID/TID with meals if smaller body weight or GI intolerance. Higher doses are usually used to help get better CNS penetration. Tetracyclines should not be used while pregnant, or with children under eight years old, to avoid staining the teeth. A short course will occasionally be used by some pediatricians (ten days or less) in children under eight years old if the benefit outweighs the risk, but it is prudent to avoid the use of tetracyclines until most of the adult teeth have developed (usually by eleven to twelve years old). Don't mix with dairy, antacids, or vitamins with minerals. Avoid direct sun; wear a 45 SPF or higher sunblock. Do not lie down within one hour of ingestion to avoid reflux esophagitis. Consider Doryx if there is severe gastrointestinal intolerance to tetracyclines, or Monodox, as these may be better tolerated forms of doxycycline.

Minocycline: 50 to 100 mg PO BID. Watch for staining of skin and autoimmune reactions. Higher doses may cause dizziness.

Tetracycline: 250 mg or 500 mg capsules: one to two g per day total, BID–QID. GI intolerance may be higher with this form of a tetracycline, which is taken on an empty stomach, and therefore other forms of tetracyclines may be preferable.

Quinolones: (PO/IV). Cipro 500 mg one PO BID, Levaquin 500 mg one PO QD, Avelox 400 mg QD, Factive 320 mg one PO QD. Cautions with quinolones: prolonged QT intervals on the electrocardiogram with the potential for arrhythmias. Check with a PDR drug checker, and do not mix with certain drugs, such as macrolides, Diflucan, Sporanox, Lariam, Coartem, certain SSRIs such as Celexa, PPIs, such as Prilosec, and any other drugs affecting QT intervals. Advise patients of possible tendonitis/tendon rupture and that they should be avoiding strenuous exercise to prevent overuse of tendons during the use of a quinolone drug. Discontinue immediately if any pain is felt over the sites of tendons in the body. Antioxidants, such as alpha-lipoic acid and curcurmin, as well as magnesium, which relaxes smooth muscle and skeletal muscle, should be considered to decrease potential side effects. The higher the generation the quinolone, often the more effective the drug. Pulsing quinolones such as Factive, which is the highest generation quinolone (fourth generation) in five-day cycles may also be effective and reduces the risk of tendon damage. When patients follow these instructions, we have found the use of quinolones to be safe and effective, especially in patients co-infected with *Bartonella*. The same precautions for quinolones apply as with the tetracyclines: Do not use in pregnancy; do not mix with antacids, or vitamins with minerals; and there may be some sun sensitivity, although usually less than is seen with tetracyclines.

Rifampin: 150 mg (if smaller body weight/children) to 300 mg PO BID with meals. Do not use when pregnant. Watch for drug interactions, as rifampin often may lower or raise levels of other medications being administered. Rifampin should be used in combination with other intracellular antibiotics to avoid resistance, and it is particularly useful in the Lyme-MSIDS patient who is suffering with multiple intracellular co-infections, such as *Bartonella*, or *Brucella*.

Designing Combination Treatment Therapies		
LYME DISEASE	*BARTONELLA*	*BABESIA*
*Amoxicillin+Probenecid + Macrolide + Plaquenil *Bicillin+Macrolide+Plaquenil *Cephalosporin (oral or IV) +Macrolide+Plaquenil	+ Septra	+Mepron/Artemesia +Malarone/Artemesia +Lariam/Artemesia +Cryptolepis/or Neem
*Doxy + Plaquenil	+ Quinolone + Rifampin	+Lariam/Artemesia +Malarone/Cryptolepis
*Macrolide + Plaquenil	+ Septra + Quinolone	+Mepron+/−herbal tx +Malarone+/−herbal tx +Lariam+/−herbal tx +Artemesia or Neem +Cryptolepis

*+/−Flagyl or Tinidazole (? pulsed), +/− GSE, + Serrapeptase (or other biofilm protocol if no contraindi-cation, i.e., bleeding tendency). Do not mix macrolides, quinolones, and/or Lariam together.
*When multiple intracellular infections are present (*Mycoplasma, Chlamydia, Brucella*, etc.), consider two intracellular antibiotics simultaneously (i.e., Plaquenil-Doxy-Quinolones). Cleocin + macrolides can also be a first-line therapy for babesiosis Cleocin + Quinine is infrequently used due to side effects.

Examples of combining cell wall/cystic/and intracellular antibiotics to treat Lyme

-Amoxicillin/probenecid/Plaquenil/Zithromax
-Ceftin or Omnicef/probenecid/Plaquenil/Biaxin
-IM Bicillin/Plaquenil/Zithromax
-IV Rocephin/Plaquenil/Zithromax

The above medications should be used with Mepron or Malarone if the patient also has babesiosis or another piroplasm. Nystatin 500,000 units 2 PO BID/TID should be used routinely to decrease yeast with a sugar-free/yeast-free diet with high-dose acidophilus/probiotics. Do not mix macrolides and quinolones and/or Lariam or other drugs that may affect the QT interval on the electrocardiogram. Consider checking an EKG in appropriate clinical circumstances. Flagyl or Tinidazole and/or GSE can be added to extend coverage for cystic forms, as well as simultaneously using a biofilm protocol (i.e. Serrapeptase).

BIOFILM FORMS

Lyme disease spirochetes have also been found to survive in biofilm forms. There are several mechanisms to prevent the formation of *Borrelia* biofilm, including using natural enzymes such as nattokinase (for maximum effect), and the destruction of *Borrelia* biofilms can be accomplished with the enzyme lumbrokinase (for maximum effect). The antibiotic doxycycline in high concentrations also has an effect on the destruction of biofilms, but there is no synergistic effect when enzymes and doxycycline are used together.

Serrapeptase, which is another proteolytic enzyme, has the added advantage of both preventing the formation of biofilms and destroying them. It is also capable of digesting blood clots (some researchers believe that *Borrelia* can persist in fibrin clots in the body), cysts, and reducing inflammation. We therefore will use enzymes like Serrapeptase, one to two capsules two times per day (NutraMedix) in select patients during and after antibiotic therapy for Lyme disease. There have been no controlled clinical trials to date on the effectiveness of using biofilm protocols in Lyme disease.

General recommendations regarding diet and the need for probiotics (acidophilus) with the use of antibiotics

It is necessary to follow a sugar-free diet, and occasionally a stricter yeast-free diet, depending on the number of antibiotics prescribed. That is because antibiotics can cause an overgrowth of yeast and deplete beneficial bacteria in the GI tract, which can lead to diarrhea. To avoid the possibility of the overgrowth of yeast and *Clostridium*, it is necessary to try and avoid all simple sugars (candies, cakes, pies, honey, molasses, white bread, white pasta, white rice, sweet fruits, such as, for example, bananas, raisins, grapes, dates, melons, mangoes) and to take an adequate amount of beneficial probiotics. Examples of commercial probiotics include Ultra Flora, *Saccharomyces boulardii*, Probiomax, and Theralac, one dose, two times per day, away from the antibiotics (one hour before or several hours later); this will generally prevent the occurrence of yeast or diarrhea. Occasionally patients will break through with loose stools and/or yeast and require the addition of another probiotic, such as VSL3, which can be ordered online. A prescription for VSL3 DS (double strength) may be provided by a health-care practitioner, if the patient's insurance covers it.

If a patient happens to develop diarrhea or yeast despite following these guidelines, they should stop taking the antibiotics until the diarrhea resolves, and call their health-care provider for further instructions. Any diarrhea that persists for more than one or two days should be evaluated with a stool specimen to check for the presence of *Clostridium difficile*. Other natural supplements, such as oregano oil (Oregacyn or OregaRESP), garlic (allicin), and GSE may also be used concomitantly two times a day to help control yeast. These can be taken at the same time as antibiotics. A prescription for Diflucan may be necessary if yeast continues to be an issue, but we usually find that it is the failure to follow a strict sugar-free diet that is often the cause of recurrent yeast. If it is necessary to take Diflucan, it should not be taken at the same time as other drugs that can affect QT intervals, so occasionally we may prescribe it only on the weekends, away from those drugs with potential interactions, if it is absolutely necessary (excluding Lariam, which has a long half-life). Other dietary restrictions, in addition to avoiding sugar and yeast, may also be necessary if the patient has tested positive for celiac disease and food allergies/sensitivities. These dietary modifications should be integrated into the treatment plan to ensure optimal health, and to minimize any side effects of the medications.

Treatment of Bacterial Co-infections

Ehrlichiosis/anaplasmosis:

Doxycycline 100 mg, one to two BID for seven to ten days is usually adequate to treat *Ehrlichia* and *Anaplasma*. If there is an allergy, intolerance, or contraindication to using tetracyclines, then rifampin can be used instead (150 mg PO BID to 300 mg PO BID), depending on body weight. Precautions described above should be followed with the use of these medications. *Ehrlichia* can be life-threatening in the very young and elderly, so prompt therapy is essential when there is a high clinical suspicion.

Bartonella: B. henselae (cat scratch disease, ticks); B. Quintana (trench fever, lice); B. bacilliformis (Carrion's disease, sand flies):

Treatment regimens generally include rotations of intracellular antibiotics, using dosages previously described for the treatment of Lyme disease.

Combination Antibiotic Regimens for *Bartonella* and Other Intracellular Organisms

- Plaquenil/doxycycline/rifampin/nystatin
- Plaquenil/doxycycline/Zithromax/nystatin
- Plaquenil/doxycycline/Levaquin/nystatin
- Plaquenil/Zithromax/Septra
- Plaquenil/Zithromax/rifampin
- Plaquenil/rifampin/Factive
- Plaquenil/rifampin/Factive/tetracyclines (doxycycline, minocycline)

-Malarone (and Mepron) may be added to the above regimens if there is associated babesiosis, but its use in regimens with rifampin may lead to lower drug levels (the same is true for tetracyclines, but may still be efficacious if dosed at higher levels).

Several patients in our practice have remained PCR positive for *Bartonella* months after treatment with single-drug therapy, so combination therapy with at least two intracellular antibiotics for several months is preferable in the treatment-resistant patient.

Mycoplasma spp.:

We have had patients test positive for *Mycoplasma* infections such as *M. fermentans* with single-drug therapy after almost one year of continuous treatment. Therefore, combination therapy with at least two intracellular antibiotics is preferable when there is proof of active *Mycoplasma* infection.

Chlamydia spp.:

Chlamydia is an intracellular bacteria, so the same treatment regimens apply as with *Bartonella* and *Mycoplasma*.

Rickettsial spp.:

Rocky Mountain spotted fever (*Rickettsia rickettsii*), typhus, Q fever (*Coxiella burnetii*): These are all gram-negative intracellular bacteria and are treated effectively in the acute stages with tetracyclines such as doxycycline 100 mg PO BID. As with ehrlichiosis, RMSF can be life-threatening in immunocompromised individuals, so prompt therapy is essential if there is a high clinical suspicion. Neither tetracyclines nor chloramphenicol (second-line therapy) are rickettsicidal, so an adequate immune system is required to use them effectively. Any high clinical suspicion (tick bite, exposure in a highly tick-endemic area) and laboratory testing showing an abnormal WBC count, thrombocytopenia, and/or elevated liver functions (similar to abnormal laboratory testing seen with *Ehrlichia/Anaplasma*) should prompt immediate treatment. Q fever titers are not specific, and false positives can be seen with other rickettsial infections and viruses. Chronic Q fever endocarditis requires long-term treatment with antibiotics. Several regimens that have been published in the medical literature include the use of doxycycline and Plaquenil for up to three years and doxycycline and quinolones (or rifampin) for several years. Use the same dosages previously described for Lyme disease and associated co-infections. These cases are best managed in conjunction with a cardiologist and infectious disease specialist.

Tularemia

Treatment regimens for Lyme patients with MSIDS infected with tularemia include IV/PO doxycycline (200 mg to 400 mg per day), quinolones, such as IV/PO Cipro (dosage based on body weight), IM/IV streptomycin (1 gram Q 12 x ten days in adults, lower dosing in children, i.e,. 20 to 40 mg/kg day in divided doses), IV gentamycin (5 mg/kg per day in three divided doses), and rarely, chloramphenicol in treatment-resistant cases (50 mg/kg per day, up to 100 mg/kg per day in four divided doses). There have been treatment failures reported with beta lactam antibiotics and with intracellular antibiotics, including ciprofloxacin, tetracyclines, and macrolide antibiotics used alone. These resistant patients often required combination therapy such as doxycycline or chloramphenicol plus streptomycin or gentamycin treatment, or they responded to IV gentamycin alone for seven to ten days.

Brucellosis

Treatment for *Brucella* needs to be for a minimum of six weeks, and relapses are common if it is not caught early. Tetracyclines (500 mg PO QID) or doxycycline (100 mg to 200 mg PO BID) plus streptomycin 1 g IM QD-BID helps to decrease relapse rates. IV gentamycin (5 mg/kg per day in three divided doses) has also been effective in decreasing relapses, as has been the addition of Septa DS, one tab TID-QID, or rifampin 300 mg PO BID to a tetracycline regimen, especially in patients with CNS involvement (meningoencephalitis). In the case of *Brucella endocarditis*, triple antibiotic regimens (doxy, rifampicin, and streptomycin; or doxy, rifampicin, and cotrimoxazole) are recommended for at least six months, until titers decrease to a minimum of 1:160.

Treatment of Parasitic Infections

Babesiosis:

First-line treatment protocols include Mepron 750 mg one to two tsp PO BID, with a high-fat meal, and Zithromax 500 mg per day (or Biaxin 500 mg PO BID), Plaquenil 200 mg PO BID, and nystatin tablets 500,000 U PO BID. Septra DS one PO BID may be added to that regimen if there are resistant or severe symptoms, and if the patient does not have a sulfa allergy. If there is an overlapping *Bartonella* infection, adding Septra DS may also be useful. Antimalarial herbs, such as artemesinin, cryptolepis, or neem may also be layered onto this regimen if the patient's malarial-type symptoms persist. Dosing varies by body weight, but average doses of artemesia are one three times per day (liposonal artemesia is one twice a day), cryptolepis one teaspoon TID (start ½ teaspoon or less, if sensitive, TID), and neem dosing may vary between thirty drops, three to four times per day. Antimalarial herbs are generally used one at a time and may be rotated, depending on the patient's clinical response. Layering up *Babesia* medications and herbs in this manner can be very helpful in treating resistant malaria-type symptoms.

Malarone is also a good choice for patients with babesiosis as there is now Mepron resistance in the United States. Malarone is usually dosed at four tablets a day for three days as a loading dose, followed by one tablet two times per day. Some MSIDS patients with severe malarial symptoms require two tablets PO BID to control their symptoms. We have seen clinical and laboratory evidence of persistent and relapsing babesiosis at lower doses and have not seen adverse effects in patients using this regimen. Patients should avoid taking CoQ10 as a vitamin supplement while on Malarone or Mepron, as it can interfere with its clinical efficacy. Malarone can be used alone as a single agent, but Mepron should always be used with a macrolide to prevent drug resistance.

Patients who previously failed regimens of Mepron or Malarone, or have intolerances to the drugs, should be rotated to clindamycin. Cleocin 300 mg, 2 PO BID-TID with Plaquenil 200 mg, 1 PO BID, Zithromax 250 mg PO BID, and nystatin 500,000 U PO BID +/– Septra DS 1 PO BID is one commonly used effective combination. Mepron, Malarone, and/or antimalarial herbs can be layered onto this treatment regimen if the patient has severe or resistant symptoms. We use IV Cleocin, 600 mg to 900 mg BID in patients with severe GI intolerance to oral clindamycin (dosing depends on body weight), or in those with severe malarial symptoms who have failed oral regimens. We do not often use the classic *Babesia* therapy of Cleocin 600 mg PO TID and quinine 325 mg two PO TID as a first-line therapy (although it may be helpful) because of the severe side effects of quinine, which include nausea, vomiting, tinnitus, and rashes in up to 50 percent of the patients. Cleocin and quinine may be reserved for babesiosis in late-stage pregnancy, as it is one of the few regimens that have been proven safe for the fetus.

Many patients who were not treated early relapse once treatment is stopped. Many of these patients still have positive PCRs (DNA probes) and positive FISH testing (RNA probes), despite months of antibabesial therapy. In those patients we often have to rotate to other antimalarial regimens, such as Coartem, four tablets PO BID for three days (day one, 7:00 A.M. and 3:00 P.M., days two and three, 7:00 A.M. and 7:00 P.M.), or Lariam 250 mg, 1 PO HS every five to seven days. Coartem is an antimalarial combination of lumafantine and artemether, and has some clinical efficacy in babesiosis. It can be used alone or with Daraprim 25 mg, 2 PO QD for three days in severely ill patients, and/or in combination with doxycycline.

Lariam is an older drug used for malarial prophylaxis but which also has clinical efficacy against babesiosis. Both Coartem and Lariam can affect the QT interval on the electrocardiogram, so they should not be used with each other, or in combination with other drugs affecting QT intervals (macrolides, quinolones, fluconazole, itriconazole, certain SSRIs, and PPIs). Lariam has possible neuropsychiatric side effects, such as seizures, hallucinations, psychosis, increased depression and paranoia, as well as frequently causing vivid dreams with occasional nausea and dizziness (usually at higher doses, not clinically significant for most patients at a half tablet every three days, or one tablet every five to seven days). Its use must therefore be limited to patients who are neuropsychologically stable and who have failed other *Babesia* regimens. It may be combined with doxycycline, Plaquenil, and artemesinin for increased clinical efficacy. Lariam has an extremely long half-life (three weeks), so it is necessary to avoid medications with effects on QT intervals for up to fifteen weeks post-Lariam in select patients.

We have found all of these combinations to be helpful and generally well tolerated, but none are 100 percent effective. Clinically lowering down the parasitic load by rotating the drug regimens is useful, as it helps many patients with resistant Lyme-MSIDS symptoms. A recent 2013 FDA warning for Lariam noted possible persistent neurological and psychiatric effects, so the drug should only be used in treating resistant babesiosis with an informed consent. In patients with life-threatening babesiosis, who are immunocompromised and have failed all other regimens, exchange transfusion is a last resort to decrease the parasitic load.

Other parasitic infections are also occasionally found in the MSIDS patient, especially intestinal parasites, such as giardia, amoeba, pinworm, and hookworm, with patients occasionally testing positive for parasites such as schistosomiasis, and strongyloides. These infections are found on both serum antibody testing and stool cultures (Metametrix GI Effects, stool CDSA). Regimens including biltricide, ivermectin, pyrantel pamoate (PinX), and Alinia have been effective in certain patients with not only persistent GI symptoms, but also fatigue, headaches, and myalgias resistant to classical tick-borne therapy. Dosing for these regimens is based on the patient's body weight.

LYME AND PREGNANCY:

Borrelia burgdorferi may be transmitted transplacentally to the fetus, as may associated coinfections. *Borrelia burgdorferi* has also been isolated from breast milk in a study published in 1995 by Schmidt et al. Although the incidence of transmission through breast-feeding has been debated in the scientific literature, there is nevertheless a potential risk. An open and informed dialogue with expectant mothers regarding the risks and benefits of antibiotics during pregnancy and breast-feeding should routinely take place.

Antibiotics such as penicillins, cephalosporins, and macrolides are all category B, and proven to be safe in pregnancy. Flagyl is FDA category B, but trimester and population-specific risks exist, and it should not be routinely used unless clinically indicated. Dosages, side effects, and contraindications are the same as previously discussed. Examples of antibiotic regimens used in pregnancy include oral cell wall antibiotics such as Amoxicillin 500 mg two to three PO TID to QID, or 875 mg, two to three PO BID (based on body weight and/or peak serum levels), Omnicef 300 mg one PO BID, or other oral cephalosporins such as Suprax 400 mg, one PO BID. Intramuscular injections of Bicillin LA, 1.2 million units two to three times per week are also very effective, and are useful in women with severe symptoms unresponsive to oral medication, and/or significant nausea. The long-acting effect of Bicillin may also potentially decrease the risk of maternal-fetal transmission, as regular injections avoid some of the variations seen in peak and trough levels with oral medications. We have seen positive PCRs for *Borrelia burgdorferi* on specimens of the placenta and/or cord blood post-partum, despite women remaining on PO antibiotics, although the babies were healthy at birth. Macrolides such as Zithromax and Biaxin do not penetrate well into the placenta, but may be useful for controlling symptoms in the mother. Rarely IV medication like Rocephin is needed for maternal neurologic and/or cardiac involvement, or will be considered in the first trimester when the fetal organs are forming, especially if a woman has a history of frequent miscarriages associated with Lyme disease.

Pregnant women with active tick-borne infections should be managed in conjunction with a high-risk OB-GYN, and all medication and nutritional regimens should be coordinated with the patient's gynecologist.

VIRAL INFECTIONS:

There is no specific treatment for tick-borne viral encephalopathies like Powassan encephalitis, except supportive treatment. HIV medications are being studied as a possible option for these patients. Fortunately, most infections do not result in disease, as the fatality rate can be between 10 percent and 30 percent in certain studies.

Any patient who does not adequately respond to appropriate antibiotic protocols while addressing the 16 point differential on the MSIDS map, and who has high viral titers and/or a positive PCR, may suffer from chronic viral infections (which may have been present and/or reactivated), and a trial of antiviral medication is warranted. This could include a trial of Valtrex, Famvir, acyclovir, or Valcyte in severe cases. In our experience, classical antiviral drugs such as Valtrex and Famvir do not have a significant clinical effect in the majority of MSIDS patients. Valtrex was used successfully in clinical trials at Stanford University for patients with elevated titers of HHV-6 whose chronic fatigue started shortly after a viral illness. Valcyte has significant hematological side effects and should be used with caution.

Neutraceuticals such as transfer factors, and mushroom derivatives that increase NK and T cells (which are antiviral) such as 3–6 beta-glucan, are safer alternatives with scientific studies showing efficacy. Oleuropein, the active compound in olive leaf extract, has also scientifically been shown to be virucidal against many viruses.

FUNGAL INFECTIONS/*CANDIDA*:

Protecting against yeast/*Candida* is extremely important while patients are on antibiotics. Oral nystatin (and occasionally Diflucan, in severe cases), neutraceuticals such as oregano oil, garlic, berberine, and grapefruit seed extract, and low-carbohydrate diets combined with high doses of probiotics can be beneficial. Nystatin is usually dosed at two 500,000 U tablets PO BID in our patients, taken at the same time as antibiotics, with probiotics including *Saccharomyces boulardi* taken in-between doses of nystatin. In resistant cases, Diflucan or other antifungal drugs may be added QD or pulsed one to two days a week (away from medications which affect the QT interval). Nystatin in powder, liquid, or capsules is also an option for patients with more severe clinical manifestations. A trial off antibiotics and treating for systemic yeast is occasionally warranted for patients whose antibiotics are failing and who present with symptoms consistent with a *Candida* syndrome.

Immune Dysfunction

We regularly use drugs like Plaquenil (hydroxychloroquine) 200 mg PO BID to modulate an overstimulated immune system, except in patients with psoriasis, when the drug is contraindicated. Regular eye exams once a year are advised, but we have never seen a Plaquenil-induced retinopathy.

Inflammation

Classical therapies include immune modulators (Plaquenil, DMARDs), drugs with anti-inflammatory effects (macrolides, tetracyclines), NSAIDS and COX-2 inhibitors, and 2 to 4 gms IVIG for decreased immunoglobulin levels or severe neuropathy, as in small-fiber neuropathy and CIDP (chronic inflammatory demyelinating polyneuropathy). Properly treating Lyme disease and associated co-infections and lowering down the total load of organisms in the body is essential in order to significantly decrease inflammation and control symptom flares. This can be accomplished with the antibiotics and classical therapies discussed above, as well as integrative therapies that focus on the down-regulation of the nitric oxide pathway to help decrease inflammatory cytokines, prostaglandins, and leukotrienes. This would include the use of LDN combined with various antioxidants (especially curcurmin, up to 2 to 4 gms per day, resveratrol, green tea extract, 200 mg per day), CoQ10 (100 mg to 200 mg per day, starting dose), B vitamins (especially B_1, B_2, B_6, methyl B_{12}), α-lipoic acid (300 mg to 600 mg two times per day), minerals such as Mag++ (average dose: 500 mg per day) and Zn++ (average dose: 15 to 30 mg per day), omega-3 FAs (minimum 2 gm per day), glutathione precursors, such as NAC (600 mg two times per day), glycine, and oral liposomal glutathione (Wellness Pharmacy) 500 mg per day.

An alkaline Mediterranean-style anti-inflammatory diet (low levels of meat, eggs, dairy, sugar, and high in healthy fruits and vegetables, with olive oil) combined with the above medications and neutraceuticals can be of significant benefit in controlling inflammation. LDN is obtained through specialty pharmacies and is dosed at 2 mg PO HS for one month, 3 mg PO HS the next month, and 4 to 4.5 mg PO HS as a final dose. Side effects include insomnia, so dosing may need to go at a slower pace for certain patients, or taken on an empty stomach upon awakening if the drug interferes with sleep. LDN should not be used in patients with frequently dosed or long-acting narcotics since it interferes with their effects and may induce narcotic withdrawal. Using two Alka-Seltzer Gold tablets (or equivalent sodium bicarbonate) to alkalize the body, combined with 1,500 mg to 2,000 mg of oral liposomal glutathione, has been effective with or without LDN in decreasing inflammation and Jarish-Herxheimer flares in up to 70 percent of patients.

Chemical Sensitivity, Environmental Illness, Heavy Metals, Mold, and Neurotoxins (external and internal biotoxins):

Many patients test positive for heavy metals. Chelation can be performed by using an oral chelation regimen (DMSA, DMPS, D-penicillamine), transdermal chelation (for children), IV chelation (DMPS, EDTA), and rectal suppositories (Detoxamine, EDTA). We generally use low-dose oral DMSA at bedtime every several days (100 mg to 200 mg) or pulsed DMSA two days in a row on the weekends (5 mg/kg to 10 mg/kg PO BID, one hour before meals), as some Lyme disease patients do not tolerate standard dosages of oral chelating agents due to Jarish-Herxheimer flares. IV chelation therapy with Disodium EDTA has also been used to treat atherosclerosis and was recently found to modestly reduce the risk of adverse cardiovascular outcomes (*JAMA*, 2013).

Nutritional supplements used Q3rd night with DMSA include *Chlorella* (split cell, seven tablets) with 600 mg NAC, alpha-lipoic acid (600 mg), and occasionally Med Caps DPO (Xymogen) if phase I and phase II liver detoxification pathways are not functioning efficiently. EDTA suppositories (750 mg) can also be added, if the patient has very high levels of lead. It is essential to use a good multimineral supplement on days the patient is not chelating (with a minimum of

800 mg to 1,000 mg calcium per day, 400 mg to 600 mg magnesium per day, zinc 30 mg per day, with trace minerals), since the chelation process removes essential minerals. Blood levels of trace minerals should therefore be checked intermittently during or after chelation (such as se-rum Mag++, RBC Mag++, zinc, copper, iodine, selenium, etc.) or if the patient complains of muscle cramps. These mineral supplements should be taken at least several hours away from the antibiotics to avoid interfering with absorption. Higher dose DMSA 5 to 10 mg/kg TID, one hour before meals, three days on, eleven days off (standard chelation protocols) can be used in patients with very high levels of heavy metals, usually once they are off antibiotics. The above protocols have been proven to be safe and effective for our patients.

Those individuals with chemical sensitivity/EI, and/or high levels of internal biotoxins (such as quinolinic acid) or mold neurotoxins (testing can be done through Real Time Labs) may require other detoxification protocols. This may include the use of infrared saunas, the use of binding formulas (bentonite clay, charcoal, zeolite), high-dose oral liposomal glutathione (GSH), IV GSH, increased nutritional supplementation to support detoxification (Mag++, NAC, GLY, α-lipoic acid, DIM, sulforaphane glucosinalate, methylation cofactors, and/or a phosphati-dylcholine (PC) exchange) in conjunction with a diet high in protein and cruciferous vegetables. Other patients may require a modified Shoemaker protocol (cholestyramine, Welchol) as toler-ated for mold toxins, apart from eliminating the sources of toxicity.

Allergies: Foods, Drugs, Environmental

Many Lyme disease patients have overlapping food allergies and sensitivities, usually second-ary to an associated problem with *Candida* and a leaky gut. Classical treatment includes avoidance of allergens, rotation diets, and occasional immunizations against offending allergens. Integra-tive treatment includes treating an underlying *Candida* syndrome or leaky gut with dysbiosis if present, and using enzyme therapy if the patient is deficient. Some patients have reported benefits from using techniques such as Nambudripad's Allergy Elimination Techniques (NAET) to clear resistant food allergies, but we have not had enough experience with the technique to validate its effectiveness in our patient population.

NUTRITIONAL AND ENZYME DEFICIENCIES

Treatment: Replace vitamins, minerals, amino acids (AA), essential fatty acids (EFA), and enzymes (plant or pancreatic with amylase, lipase, proteases) as per test results.

MITOCHONDRIAL DYSFUNCTION

Treatment: NT factors (glycosylated phospholipids, such as those from Researched Nutri-tionals) three tablets two times per day, for two months, followed by three per day. Also use CoQ10, 200 mg to 400 mg per day (if not on Mepron or Malarone), and acetyl L-carnitine (1,000 mg PO BID). Other options include NADH (5 mg per day) and D-ribose, 5 gm scoops, two to three times per day for several months if there is an inadequate response. Avoid D-ribose for prolonged periods of time, due to possible effects of increasing glycosylation in patients with blood sugar problems.

NEUROPSYCHOLOGICAL DISORDERS

Health-care providers should ask about the patient's previous psychiatric history, and refer for counseling or psychiatric help, including cognitive processing therapy, *Journey* work (Bran-don Bays), EMDR, or EFT (emotional freedom technique). Medications include SSRIs such as Zoloft 100 mg to 200 mg per day, buproprion (Wellbutrin XR 150 mg PO BID, Remeron 15 mg HS, and anxiolytics such as Xanax, Klonopin, and Ativan). Stress-reduction techniques include yoga, meditation, Tai Chi. Individualized herbal treatments include St. John's Wort, 5-HTP, SAM-e valerian root, kava kava, and L-theanine (typically dosed 100 to 200 mg per day).

Endocrine Abnormalities

The hypothalamic-pituitary axis may be affected in Lyme disease-MSIDS. Check FSH, LH, GH, and IgF1, antithyroid antibodies, TSH, T3 and T4, FT3/4, DHEA/cortisol, sex hormones, and occasionally leptin, MSH, ADH, and VIP levels. Use replacement dosages of hormones and correct underlying abnormalities to return levels to normal ranges.

Sleep disorders

Treatment: Activating agents in the A.M. (Provigil 100 mg to 200 mg, Nuvigil 150 mg PO QD) and/or sleep-promoting agents in the P.M., especially those that encourage deep, slow wave sleep (Lyrica 50 mg to 150 mg HS, Trazadone 50 mg to 150 mg HS, Gabitril 4 mg to 12 mg HS, Seroquel 25 mg HS, Xyrem 3 grams to 4.5 grams (6ml to 9 ml), taken twice per night, four hours apart). Ambien and Lunesta may also be used with the above medications if necessary. Refer to the PDR for possible side effects and interactions.

Other options include balancing neurotransmitter levels (i.e., low serotonin) with 5-HTP 100 mg HS, and also using GABA for sleep. SeriPhos (phosphaditylserine) may be helpful if there are elevated levels of cortisol HS. We have also found valerian root (1,000 mg to 1,500 mg HS), L-theanine (100 mg HS), and melatonin (1 to 6 mg HS) to be effective, and they can all be mixed with classical sleep medications to increase efficacy.

Autonomic Nervous System (ANS) Dysfunction/POTS

Treatment: Salt (minimum 3 gm to 4 gm per day), increase fluids (3 liters +), consider Florinef (0.1 mg to 0.2 mg per day), Midodrine (starting dose 2.5 PO TID, maximum 5 mg to 10 mg PO TID), Cortef (5 mg PO QD starting dose, but dosing depends on level of symptoms and adrenal insufficiency), and/or B blockers (Toprol XL). Occasionally Catapres (oral 0.1 mg PO BID starting dose, or Catapres TTS patches), and SSRIs such as Zoloft are needed for an inadequate response.

Elevated LFTs

Treatment: Treat symptomatically once underlying etiologies have been ruled out and addressed. Herbal therapies can include milk thistle (silymarin) PO BID, Hepa #2 (Zhang, TCM) two capsules PO BID, NAC 600 mg PO BID, alpha-lipoic acid 600 mg PO BID.

Pain

High-dose narcotics should be avoided if possible (or used in limited quantity unless absolutely necessary, i.e., the patient has failed other therapeutic trials for pain), due to tolerance/addiction and possible effects on sleep and hormones. Low-dose Ultram may be a useful alternative in combination with other nonnarcotic drug regimens to control pain if necessary. Narcotics also interfere with the use of LDN, which is a very useful medication in controlling inflammation and pain in the Lyme-MSIDS patient. Treating the underlying cause of the pain using the MSIDS map often helps to decrease levels of narcotics.

Appendix B

Glossary of Pharmaceutical Names

Brand Name	Generic Name
Actigall	ursodiol
Adderall (XR)	dextroamphetamine/amphetamine
Aldactone	spironolactone
Aleve	naproxen sodium
Allegra	fexofenadine
Allegra-D	fexofendadine/pseudoephedrine
Altace	ramipril
Ambien	zolpidem
Amoxicillin	amoxicillin (generics are generally used).
Anafranil	clomipramine
Arava	leflunomide
Arimidex	anastrazole
Ativan	lorazepam
Augmentin	amoxicillin/clavulanate
Avelox	moxifloxacin
Avonex	interferon beta 1 α
Baraclude	entecavir
Benadryl	diphenhydramine
Benicar	olmesartan
Betaseron	interferon beta 1b
Biaxin	clarithromycin
Bicillin	penicillin G benzathine
Biest	estradiol/estriol (compounded)
BuSpar	buspirone
Catapres	clonidine
Cedax	ceftibuten
Ceftin	cefuroxime axetil
Celebrex	celecoxib

Brand Name	Generic Name
Celexa	citalopram
Chemet	DMSA
Cimzia	certolizumab pegol
Cipro	ciprofloxacin
Claforan	cefotaxime
Claritin	loratadine
Claritin-D 24 Hr.	loratadine/pseudoephedrine
Cleocin	clindamycin
Climara	estradiol transdermal
Clomid	clomiphene
Coartem	artemether/lumefantrine
Copaxone	glatiramer
Cortef	hydrocortisone
Coumadin	warfarin
Cuprimine	penicillamine
Cymbalta	duloxetine HCl
Cytomel	liothyronine
Cytovene	ganciclovir
Daraprim	pyrimethamine
DDAVP Nasal	desmopressin nasal
Decadron	dexamethasone
Depakote	divalproex sodium
Deplin	methyltetrahydrofolate
Detrol LA	tolterodine
Diamox	acetazolamide
Dificid	fidaxomicin
Diflucan	fluconazole
Dilaudid	hydromorphone
DMSA	dimercaptosuccinic acid
Dynabac	dirithromycin
EDTA	ethylenediaminetetraacetic acid
Elavil	amitriptyline
Enbrel	etanercept
Epivir	lamivudine
Factive	gemifloxacin
Famvir	famciclovir
Fioricet	butalbital/acetaminophen/caffeine
Flagyl	metronidazole
Flexeril	cyclobenzaprine
Florinef	fludrocortisone
Fosamax	alendronate
Gabitril	tiagabine
Glucophage	metformin
Hepsera	adefovir
Humira	adalimumab
Imitrex	sumatriptan
Imuran	azathioprine
Incivek	telaprevir

Brand Name	Generic Name
Klonopin	clonazepam
Lanoxin	digoxin
Lariam	mefloquine
Lasix	furosemide
LDN	low-dose naltrexone
Levaquin	levofloxacin
Lexapro	escitalopram
Lunesta	eszopiclone
Lyrica	pregabalin
Malarone	atovaquone/proguanil
Medrol	methylprednisolone
Mepron	atovaquone
Mestinon	pyridostigmine
Mevacor	lovastatin
Minocin	minocycline
Mobic	meloxicam
Motrin	ibuprofen
MS Contin	morphine sulfate
Naprosyn	naproxen
Neurontin	gabapentin
Nuvigil	armodafinil
Oleptro	trazodone
Omnicef	cefdinir
Pamelor	nortriptyline
Parlodel	bromocriptine
Paxil	paroxetine
Percocet	oxycodone/acetaminophen
Phenobarbital (only generic)	phenobarbital
Plaquenil	hydroxychloroquine
PredForte (eye drops)	prednisolone acetate ophthalmic
Prilosec	omeprazole
Primaxin	imipenem/cilastatin
ProAmatine	midodrine
Procrit	epoetin alpha
Provigil	modafinil
Prozac	fluoxetine
Qualaquin	quinine sulfate
Questran	cholestyramine
Rebif	interferon beta 1 α
Reglan	metoclopramide
Remeron	mirtazipine
Restoril	temazepam
Rheumatrex	Methotrexate
Ribasphere	ribavirin
Rifampin	rifampin
Rilutek	riluzole
Risperdal	risperidone
Ritalin	Methylphenidate

Brand Name	Generic Name
Rocephin	ceftriaxone
Septra DS	trimethoprim/sulfamethoxazole
Seroquel	quetiapine
Solu-Medrol	methylprednisolone sodium succinate
Sonata	zaleplon
Sporanox	itraconazole
Strattera	atomoxetine
Sudafed	pseudoephedrine
Sumycin	tetracycline
Suprax	cefixime
Synthroid	levothyroxine
Tegretol	carbamazepine
Tenormin	atenolol
Tindamax	tinidazole
Topamax	topiramate
Toprol XL	metoprolol succinate
Tylenol	acetaminophen
Tyzeka	telbivudine
Ultram	tramadol
Valcyte	valganciclovir
Valium	diazepam
Valtrex	valacyclovir
Vancocin	vancomycin
Viread	tenofovir disoproxil
Victrelis	boceprevir
Vivelle-Dot	estradiol transdermal
Voltaren	diclofenac sodium
Vyvanse	lisdexamfetamine dimesylate
WelChol	colesevelam
Wellbutrin	bupropion HCl
Xanax	alprazolam
Xifaxan	rifaximin
Xyrem	sodium oxybate
Zanaflex	tizanidine
Zantac	ranitidine
Zipsor	diclofenac sodium
Zithromax	azithromycin
Zocor	simvastatin
Zofran	ondansetron
Zoloft	sertraline
Zovirax	acyclovir
Zyrtec	cetirizine
Zyrtec-D	certirizine/pseudoephedrine

Appendix C

Journal Names and Abbreviations

AAOHN Journal (American Association of Occupational Health Nurses)

Acta Neurol Scand: Acta Neurologica Scandinavica

Acta Paediatr: Acta Paediatrica

Adv Exp Med Biol: Advances in Experimental Medicine and Biology

Adv Neuroimmunol: Advances in Neuroimmunology

Alternative Medicine Review

Am Fam Physician: American Family Physician

Am J Clin Nutr: American Journal of Clinical Nutrition, The

Am J Clin Pathol: American Journal of Clinical Pathology

Am J Dig Dis: American Journal of Digestive Diseases, The

Am J Gastro: American Journal of Gastroenterology, The

Am J Gastroenterol: American Journal of Gastroenterology, The

Am J Med: American Journal of Medicine, The

Am J Ophthalmol: American Journal of Ophthalmology

Am J Physiol Cell Physiol: American Journal of Physiology—Cellular and Molecular Physiology

Am J Physiol Lung Cell Mol Physiol: American Journal of Physiology—Lung Cellular and Molecular Physiology

Am J Psychiatry: American Journal of Psychiatry, The

Am J Respir Crit Care Med: American Journal of Respiratory and Critical Care Medicine

Am J Trop Med Hyg: American Journal of Tropical Medicine and Hygiene, The

Amer Jnl Gastroenterology: American Journal of Gastroenterology, The

American Journal of Dermatopathology

American Journal of Epidemiology

American Journal of Physiology

American Journal of Public Health

Ann Allergy: Annals of Allergy, Asthma & Immunology

Ann Behav Med: Annals of Behavioral Medicine

Ann Intern Med: Annals of Internal Medicine

Ann NY Acad Sci: Annals of the New York Academy of Sciences

Ann Neurol: Annals of Neurology

Ann Rheum Dis: Annals of the Rheumatic Diseases

Ann. Clin. Lab. Sci: Annals of Clinical & Laboratory Science

Annals of Agricultural and Environmental Medicine

Annals of Pharmacotherapy

Annals of Tropical Medicine and Parasitology

Annu Rev Med: Annual Review of Medicine

Annu. Rev. Genet: Annual Review of Genetics

Annual Review of Immunology

Antibiotics and Chemotherapy

Antimicrobial Agents and Chemotherapy

APMIS (Acta Pathologica Microbiologica et Immunilogica Scandinavica)

Arch Dermatol: Archives of Dermatological Research

Arch Dis Child: Archives of Disease in Childhood

Arch Intern Med: Archives of Internal Medicine

Arch Neurol: Archives of Neurology

Arch Pediatr Adolesc Med: Archives of Pediatrics & Adolescent Medicine

Arch Phys Med Rehabil: Archives of Physical Medicine and Rehabilitation

Arch Surg: Archives of Surgery

Arthritis Res Ther: Arthritis Research & Therapy

Arthritis Rhem: Arthritis & Rheumatism

Asthma

Autoimmun Rev: Autoimmunity Reviews

Autoimmunity

Auton Neurosci: Autonomic Neuroscience

Behav. Brain. Res: Behavioural Brain Research

Behavioural Pharmacology

Biochem Int: Biochemistry International

Biochemical Journal

Biol Psychiatry: Biological Psychiatry

BioMedCentral Neurology

Bioorg Med Chem Lett: Bioorganic & Medicinal Chemistry Letters

BJMP: British Journal of Medical Practitioners

Blood

BMC Neurol: BMC Neuroscience

BMJ: British Medical Journal

Br J Dermatol: British Journal of Dermatology

Brain Behav Immun: Brain, Behavior, and Immunity

Brit Jnl Derm: British Journal of Dermatology

Brit. J. Med. Practit: British Journal of Medical Practitioners

British Journal of Nutrition

Can Med Assoc: Canadian Medical Association Journal

Cardiology

Case Reports in Immunology

Cell

Cell Immunology: Cellular Immunology

Cell Physiology: American Journal of Physiology

Chest

Circulation

Cleve. Clin. J. Med: Cleveland Clinic Journal of Medicine

Clin Biochem: Clinical Biochemistry

Clin Exp Allergy: Clinical & Experimental Allergy

Clin Exp Immunol: Clinical & Experimental Immunology

Clin Exp Rheum: Clinical and Experimental Rheumatology

Clin Inf Dis: Clinical Infectious Diseases

Clin Infect Dis: Clinical Infectious Diseases

Clin Microbiol Infect: Clinical Microbiology and Infection

Clin Microbiol Rev: Clinical Microbiology Reviews

Clin Orthop: Clinical Orthopaedics and Related Research

Clin Ped: Clinical Pediatrics

Clin Pediatr: Clinical Pediatrics

Clin Prac of Alt Med: Clinical Practice of Alternative Medicine

Clin Rheumatol: Clinical Rheumatology

Clin Sci (Lond): Clinical Science (London)

Clin Vaccine Immunol: Clinical and Vaccine Immunology

Clin. Gastroenterol. Hepatol: Clinical Gastroenterology and Hepatology

Clinical and Developmental Immunology

Clinical Diabetes

Clinical Rheum: Clinical Rheumatology

Cochrane Database of Systematic Reviews

Contemporary Clinical Trials

CRC Crit Rev Food Sci Nutr: Critical Reviews in Food Science and Nutrition

Critical Reviews in Toxicology

Curr Allergy Asthma Rep: Current Allergy and Asthma Reports

Curr Biol: Current Biology

Current Directions in Psychological Science

Current Medical Diagnosis & Treatment

Current Medicinal Chem: Current Medicinal Chemistry

Curr Mol Med: Current Molecular Medicine

Curr Opin Biotechnol: Current Opinion in Biotechnology

Curr Opin Investig Drugs: Current Opinion in Investigational Drugs

Curr Opin Pulm Med: Current Opinion in Pulmonary Medicine

Curr Opin Rheum: Current Opinion in Rheumatology

Current Opinion in Genetics & Development

Current Opinion in Neurology

Curr. Opin. Struct. Biol: Current Opinion in Structural Biology

Curr Pharm Des: Current Pharmaceutical Design

Curr Rheumatol Rep: Current Rheumatology Reports

Cytokine

Diabetologia

Diagn Microbiol and Infect Dis: Diagnostic Microbiology and Infectious Disease

Dig Dis Sci: Digestive Diseases and Sciences

Directions in Psychiatry

EASD—European Association for the Study of Diabetes

EID: Emerging Infectious Diseases

Emerg Infect Dis: Emerging Infectious Diseases

Endocr Rev: Endocrine Reviews

Environment International

Epigenetics

Eur Infect Dis: European Journal of Clinical Microbiology & Infectious Diseases

Eur J Cancer: European Journal of Cancer

Eur J Clin Microbiol Infect Dis: European Journal of Clinical Microbiology & Infectious Diseases

Eur J Endocrinol: European Journal of Endocrinology

Eur J Gastroenterol Hepatol: European Journal of Gastroenterology & Hepatology

Eur J Heart Fail: European Journal of Heart Failure

Eur J Pediatr: European Journal of Pediatrics

Eur J Pharmacol: European Journal of Pharmacology

Eur Soc of Clin Microbiol and Inf Dis: European Society of Clinical Microbiology and Infectious Diseases

Eurosurveillance

Evidence-Based Complementary and Alternative Medicine

Expert Rev Anti Infect Ther: Expert Review of Anti-Infective Therapy

FEBS J: FEBS Journal (Federation of European Biochemical Societies)

Fortschritte der Medizin

Free Radic Biol Med: Free Radical Biology & Medicine

Future Microbiol: Future Microbiology

Ghana Med Jnl: Ghana Medical Journal

Health Services Research

Hepatology

Homeostasis

Hormone and Metabolic Research

Hypertension

IAMM: Indian Association of Microbiologists

IMAJ: Israel Medical Association Journal, The

Immunol Today: Immunology Today

Immunology

Indian Journal of Experimental Biology

Indian Journal of Pharmacology

Indian Pacing Electrophysiol J: Indian Pacing and Electrophysiology Journal

Infect Immun: Infection and Immunity

Infection

Infectious Agents and Disease

Infectious Disease: Infectious Disease Clinics of North America

Int J Immunopharmacol: International Journal of Immunopharmacology

Int J Infect Dis: International Journal of Infectious Diseases

Int J Neurosci: International Journal of Neuroscience

Int J Pharmalcol: International Journal of Pharmacology

Int Jnl Med: International Journal of Medicine

Int Microbiol: International Microbiology

Intern Med: Internal Medicine News

Internal Medicine (Japanese Society of Internal Medicine)

International Journal of Clinical Medicine

International Journal of Medical Sciences

International Journal of Pharmacy Practice

J Agric Food Chem: Journal of Agricultural and Food Chemistry

J Allergy Clin Immunol: Journal of Allergy and Clinical Immunology

J Alzheimers Dis: Journal of Alzheimer's Disease

J Am Acad Psychiatry Law: Journal of the American Academy of Psychiatry and the Law, The

J Am Coll Cardiol: Journal of the American College of Cardiology

J Am Diet Assoc: Journal of the American Dietetic Association

J Am Vet Med Assoc: Journal of the American Veterinary Medical Association

J Androl: Journal of Andrology

J App Physiol: Journal of Applied Physiology

J Appl Microbiol: Journal of Applied Microbiology

J Assoc Physicians India: Journal of the Association of Physicians of India

J Biol Chem: Journal of Biological Chemistry, The

J Clin Endocrinol Metab: Journal of Clinical Endocrinology & Metabolism, The

J Clin Gastroenterol: Journal of Clinical Gastroenterology

J Clin Invest: Journal of Clinical Investigation

J Clin Microbiol: Journal of Clinical Microbiology

J Clin Psychiatry: Journal of Clinical Psychiatry

J Clin Sleep Med: Journal of Clinical Sleep Medicine

J Degenerative Dis: Journal of Degenerative Diseases, The

J Endocrinol Invest: Journal of Endocrinological Investigation

J Ethnophamacol: Journal of Ethnopharmacology

J Helminthol: Journal of Helminthology

J Immunol Methods: Journal of Immunological Methods

J Immunol: Journal of Immunology, The

J Inf Dis: Journal of Infectious Diseases, The

J Infect Dis: Journal of Infectious Diseases, The

J La State Med Soc: Journal of the Louisiana State Medical Society, The

J Med Microbiol: Journal of Medical Microbiology

J Med Toxicol: Journal of Medical Toxicology

J Musculoskel Pain: Journal of Musculoskeletal Pain

J Musculoskeletal Pain: Journal of Musculoskeletal Pain

J Neuroimmunol: Journal of Neuroimmunology

J Neuroinflammation: Journal of Neuroinflammation

J Neurol Sci: Journal of Neuroscience Research

J Neuropathol Exp Neurol: Journal of Neuropathology & Experimental Neurology

J Nutr: Journal of Nutrition

J Pain: Journal of Pain, The

J Parasitol: International Journal for Parasitology

J Pharm Pharmacol: Journal of Pharmacy and Pharmacology

J Pharmacol Exp Ther: Journal of Pharmacology and Experimental Therapeutics

J Psychosom Res: Journal of Psychosomatic Research

J R Soc Med: Journal of the Royal Society of Medicine

J Rheumatol: Journal of Rheumatology, The

J Steroid Biochem Mol Biol: Journal of Steroid Biochemistry and Molecular Biology, The

J Urol: Journal of Urology

J Vet Med Sci: Journal of Veterinary Medical Science, The

J. Appl. Bacteriol: Journal of Applied Bacteriology

J. Chronic Fatigue Syndr: Journal of Chronic Fatigue Syndrome

J. Clin Microbiology: Journal of Clinical Microbiology

J. Clin. Neurosci: Journal of Clinical Neuroscience

J. Mol. Microbiol. Biotechnol: Journal of Molecular Microbiology and Biotechnology

J. Neurol and Psychopathol: Journal of Neurology and Psychopathology, The

J. Neuropath. and Exp Neur: Journal of Neuropathology & Experimental Neurology

J. Physiol: Journal of Physiology, The

JAMA: Journal of the American Medical Association, The (JAMA)

JANA: Journal of the American Nutraceutical Association (JANA)

JEM: Journal of Experimental Medicine, The (JEM)

Jnl of Applied Bacteriology: Journal of Applied Bacteriology

Jnl of Chr Fatigue Syndrome: Journal of Chronic Fatigue Syndrome

Jnl of Neurosci: Journal of Neuroscience, The

Journal of Advanced Nursing

Journal of Aging and Phys Activ: Journal of Aging and Physical Activity

Journal of Alternative and Complementary Medicine, The

Journal of Antimicrobial Chemotherapy

Journal of Bacteriology

Journal of Cardiopulmonary Rehabilitation & Prevention

Journal of Cellular Biochemistry

Journal of Clin Microbiol: Journal of Clinical Microbiology

Journal of Clinical Oncology

Journal of Clinical Psychology

Journal of Consulting and Clinical Psychology

Journal of Diabetes

Journal of Internal Medicine

Journal of Nephrology

Journal of Neurochem: Journal of Neurochemistry

Journal of Nutritional and Environmental Medicine

Journal of Occupational Medicine

Journal of Perinatology

Journal of Personality and Social Psychology

Journal of Pharmacy Practice

Journal of Psychiatric Practice

Journal of Sports Medicine and Physical Fitness, The

Journal of the National Cancer Institute

Journal of the Neurological Sciences

Lancet Neurology, The

Lancet, The

Lupus

Mayo Clin Proc: Mayo Clinic Proceedings

Med /Clin (Bare): Medicina Clínica (Barcelona)

Med GenMed: Medscape General Medicine

Med Hypotheses: Medical Hypotheses

Med Mal Infect: Médecine et Maladies Infectieuses

Med Sci Monitor: Medical Science Monitor

Metabolism

Microbiol Rev: Microbiological Reviews

Microbiology

MMWR: Morbidity and Mortality Weekly Report (MMWR)

Mol Microbiol: Molecular Microbiology

Mol. Biol. Rev: Microbiology and Molecular Biology Reviews

Mol. Nutr. Food Res: Molecular Nutrition & Food Research

Mol. Psychiatry: Molecular Psychiatry

Morb Mortal Wkly Rep: Morbidity and Mortality Weekly Report (MMWR)

Mucosal Immunity: Mucosal Immunology

Multiple Sclerosis

Multiple Sclerosis Journal

Muscle & Nerve

N Engl J Med: New England Journal of Medicine, The

Nat Clin Pract Gastroenerol Hepatol: Nature Clinical Practice Gastroenterology & Hepatology

Nat. Prod. Rep: Natural Product Reports

Nature

Nature Neuroscience

Nature Reviews Neuroscience

NEJM: New England Journal of Medicine, The

Neoplasia

Nervenarzt: Nervenarzt, Der

Neurobiology of Disease

NeuroImmunoModulation

Neurology

Neurology Research International

Neuroscience & Biobehavioral Reviews

Neuroscience Letters

NeuroToxicology

New York Times, The

Novartis Found Symp: Novartis Foundation Symposia

Nutr Cancer: Nutrition and Cancer

Nutr Hosp: Nutricion Hospitalaria

Obstet Gynecol Surv: Obstetrical & Gynecological Survey

Occup Environ Med: Journal of Occupational and Environmental Medicine

Oncology Nursing Forum

Open Access

Ophthalmology

Otolaryngology—Head and Neck Surgery

PACE

Pain Med: Pain Medicine

Parasitology Today

Pediatr Infect Dis J: Pediatric Infectious Disease Journal, The

Pediatrics

Phys Ther: Physical Therapy

Phytother Res: Phytotherapy Research

Planta Med: Planta Medica

PLOS ONE

PLOS Pathogens

Polish Journal of Pharmacology

Postgrad Med: Postgraduate Medicine

Preventive Medicine

Prog Neuropsychopharmacol Biol Psychiatry: Progress in Neuro-Psychopharmacology & Biological Psychiatry

Psych Bulletin: Psychological Bulletin

Psychiatr Clin North Am: Psychiatric Clinics of North America

Psychiatric Quarterly

Psychiatric Times

Psycho-Oncology

Psychosomatic Medicine

Psychosomatics

Ren Fail: Renal Failure

Respirology

Rev Neurol (Paris): Revue Neurologique

Rheum Dis Clin North Am: Rheumatic Disease Clinics of North America

Rheumatol Int: Rheumatology International

Rocz Akad Med Bialymst: Roczniki Akademii Medycznej w Bialymstoku

Scand J Rheumatol Supp: Scandinavian Journal of Rheumatology

Scanning Electron Microscopy

Schizophr Bull: Schizophrenia Bulletin

Sci. Transl. Med: Science Translational Medicine

Science

Scientific American

Semin Neurol: Seminars in Neurology

Sleep

South Med J: Southern Medical Journal

Stress

Ticks and Tick-Borne Diseases

Trends Endocrinol Metab: Trends in Endocrinology & Metabolism

Trends Neurosci: Trends in Neurosciences

Trop Doct: Tropical Doctor

Turkish Journal of Pediatrics, The

Urology

Veterinary Parasitology

Wilderness & Environmental Medicine

Wilderness Medicine

World J Gastroenterol: World Journal of Gastroenterology

Yale J Biol Med: Yale Journal of Biology and Medicine, The

Zentralbl Bakteriol Mikrobiol Hyg A: Zentralblatt für Bakteriologie, Mikrobiologie und Hygiene: Serie A

Zh Mikrobiol Epidemiol Immunobiol: Zhurnal Mikrobiologii Epidemiologii I Immunobiologii

Recommended Reading

Buhner, Stephen Harrod. *Healing Lyme: Natural Prevention and Treatment of Lyme Borreliosis and Its Co-infections.* Randolph, VT: Raven, 2005.

Connolly, Pat. *The Candida Albicans Yeast-Free Cookbook: How Good Nutrition Can Help Fight the Epidemic of Yeast-Related Diseases.* Los Angeles: Keats, 2000.

Cooper, David A. *God Is a Verb.* New York: Putnam, 1997.

A Course in Miracles: Combined Volume. Glen Elen, CA: Foundation for Inner Peace, 1992.

Crook, William F. MD. *The Yeast Connection.* Jackson, TN: Professional, 1983.

Lipton, Bruce H. *The Biology of Belief.* Memphis: Spirit 2000, 2003.

Murray, Polly. *The Widening Circle: A Lyme Disease Pioneer Tells Her Story.* New York: St. Martin's Press, 1996.

Pert, Candace B. *Molecules of Emotion: Why You Feel the Way You Feel.* New York: Scribner, 1997.

Semon, Bruce, and Lori Kornblum. *An Extraordinary Power to Heal.* Milwaukee: Wisconsin Institute of Nutrition, 2003.

Thrangu, Gangshar, and David Karma Choephel. *Vivid Awareness: The Mind Instructions of Khenpo Gangshar.* Boston: Shambhala, 2011.

Weintraub, Pamela. *Cure Unknown: Inside the Lyme Epidemic.* New York: St. Martin's Press, 2008.

References

Introduction

Smith, R., et al. "Lyme borreliosis: Europe-wide coordinated surveillance and action needed?" *Euro Surveill*. 2006;11(25):pii=2977.

One: Identifying Lyme Disease

Ford, E. S., et al. "Prevalence and correlates of metabolic syndrome based on a harmonious definition among adults in the U.S." *Journal of Diabetes* 2010; 2(3): 180–93.

Macdonald, A. "Spirochetal cyst forms in neurodegenerative disorders, . . . hiding in plain sight." *Medical Hypotheses* 67 no. 4 (2006): 819–32.

Shadick, N. A., et al. "Musculoskeletal and neurologic outcomes in patients with previously treated Lyme disease." *Annals of Internal Medicine* 1999 no. 131 (12): 919–26.

Tai-Seale, M. et al. "Time allocation in primary care office visits." *Health Services Research* vol. 42, issue 5, pages 1871–1894, October 2007.

Two: The Horowitz Sixteen-Point Differential Diagnostic Map

Aberer, E., Kersten, A., Klade, H., et al. "Heterogeneity of *Borrelia burgdorferi* in the skin." *American Journal of Dermatopathology* 18 no. 6 (1996): 571–79.

Aguero-Rosenfeld, M. E., Wang, G., Schwartz, I., and Wormser, G. P. "Diagnosis of Lyme borreliosis." *Clin Microbiol Rev* 18 (2005): 484–509.

Ang, C. W., Notermans, D. W., Hommes, M., et al. "Large differences between test strategies for the detection of anti-*Borrelia* antibodies are revealed by comparing eight ELISAs and five immunoblots." *Eur J Clin Microbiol Infect Dis* 30 no. 8 (2011): 1027–32.

Bakken, L. L., Callister, S. M., Wand, P. J., and Schell, R. F. "Intralaboratory comparison of test results for detection of Lyme disease by 516 participants in the Wisconsin State Laboratory of Hygiene/College of American Pathologists Proficiency Testing Program." *J Clin Microbiol* 35 no. 3 (1997): 537–43.

Barbour, A. G. "Isolation and cultivation of Lyme disease spirochetes." *Yale J Biol Med* 57 (1984): 521–25.

Barnett, W., Sigmund, D., Roelcke, U., and Mundt, C. "Endogenous paranoid-hallucinatory syndrome caused by *Borrelia encephalitis.*" *Nervenarzt* 62 no. 7 (July 1991): 445–47.

Benke, T., Gasse, T., Hittmair-Delazer, M., and Schmutzhard, E. "Lyme encephalopathy: Long-term neuropsychological deficits years after acute neuroborreliosis." *Acta Neurol Scand* 91 no. 5 (May 1995): 353–57.

Berman, D. S., and Wenglin, B. D. "Complaints attributed to chronic Lyme disease: Depression or fibromyalgia?" *Am J Med* 99 no. 4 (October 1995): 440.

Bloom, B. J., Wyckoff, P. M., Meissner, H. C., and Steere, A. C. "Neurocognitive abnormalities in children after classic manifestations of Lyme disease." *S: Pediatr Infect Dis J* 17 vol. 3 (March 1998): 189–96.

Breier, F., Khanakah, G., Stanek, G., et al. "Isolation and polymerase chain reaction typing of *Borrelia afzelii* from a skin lesion in a seronegative patient with generalized ulcerating bullous lichen sclerosus et atrophicus." *Br J Dermatol* 144 no. 2 (February 2001): 387–92.

Brown, J. S., Jr. "Geographic correlation of schizophrenia to ticks and tick-borne encephalitis." *Schizophr Bull* 20 no. 4 (1994): 755–75.

Brown, S. L., Hansen, S. L., Langone, J. J. (FDA Medical Bulletin) "Role of serology in the diagnosis of Lyme disease." *JAMA* 282 no. 1 (July 1999): 62–66.

Brunner, M. "New method for detection of *Borrelia burgdorferi* antigen complexed to antibody in seronegative Lyme disease." *J Immunol Methods* 249 nos. 1–2 (March 1, 2001): 185–90.

Buechner, S. A., et al. "Lymphoproliferative responses to *Borrelia burgdorferi* in patients with erythema migrans, acrodermatitis chronica atrophicans, lymphadenosis benigna cutis and morphea." *Arch Dermatol,* 131 (1995): 673–77.

Cameron D., Horowitz R., et al. "Evidence-based guidelines for the management of Lyme disease." *Expert Review of Anti Infective Therapy* 2 no. 1 (February 2004).

Casjens, S., Palmer, N., van Vugt, R., et al. "A bacterial genome in flux: The twelve linear and nine circular extrachromosomal DNAs in an infectious isolate of the Lyme disease spirochete *Borrelia burgdorferi.*" *Mol Microbiol* 35 (2000): 490–516.

Centers for Disease Control Prevention. Accessed April 6, 2013. http://www.cdc.gov/osels/ph_sur veillance/nndss/casedef/lyme_disease_current.htm.

Centers for Disease Control Prevention. *Morbidity and Mortality weekly report* 56(23) 573–76, June 15, 2007. http://www.cdc.gov/ncphi/disss/nndss/casedef/lyme_disease_2008.htm.

Cerar, T., Rusic-Sabljic, E., Glinsek, U., et al. "Comparison of PCR methods and culture for the detection of *Borrelia spp.* in patients with erythema migrans." *Clin Microbiol Infect* 14 (2008): 653–58.

Chmielewska, A. "Comparison of sensitivity and PCR." *Agric Environ Med* (2006).

Coulter, P., Lema, C., et al. "Two-year evaluation of *Borrelia burgdorferi* culture and supplemental tests for definitive diagnosis of Lyme disease." *J. Clin. Microbiol* 43 (2005): 5080–84.

Coyle, P. K., Schutzer, S. E., Deng, Z., et al. "Detection of *Borrelia burgdorferi*–specific antigen in antibody-negative cerebrospinal fluid in neurologic Lyme disease." *Neurology* 45 no. 11 (November 1995): 2010–15.

Dattwyler, R. J., et al. "Seronegative Lyme disease. Dissociation of specific T- and B-lymphocyte responses to *Borrelia burgdorferi.*" *N Engl J Med* 319 (1988): 1441–46.

Dattwyler, R. J., Volkman, D. J., Luft, B. J., et al. "Seronegative Lyme disease. Dissociation of specific T- and B-lymphocyte responses to *Borrelia burgdorferi.*" *N Engl J Med* 319 no. 22 (December 1, 1988): 1441–46.

de Martino, S. J., "Role of biological assays in the diagnosis of Lyme borreliosis presentations. What are the techniques and which are currently available?" *Med Mal Infect* 37 nos. 7–8 (2007): 496–506.

Dejmkova, H., Hulinska, D., Tegzova, D., et al. "Seronegative Lyme arthritis caused by Borrelia garinii." *Clin Rheumatol* 21 no. 4 (August 2002): 330–34.

Dorward, D. W., Fischer E. R., and Brooks, D. M. "Invasion and cytopathic killing of human lymphocytes by spirochetes causing Lyme disease." *Clin Infect Dis* 25 supp. 1 (July 1997): 52–58.

Dressler, F., et al. "The T-cell proliferative assay in the diagnosis of Lyme disease." *Ann Intern Med 1991* 115: 533–39.

Eshoo, M. W., et al. "Direct molecular detection and genotyping of Borrelia burgdorferi from whole blood of patients with early Lyme disease." *PLoS ONE* 7 iss. 5 (May 2012).

Fallon, B. "Neuropsychiatric Lyme disease: The new great imitator." *Psychiatric Times* (June 2004).

Fallon, B. A., Kochevar, J. M., Gaito, A., and Nields, J. A. "The underdiagnosis of neuropsychiatric Lyme disease in children and adults." *Psychiatric Clinics of North America* 21 (1998): 693–703.

Fallon, B. A., and Nields, J. A. "Lyme disease: A neuropsychiatric illness." *Am J Psychiatry* 15 no. 11 (November 1994): 157–83.

Garcia Monco, J. C., et al. "Reactivity of neuroborreliosis patients to cardiolipin and gangliosides." *J Neurol Sci* 117 nos. 1–2 (July 1993): 206–14.

Gaudino, E. A., Coyle, P. K., and Krupp, L. B. "Post-Lyme syndrome and chronic fatigue syndrome. Neuropsychiatric similarities and differences." *Arch Neurol* 54 no. 11 (November 1997): 1372–76.

Girschick, H. J., Huppertz, H. I., Russmann, H., et al. "Intracellular persistence of Borrelia burgdorferi in human synovial cells." *Rheumatol Int* 16 no. 3 (1996): 125–32.

Hajek, T., Paskova, B., Janovska, D., et al. "Higher prevalence of antibodies to Borrelia burgdorferi in psychiatric patients than in healthy subjects." *Am J Psychiatry* 159 (February 2002): 297–301.

Hess, A., Buchmann J., Zettl, U. K., et al., "Borrelia burgdorferi central nervous system infection presenting as an organic schizophrenia-like disorder." *Biol Psychiatry* 45 no. 6 (March 15, 1999): 795.

Huppertz, H. I., et al. "Lymphoproliferative responses to Borrelia burgdorferi in the diagnosis of Lyme arthritis in children and adolescents." *Eur J Pediatr* 155 (1996): 297–302.

Johnson, L., and Stricker, R. B. "Treatment of Lyme disease: A medicolegal assessment." *Expert Rev Anti Infect Ther* 2 no. 4 (August 2004): 533–57.

Kaiser, R. "False-negative serology in patients with neuroborreliosis and the value of employing of different borrelial strains in serological assays." *J Med Microbiol* (2000). Oct (49): 911–15.

Kaplan, A. "Neuropsychiatric masquerades." *Psychiatric Times* 26 no. 2 (February 2009): 1–8.

Krause, P., et al. "T cell proliferation induced by Borrelia burgdorferi in patients with Lyme borreliosis. Autologous serum required for optimum stimulation." *Arthritis Rheum* 34 (1991): 393–402.

Liveris, D., Schwartz, I., McKenna, D., et al. "Comparison of five diagnostic modalities for direct detection of Borrelia burgdorferi in patients with early Lyme disease." *Diagn Microbiol and Infect Dis* 73 (2012): 243–45.

Liveris, D., Wang, G., Girao, G., et al. "Quantitative detection of Borrelia burgdorferi in 2-millimeter skin samples of erythema migrans lesions: Correlation of results with clinical and laboratory findings." *J Clin Microbiol* 40 (2002): 1249–53.

Ma, Y., Sturrock, A., and Weis J. J. "Intracellular localization of Borrelia burgdorferi within human endothelial cells." *Infect Immun* 59 no. 2 (February 1991): 671–78.

MacDonald, A. B. "Review: Concurrent neocortical borreliosis and Alzheimer's disease: Demonstration of a spirochetal cyst form." *Ann NY Acad Sci* 539 (1988): 468–70.

Marangoni, A., Sparacino, M., Cavrini, F., et al. "Comparative evaluation of three different ELISA methods for the diagnosis of early culture-confirmed Lyme disease in Italy." *J Med Microbiol* 54 pt. 4 (April 2005): 361–67.

Marques, A. R. "Lyme disease: A review." *Curr Allergy Asthma Rep* 10 (2010): 13–20.

Miklossy, J. "Chronic inflammation and amyloidogenesis in Alzheimer's disease—role of spirochetes." *J Alzheimers Dis* 13 no. 4 (May 2008): 381–91.

Miklossy, J., Khalili, K., Gern, L., et al. "Borrelia burgdorferi persists in the brain in chronic Lyme neuroborreliosis and may be associated with Alzheimer's disease." *J Alzheimers Dis* 6 no. 6 (December 2004): 639–81.

Montgomery, R. R., Nathanson, M. H., and Malawista, S. E. "The fate of *Borrelia burgdorferi*, the agent for Lyme disease, in mouse macrophages. Destruction, survival, recovery." *J Immunol* 150 no. 3 (February 1993): 909–15.

Nowakowski, J., Schwartz, I., Liveris, D., et al. "Laboratory diagnostic techniques for patients with early Lyme disease associated with erythema migrans: A composition of different techniques." *Clin Infect Dis* 33 (2001): 2023–27.

Pachner, A. R. "Neurological manifestations of Lyme disease, the new "great imitator." *Infectious Disease* 11 Suppl. 6 (1989): 1482–86.

Pfister, H. W., Preac-Mursic, V., Wilske, B., et al. "Catatonic syndrome in acute severe encephalitis due to *Borrelia burgdorferi* infection." *Neurology* 43 no. 2 (February 1993): 433–35.

Pikelj, F., Strle, F., and Mozina, M. "Seronegative Lyme disease and transitory atrioventricular block." *Ann Intern Med* 111 no. 1 (July 1, 1989): 90; 49 no. 10 (October 1989): 911–15.

Pollack, R. J., Telford, S. R., III, and Spielman, A. "Standardization of medium for culturing Lyme disease spirochetes." *J Clin Microbiol* 31 (1993): 1251–55, 9.

Riedel, M., Straube, A., Schwarz, M. J., et al. "Lyme disease presenting as Tourette's syndrome." *Lancet* 35 no. 9100 (February 1998): 418–19.

Sapi, E., Pabbati, N., Datar, A., Davies, E. M., Rattelle, A., and Kuo, B. A. "Improved culture conditions for the growth and detection of Borrelia from human serum." *International Journal of Medical Sciences* 2013; 10(4): 362–376. doi:10.7150/ijms.5698.

Schutzer, S. E., Coyle, P. K., Belman, A. L. et al., "Sequestration of antibody to *Borrelia burgdorferi* in immune complexes in seronegative Lyme disease." *Lancet* 335 no. 8685 (February 10, 1990): 312–15.

Sherr, V. T. "Panic attacks may reveal previously unsuspected chronic disseminated Lyme disease." *Journal of Psychiatric Practice* 6 (November 2000): 352–56.

Sigal, L. H., et al. "Cellular immune findings Lyme disease." *Yale J Biol Med* 57 (1984): 595–98.

Skogman, B. H., et al. "Adaptive and innate immune responsiveness to *Borrelia burgdorferi* sensu lato in exposed asymptomatic children and children with previous clinical Lyme borreliosis." *Clinical and Development Immunology* 2012, 1–10.

Steere, A. C. "Seronegative Lyme disease." *JAMA* 270 no. 11 (September 15, 1993): 1369.

Stricker, R. B., and Johnson, L. "Lyme wars: Let's tackle the testing." *British Medical Journal* 335 no. 7628 (November 17, 2007): 1008.

Valentine-Thon, E., et al. "A novel lymphocyte transformation test for Lyme borreliosis." *Diagn Microbiol Infect Dis* 57 (2007): 27–34.

Woessner, R. A., and Trieb, J. "Pain, fatigue, depression after borreliosis. Antibiotics used up—what next?" *Morbidity and Mortality Weekly Fortschr Med.* 145 no. 38 (September 18, 2003): 45–48.

Zhang, X, Meltzer, M. I., Pena, C.A., et al. "Economic impact of Lyme disease." *Emerg Infect Dis* 12 no. 4 (2006): 653–60.

Ziska, M .H., Donta, S. T., and Demarest, F. C. "Physician preferences in the diagnosis and treatment of Lyme disease in the United States." *Infection* 24 no. 2 (March–April 1996): 182–86.

Three: Detecting and Treating Lyme Disease

Alban, P. S., et al. "Serum-starvation induced changes in protein synthesis and morphology of *Borrelia burgdorferi*." *Microbiology* 146 (2000): 119–27.

Brorson, O., et al. "Transformation of cystic forms of *Borrelia burgdorferi* to normal, mobile spirochetes." *Infection* 25 no. 4 (1997): 240–45.

———. "A rapid method for generating cystic forms of *Borrelia burgdorferi*, and their reversal to mobile spirochetes." *APMIS* 106 (1998): 1131–41.

DeLong, A. K., Blossom, B., Maloney, E. L., Phillips, S. E. "Antibiotic retreatment of Lyme disease in patients with persistent symptoms: A biostatistical review of randomized, placebo-controlled, clinical trials," *Contemporary Clinical Trials* 33 iss. 6 (November 2012): 1132–42, 10.1016/j.cct.2012.08.009.

Kung, F., et al. "*Borrelia burgdorferi* and tick proteins supporting pathogen persistence in the vector." *Future Microbiol* 8 no. 1 (2013): 41–56.

Nicolson, G., et al. "Role of chronic bacterial and viral infections in neurodegenerative, neurobehavioral, psychiatric, autoimmune and fatiguing illnesses: Part I." *BJMP* 2 no. 4 (2009): 20–28.

Preac-Mursic, V., et al. "Formation and cultivation of *Borrelia burgdorferi* spheroplast-L-form variants." *Infection* 24 no. 3 (1996): 218–26.

Rollend, L., et al. "Transovarial transmission of Borrelia spirochetes by Ixodes scapularis: A summary of the literature and recent observations." *Ticks and Tick-Borne Diseases* 4 (2013) 46–51.

Sapi, E., and MacDonald, A. "Biofilms of *Borrelia burgdorferi* in chronic cutaneous borreliosis." *Am J Clin Pathol* 129 (2008): 988–989.

Four: Lyme and Common Tick-Borne Bacterial Infections

Braun J., et al. *Chlamydia pneumoniae*—a new causative agent of reactive arthritis and undifferentiated oligoarthritis." *Ann Rheum Dis* 53 (1994): 100–5.

Badger, M. S. "Tick talk: Unusually severe case of tick-borne relapsing fever with acute respiratory distress syndrome—case report and review of the literature." *Wilderness and Environmental Medicine* 19 (2008): 280–86.

Cadavid, D., et al. "Neuroborreliosis during relapsing fever: Review of clinical manifestations, pathology, and treatment of infections in human and experimental animals." *Clin Infect Dis* 26 (1998): 151–64.

Cecil, R. L., Wyngaarden, J. B., Smith, L. H., Bennett, J. C. *Cecil Textbook of Medicine.* Philadelphia: W. B. Saunders, 1992.

Centers for Disease Control and Prevention. "Cluster of tick paralysis—Colorado." *Morb Mortal Wkly Rep* 55 (September 2006): 933–35.

Diaz, J. H., "A 60-year meta-analysis of tick paralysis in the United States: A predictable, preventable, and often misdiagnosed poisoning." *J Med Toxicol* 6 (2010): 15–21.

Dittman, W. "Congenital relapsing fever (*Borrelia hermsii*)." *Blood* 96 (2000): 3333.

Fedakar, A., et al. "Treatment protocol and relapses of brucella endocarditis; cotrimoxazole in combination with the treatment of brucella endocarditis." *Trop Doct* 41 no. 4 (October 2011): 227–29.

Furr, P. M., et al. "Mycoplasmas and ureaplasmas in patients with hypogammaglobulinaemia and their role in arthritis: Microbiological observations over twenty years." *Ann Rheumatoc-Dis* 53 (1994): 183–84.

Gentile, D. A., et al. "Tick-borne diseases." P. S. Auerbach, ed., *Wilderness Medicine.* St. Louis, MO: Mosby, 2001, pp. 769–806.

Gugliotta, J. L., et al. "Meningoencephalitis from *Borrelia miyamotoi* in an immunocompromised patient." *N Engl J Med* 368 (January 17, 2013): 240.

Hashemi, S. H., et al. "Comparison of doxycycline-streptomycin, doxycycline-rifampin, and ofloxacin-rifampin in the treatment of brucellosis: A randomized trial." *Int J Infect Dis.* 16 no. 4 (April 2012): e247–51.

Herman, L., and Robinson, T. T. "Complete heart block from Lyme carditis." *American Family Physician* 52 no. 4 (September 15, 1995): 1101.

Hofmeister, E. K., Kolbert, C. P., Abdulkarim, A. S., et al. "Cosegregation of a novel *Bartonella* species with *Borrelia burgdorferi* and *Babesia microti* in *Peromyscus leucopus.*" *J Infect Dis* 177 no. 2 (February 1998): 409–16.

Inman, R. D., et al. "Heary metal exposure reverses genetic resistance to Chlamydia-induced arthritis." *Arthritis Research & Therapy* 11 (February 2009): R19.

Kaell, A. T., Volkman, D. J., Gorevic, P. D., and Dattwyler, R. J. "Positive Lyme serology in subacute bacterial endocarditis: A study of four patients." *Journal of the American Medical Association* 264 no. 22 (December 12, 1990): 2916–18.

Kaya, A., et al. "Tularemia in children: Evaluation of clinical, laboratory and therapeutic features of 27 tularemia cases." *The Turkish Jnl of Pediatrics* 54 (2012): 105–12.

Longo, D. L., et al. *Harrison's Principles of Internal Medicine.* New York: McGraw-Hill, 2012.

Marcus, L. C., Steere, A. C., Duray, P. H., et al. "Fatal pancarditis in a patient with coexistent Lyme disease and babesiosis. Demonstration of spirochetes in the myocardium." *Annals of Internal Medicine* 103 no. 3 (September 1985): 374–76.

Maurin, M., et al. "Phagolysosomal alkalinization and the bactericidal effect of antibiotics." *J. Infect Dis* 166 (1992): 1097–1102.

McMulan, L., et al. "A new phlebovirus associated with severe febrile illness in Missouri." *N Engl J Med* 367 (August 30, 2012): 834–41.

Mühlradt, P. F., Quentmeier, H., and Schmitt, E. "Involvement of interleukin-1 (IL-1), IL-6, IL-2 and IL-4 in generation of cytolytic T cells from thymocytes stimulated by a Mycoplasma fermentans-derived product." *Infect. Immun* 59 (1991): 3962–68.

Nicholson, W. L., Masters, E., et al. "Preliminary serologic investigation of 'Rickettsia amblyommii' in the aetiology of Southern tick associated rash illness (STARI)." *Eur Soc of Clin Microbiol and Inf Dis* CMI 15 supp. 2(2009): 235–36.

Nicolson, G. L., Gan, R., and Haier, J. "Evidence for *Brucella spp.* and *Mycoplasma spp.* Co-infections in the blood of chronic fatigue syndrome patients." *J. Chronic Fatigue Syndr* 12 no. 2 (2005): 5–17.

Nicolson, G., et al. "High prevalence of mycoplasmal infections in symptomatic (chronic fatigue syndrome) family members of Mycoplasma-positive Gulf War Illness patients." *Jnl of Chr Fatigue Syndrome* 11 no. 2 (2003): 21–36.

Nicolson, G., et al. "Mycoplasmal infections and fibromyalgia/chronic fatigue illness (Gulf War Illness) associated with deployment to Operation Desert Storm." *Int Jnl Med*, 1 (1998): 80–92.

Philipp, M. T., et al. "Serologic evaluation of patients from Missouri with erythema migrans-like skin lesions with the C6 Lyme test." *Clin Vaccine Immunol.* 13 no. 10 (October 2006): 1170–71.

Phillips, S., Horowitz, R., et al. "Rash decisions about southern tick-associated rash illness and Lyme disease." *Clinical Infectious Diseases* 42(2): (February 2006): 306–7.

Schnarr, S., et al. "Chlamydia and Borrelia DNA . . . in synovial fluid of patients with early undifferentiated oligoarthritis: Result of a prospective study." *Arthritis Rheum.* 44 no. 11 (2001) 2679–85.

Schouls, L. M., et al. "Detection and identification of ehrlichia, *Borrelia burgdorferi* sensu lato and *Bartonella* species in Dutch Ixodes ricinus ticks." *J. Clin Microbiology.* 37 no. 7 (July 1999) 2215–2215.

Schwan, T., et al. "Tick-borne relapsing fever and Borrelia hermsii, Los Angeles County, California, USA." *Emerging Infectious Diseases* 15, no. 7 (July 2009): 1056–31. http://wwwnc.cdc.gov /eid/article/15/7/0909-0223-t2.htm.

Schwan, T. G., et al. "Identification of the tick-borne relapsing fever spirochete *Borrelia hermsii* by using a species specific monoclonal antibody." *J Clin Microbiol* 30 (1992): 790–95.

Shah, J., and Horowitz, R. "Human babesiosis and ehrlichiosis—current status." *Eur Infect Dis* 6 iss. 1, (Spring 2012): 45–56.

Simecka, J. W., et al. "Interactions of mycoplasmas with B cells: Production of antibodies and nonspecific effects." *Clin. Infect. Dis.* 17 (suppl.); (1993): S176–82.

Snowden, J., et al. "Tularemia: Retrospective review of 10 years' experience in Arkansas." *Clin Ped* 50 no. 1 (2011): 64–68.

Five: Lyme and Other Co-infections: Parasitic, Viral, and Fungal Infections

Allred, D. R. "Babesiosis: Persistence in the face of adversity." *Parasitology Today* 19 (2003): 51–55.

Bengmark, S., et al. "Plant-derived health: The effects of turmeric and curcuminoids." *Nutr Hosp* 24 no. 3 (May–June 2009): 273–81.

Bork, S., et al. "Protein interaction networks from yeast to man." *Curr. Opin. Struct. Biol* 14 (2004): 292–99.

Brasseur, P., et al. "Human babesial infections in Europe." *Rocz Akad Med Bialymst* 41 no. 2 (1996): 117–22.

Bray, P. G., et al., "Defining the role of PfCRT in *Plasmodium falciparum* chloroquine resistance." *Molecular Microbiology* 56, iss. 2 (April 2005): 323–33.

Bugyei, K. A., et al. "Clinical efficacy of a tea-bag formulation of Cryptolepis sanguinolenta root in the treatment of acute uncomplicated falciparum malaria." *Ghana Med Jnl* 44 no. 1 (March 2010).

Conrad, P. A., et al. "Description of Babesia duncani n.sp. (Apicomplexa: Babesiidae) from humans and its differentiation from other piroplasms." *International Journal for Parasitology* 36 iss. 7 (June 2006): 779–89.

Figueroa, J. V., et al. "Nucleic acid probes as a diagnostic method for tick-borne hemoparasites of veterinary importance. "*Veterinary Parasitology* 57 iss. 1–3 (March 1995): 75–92.

Gordon, S., et al. "Adult respiratory distress syndrome in babesiosis." *Chest* 86 no. 4 (October 1984): 663–64.

Hersh, M., et al. "Reservoir competence of wildlife host species for *Babesia microti. EID* 18, no. 12 (December 2012).

Herwaldt, B. L., et al., "Babesiosis in Wisconsin: A potentially fatal disease." *Am J Trop Med Hyg.* 53(1995): 146–51.

Horowitz, et al. "Delayed onset adult respiratory distress syndrome in *Babesiosis.*" *Chest* 106 no. 4 (1994): 1299–1301.

Iacopino, V., et al. "Life-threatening babesiosis in a woman from Wisconsin." *Arch Intern Med* 50 no. 7 (July 1990): 1527–28.

Joseph, J. T., Purtill, K., Wong, S. J., et al. "Vertical transmission of *Babesia microti, United States.*" *Emerg Infect Dis.* 18 no. 8 (August 2012): 11318–21.

Juven, B., and Henis, Y. "Studies on the antimicrobial activity of olive phenolic compounds." *J. Appl. Bacteriol* 33 (1970): 721–32.

Juven, B., et al. "Studies on the mechanism of antimicrobial action of oleuropein." *Jnl of Applied Bacteriology* 35 (1970): 559–67.

Krause, P. J., et al. "Comparison of PCR with blood smear and inoculation of small animals for diagnosis of Babesia microti parasitemia." *J. Clin. Microbiol* 34 no. 11 (November 1996): 2791–94.

Krause, P. J., et al. "Concurrent Lyme disease and babesiosis evidence for increased severity and duration of illness." *JAMA* 275 no. 21 (1996): 1657–60.

Kumar, P., Marshall, B. C., Deblois, G., and Koch, W. C. "A cluster of transfusion-associated babesiosis in extremely low birthweight premature infants." *Journal of Perinatology* 32 (2012): 731–33.

Lebech, et al. "Serologic evidence of granulocytic ehrlichiosis and piroplasma WA 1 in European patients with Lyme neuroborreliosis." 7th Intl Congress on Lyme Borreliosis (1996): 390.

Matyniak, J. E., et al. "T helper phenotype and genetic susceptibility in experimental Lyme disease." *JEM* 181 no. 3 (1995): 1251–54.

McMullan, L., et al. "A New phlebovirus associated with severe febrile illness in Missouri." *N Engl J Med* 367 (August 30, 2012): 834–41.

Montoya, J., and Liesenfeld, O. "Toxoplasmosis." *Lancet* 363 no. 9425 (2004): 1965–76.

Murnigsih, T., et al. "Evaluation of the inhibitory activities of the extracts of Indonesian traditional medicinal plants against Plasmodium falciparum and Babesia gibsoni." *J Vet Med Sci* 67 no. 8 (2005): 829–31.

Murray, P. K., et al. "The nature of immunosuppression in Trypanosoma brucei infections in mice." *Immunology* 27 (5): 815–824. "The role of the T and B lymphocytes." *Immunology* 27 (1974): 825–40.

Mylonakis E. "When to suspect and how to monitor babesiosis." *Am Fam Physician* 63 no. 10 (May 15, 2001): 1969–75.

Nicolson, G. L., and Nichols, C. "Notes on Morgellons syndrome." *J Degenerative Dis* 7 no. 4 (2007): 32–34.

Persing, D. "The Cold zone: A curious convergence of tick-transmitted diseases (*Babesia, Ehrlichia*) in the Midwest." *Clin Inf Dis* 25 supp. 1 (1997): S35–42.

Persing, D. H., et al. "Babesiosis: New insights from phylogenetic analysis." *Infectious Agents and Disease* 4 no. 4 (1995): 182–95.

White, N. J. "Why is it that antimalarial drug treatments do not always work?" *Annals of Tropical Medicine and Parasitology* 92 no. 4 (1998): 449–58.

Wright, C. W. "Recent developments in research on terrestrial plants used for the treatment of malaria." *Nat. Prod. Rep* 27 (2010): 961–68.

Yadav, V. R., et al. "Novel formulation of solid lipid microparticles of curcumin for anti-angiogenic and anti-inflammatory activity for optimization of therapy of inflammatory bowel disease." *J Pharm Pharmacol* 61 (2009): 311–21.

Yamada, K., et al. "Effects and mechanisms of action of ionophorous antibiotics valinomycin and salinomycin-Na on Babesia gibsoni in vitro." *J Parasitol* 95 no. 6 (December 2009): 1532–38.

Six: Lyme and Immune Dysfunction

Aron, C. F., Dorward, D. W., and Corwin, M. D. "Structural features of Borrelia burgdorferi— the Lyme disease spirochete: Silver staining for nucleic acids." *Scanning Electron Microscopy* 3 (1989): 109–15.

Askling, J. "The safety of anti-tumor necrosis factor therapy in rheumatoid arthritis." *Curr Opin Rheum* 20 (2008): 134–44.

Beerman, C., Wunderli-Allenspach, H., et al. "Lipoproteins from Borrelia burgdorferi applied in liposomes and presented by dendritic cells induce CD8(+) T-lymphocytes in vitro." *Cell Immunology* 201 no. 2 (May 2000): 124–31.

Braun, J., et al. "Chlamydia pneumoniae—a new causative agent of reactive arthritis and undifferentiated oligoarthritis." *Ann Rheum Dis* 53 (1994): 100–5.

Brorson, O., and Brorson, S. H. "An in vitro study of the susceptibility of mobile and cystic forms of Borrelia burgdorferi to hydroxychloroquine." *Int Microbiol* 5 no. 1 (March 2002): 25–31.

Brorson, O., Brorson, S. H., et al. "Association between multiple sclerosis and cystic structures in CSF." *Infection* 29 no. 6 (December 2001): 315–19.

Buzzard, E. F. "Spirochetes in M.S." *Lancet* 11 no. 98 (1911).

Cimmino, M. A., and Trevisan, G. "Lyme arthritis presenting as adult onset Still's disease." *B Clin Exp Rheumatol.* 7 no. 3 (May–1989): 305–8.

Coblyn, J. S., and Taylor, P. "Treatment of chronic Lyme arthritis with hydroxychloroquine." *Arthritis Rhem* 24 no. 12 (December 1981): 1567–69.

Donta, S. T. "Macrolide therapy of chronic Lyme disease." *Med Sci Monitor* 9 no. 11 (November 2003): 1136–42.

Dorner, T. "B cells in autoimmunity." *Arthritis Res Ther.* (209): 11247–57.

Dorward, D., et al. "Invasion and cytopathic killing of human lymphocytes by spirochetes causing Lyme disease." *Clin Infect Dis* 25 supp. 1 (July 1997): 52–58.

Duray, P. H., and Steere, A. C. "Clinical pathologic correlations of Lyme disease by stage." *Ann NY Acad Sci* 539 (1988): 65–79.

Fritzsche, M. "Chronic Lyme borreliosis at the root of MS—is a cure with antibiotics attainable?" *Med Hypotheses* 64 vol. 3 (2005): 438–48.

Furr, P. M., Taylor-Robinson, D., and Webster, A. D. "Mycoplasmas and ureaplasmas in patients with hypogammaglobulinaemia and their role in arthritis: Microbiological observations over twenty years." *Ann Rheum Dis* 53 (1994): 183–84.

Garcia Monco, J. C., et al. "Reactivity of neuroborreliosis patients to cardiolipin and gangliosides." *J Neurol Sci.* 117 nos. 1–2 (July 1993): 206–14.

Garcia-Monco, J. C., et al. "Multiple sclerosis of Lyme disease? A diagnostic problem of exclusion." *MedClin (Barc)* 94 no. 18 (May 12 1990): 685–88.

Gerard, P., et al. "Meningopapillitis disclosing Lyme disease." *Rev Neurol (Paris)* 152 nos. 6–7 (June–July 1996): 476–78.

Goebel, K. M., et al. "Acquired transient autoimmune reactions in Lyme arthritis: Correlation between rheumatoid factor and disease activity." *Scand J Rheumatol Supp.* 75 (1998): 314–17.

Greco, T. P., Jr., Conti-Kelly, A. M., and Greco, T. P. "Antiphospholipid antibodies in patients with purported 'chronic Lyme disease'." *Lupus* 20 (2011): 1372–77.

Halperin, J. J., et al. "Lyme neuroborreliosis: Central nervous system manifestations." *Neurology* 39 no. 6 (June 1989): 753–59.

Hansen, K., et al. "Oligoclonal B burgdorferi-specific IgG antibodies in CSF in Lyme neuroborreliosis." *J Inf Dis.* 161 no. 6 (June 1990): 1194–1202.

Inman, D., et al. "Heavy metal exposure reverses genetic resistance to Chlamydia-induced arthritis." *Arthritis Research & Therapy* 11 (February 2009): R19.

Kaatz, M., et al. "Lymphocytic infiltration (Jessner-Kanof): Lupus erythematosis tumidus or a manifestation of borreliosis?" *Brit Jnl Derm* 157 (2007): 388–431.

Karma, A., et al. "Diagnosis and clinical characteristics of ocular Lyme borreliosis." *Am J Ophthalmol.* 119 no. 2 (February 1995): 127–35.

Keymeulen, B., et al. "False positive ELISA serologic test for Lyme borreliosis in patients with connective tissue diseases." *Clinical Rheum* 12 no. 4 (December 1993): 526–28.

Kohler, J., et al. "Chronic central nervous system involvement in Lyme borreliosis." *Neurology* 38 no. 6 (June 1988): 863–67.

Kologrivova, E. N., et al. "Intensity of the production of rheumatoid factor in patients with different degrees of sensitization to B. garinii antigens." *Zh Mikrobiol Epidemiol Immunobiol* 2 (March–April 2005): 80–83.

Kurtz, S. K. "Relapsing fever/Lyme disease. Multiple sclerosis." *Med Hypotheses* 21 no. 3 (November 1986): 335–43.

Lesser, R. L., Pachner, A. R., et al. "Neuro-ophthalmologic manifestations of Lyme Disease." *Ophthalmology* 97 no. 6 (June 1990): 699–706.

Ma, Y., et al. "Intracellular localization of Borrelia burgdorferi within human endothelial cell." *Infect Immun* 59 no. 2 (February 1991): 671–78.

Marshall, V. "Multiple sclerosis is a chronic central nervous system infection by a spirochetal agent." *Med Hypotheses* 25 no. 2 (February 1988): 89–92.

Munger, K., et al. "Vitamin D intake and incidence of multiple sclerosis." *Neurology* 62 no. 1 (January 13, 2004): 60–65.

Nicolson, G. L., and Haier, J. "Role of chronic bacterial and viral infections in neurodegenerative, neurobehavioral, psychiatric, autoimmune and fatiguing illnesses, Part 2." *Brit. J. Med. Practit* 3 no. 1 (2010): 301a–11.

Olivares, J. P., et al. "Lyme disease presenting as isolated acute urinary retention caused by transverse myelitis; an electrophysiological and urodynamical study." *Arch Phys Med Rehabil* 76 no. 12 (December 1995): 1171–72.

Pausa, M., et al. "Serum resistant strains of Bb evade complement mediated killing by expressing a CD 59–like complement inhibitory molecule." *J Immunol* 170 no. 6 (March 15, 2003): 3214–22.

Radolf, J. D., et al. "Analysis of Borrelia burgdorferi membrane architecture by freeze-fracture electron microscopy." *Journal of Bacteriology* 176 no. 1 (January 1994): 21–31.

Rogers, H. J. "The question of silver cells as proof of spirochetal theory of disseminated sclerosis." *J. Neurol and Psychopathol* 13 (1932): 50.

Roush, J. K., et al. "Rheumatoid arthritis subsequent to Borrelia burgdorferi infection in two dogs." *J Am Vet Med Assoc* 195 no. 7 (October 1, 1989): 951–53.

Saulsbury, F. T. "Lyme arthritis in 20 children residing in a non-endemic area." *Clin Pediatr.* 44 no. 5 (June 2005): 419–21.

Schnarr, S., et al. "*Chlamydia* and *Borrelia* DNA in synovial fluid of patients with early undifferentiated oligoarthritis: Results of a prospective study." *Arthritis and Rheumatism* 44 iss. 11 (2001): 2679–85.

Simecka, J. W., et al. "Interactions of Mycoplasmas with B cells: Antibody production and non-specific effects." *Clin Infect Dis* 17 supp. 1 (1993): S176–S82.

Sriram, S., et al. "Chlamydia pneumonia infection of the central nervous system in multiple sclerosis." *Ann Neurol* 46 (1999): 6–14.

Steere, A., et al. "Antibiotic-refractory Lyme arthritis is associated with HLA-DR molecules that bind a Borrelia burgdorferi peptide." *JEM* 203 no. 4 (April 17, 2006): 961–71.

Steere, A., et al. "Association of chronic lyme arthritis with HLA-DR4 and HLA-DR2 alleles." *N Engl J Med* 323 (1990): 219–23.

Steiner, G. "Acute plaques in M.S., their pathogenetic significance and the role of spirochetes as the etilogical factor." *J. Neuropath. and Exp Neur* 11 no. 4 (1954): 343.

Steiner, G. "Morphology of Spirocheta myelopthora in MS." *J Neuropathol Exp Neurol* 11 no. 4 (1952): 343.

Summerday, N. M., et al. "Vitamin D and multiple sclerosis: Review of a possible association." *Jnl of Pharm Practice* 25 no. 1 (2012): 75–84.

Te, A. C., Craft, J. E., Sigal, L. H., et al. "The early clinical manifestations of Lyme disease." *Ann Intern Med* 99 no. 1 (July 1983): 76–82.

Watanakunakorn, C., and Toliver, J., Jr. "Lyme arthritis with subarticular cyst formation in metacarpal and metatarsal bones." *South Med J* 85 no. 2 (February 1992): 187–8.

Weigelt, W., Schneider, T., and Lange, R. "Sequence homology between spirochete flagellin and human myelin basic protein." *Immunol Today* 13 no. 7 (July 1992): 279–80.

Weiss, N. L., Sadock, V. A., Sigal, L. H., et al. "False positive seroreactivity to Borrelia burgdorferi in systemic lupus erythematosus: The value of immunoblot analysis." *Lupus* 4 (1995): 131–37.

Whitmire, W. M., and Garon, C. F. "Specific and nonspecific responses of murine B cells to membrane blebs of Borrelia burgdorferi." *Infection & Immunity* 61 (1993): 1460–67.

Wilder, R. L., and Crofford, L. J. "Do infectious agents cause rheumatoid arthritis?" *Clin Orthop* no. 265 (April 1991): 36–41.

Seven: Lyme and Inflammation

Alaedini, A., and Latov, N. "Antibodies against OspA epitopes of Borrelia burgdorferi cross-react with neural tissue." *J Neuroimmunol* 159 (2005): 192–95.

Breeding, P. C., Russell, N. C., and Nicolson, G. L. "An integrative model of chronically activated immune-hormonal pathways important in the generation of fibromyalgia." *Brit. J. Med. Practit.* 5 no. 3 (2012): a524–a34.

Casjens, S., et al. "Borrelia genomes in the year 2000." *J. Mol. Microbiol. Biotechnol* 2 no. 4 (2000): 401–10.

Clarkson, T., and Magos, L. "The toxicology of mercury and its chemical compounds." *Critical Reviews in Toxicology* 36 (2006): 609–62.

Clauw, D. J., et al. "Chronic pain and fatigue syndromes: Overlapping clinical and neuroendocrine features and potential pathogenic mechanisms." *Neuroimmunomodulation* 4 (1997): 134–53.

Fallon, B. A., et al. "Inflammation and central nervous system Lyme disease." *Neurobiology of Disease* 37 (2010): 534–41.

Fraser, C. M., et al. "Genomic sequence of a Lyme disease spirochaete, Borrelia burgdorferi." *Nature* 390 no. 6660 (December 11, 1997): 580–86.

Haack, M., et al. "Sleep restriction increases IL-6 and pain-related symptoms in healthy volunteers." *J Pain* 5 no. 3 (April 2004): supp. 1.

Lorton, D., et al. "Bidirectional communication between the brain and the immune system: Implications for physiological sleep and disorders with disrupted sleep." *Neuroimmunomodulation* 13 nos. 5–6 (2006): 357–74: electronic publication: August 6, 2007.

Mattsson, N., Bremell, D., Anckarsater, R., et al. *BMC Neurol* 10 no. 1 (June 22, 2010): 51.

Meliker, J. R., and Gallagher, C. M. "Mercury and thyroid autoantibodies in U.S. women, National Health and Nutrition Examination Survey (NHANES) 2007–2008." *Environment International* 40 (April 2012): 39–43; electronic publication: December 27, 2011.

Moldofsky, H. "Sleep and the immune system." *Int J Immunopharmacol* 17 (1995): 649–54.

Mühlradt, P. F., Quentmeier, H., and Schmitt, E. "Involvement of interleukin-1 (IL-1), IL-6, IL-2, and IL-4 in generation of cytolytic T cells from thymocytes stimulated by a Mycoplasma fermentans-derived product." *Infect Immun* 59 no. 11 (November 1991): 3962–68.

Nielsen, J. B., and Hultman, P. "Experimental studies on genetically determined susceptibility to mercury-induced autoimmune response." *Renal Failure* 21 nos. 3–4 (May–July 1999): 343–48.

Pachner, A. R., and Steiner, I. "Lyme neuroborreliosis: Infection, immunity and inflammation." *Lancet Neurology* 6 (2007): 544–52.

Pall, M. L. "Common etiology of posttraumatic stress disorder, fibromyalgia, chronic fatigue syndrome and multiple chemical sensitivity via elevated nitric oxide/peroxynitrite." *Med Hypotheses* 57 (2001): 139–45.

Pall, M. L. "Elevated, sustained peroxynitrite levels as the cause of chronic fatigue syndrome." *Med Hypotheses* 54 (2000): 115–25.

Parks, C. G., and Cooper, G. S. "Occupational exposures and risk of systemic lupus erythematosus: A review of the evidence and exposure assessment methods in population- and clinic-based studies." *Lupus* 15 (2006): 728–36.

Prasad, A. S., et al. "Zinc supplementation decreases incidence of infections in the elderly: Effect of zinc on generation of cytokines and oxidative stress 1,2,3." *Am J Clin Nutr* 85 (2007): 837–44.

Russell, I. J. "Neurochemical pathogenesis of fibromyalgia syndrome." *J Musculoskeletal Pain* 4 (1996): 61–92.

Sommer, C., et al. "Recent findings on how proinflammatory cytokines cause pain: Peripheral mechanisms and inflammatory and neuropathic hyperalgesia." *Neuroscience Letters* 361 (2004): 184–87.

Szczepanski A., and Benach, J. L. Lyme borreliosis: Host responses to Borrelia burgdorferi. Microbiol." *Mol. Biol. Rev* 55 no. 1 (March 1991): 21–34.

Tobrinick, E., et al. "TNF-α modulation for treatment of Alzheimer's disease: A 6-month pilot study." *MedGenMed* 8 no. 2 (2006).

Weis J. J., et al. "Biological activities of native and recombinant Borrelia burgdorferi outer surface protein A: Dependence on lipid modification." *Infect. Immun* 62 no. 10 (1994): 4632.

Wolfe, F., et al. "The prevalence and characteristics of fibromyalgia in the general population." *Arthritis Rheum* 38 (1995): 19–28.

Eight: Lyme and Environmental Toxins

Braidy, N., Grant, R., Adams, S., Guillemin, G. J. "Neuroprotective effects of naturally occurring polyphenols on quinolinic acid-induced excitotoxicity in human neurons." *FEBS J* 277 no. 2 (January 2010): 368–82.

Bralley, A., et al. "Laboratory evaluations in molecular medicine." *IAMM*, Norcross, GA. (2001).

Cascinu, S. "Neuroprotective effect of reduced glutathione on oxaliplatin-based chemotherapy in advanced colorectal cancer: A randomized, double-blind, placebo-controlled trial." *Journal of Clinical Oncology* 20 no. 16 (August 15, 2002): 3478–83.

Clarkson, T. W., et al. "The toxicology of mercury and its chemical compounds." *Critical Reviews in Toxicology* 36 (2006): 609–62.

Cooper, G. S., et al. "Occupational risk factors for the development of systemic lupus erythematosus." *J Rheumatol* 31 (2004): 1928–33.

Guillemin, G. "Expression of the kynurenine pathway enzymes in human microglia and macrophages." *Adv Exp Med Biol* 527 (2003).

Guillemin, G. "Quinolinic acid selectively induces apoptosis of human astocytes: Potential role in AIDS dementia complex." *J Neuroinflammation* 2 no. 16 (2005).

Hibberd, A. R., et al. "Mercury from dental amalgam fillings: Studies on oral chelating agents for assessing and reducing mercury burdens in humans." *Journal of Nutritional and Environmental Medicine* 8 no. 3 (January 1998): 219–31.

http://www.fda.gov/ForConsumers/ConsumerUpdates/ucm319827.htm.

Kalonia, H., Kumar, P., Kumar, A., and Nehru, B. "Protective effect of rofecoxib and nimesulide against intra-striatal quinolinic acid-induced behavioral, oxidative stress and mitochondrial dysfunctions in rats." *Neurotoxicology* 31 no. 2 (March 2010): 195–203.

Lee, B. K., et al. "Provocative chelation with DMSA and EDTA: Evidence for differential access to lead storage sites." *Occup Environ Med* 52 no. 1 (1995): 13–9.

Müller, N. "COX-2 inhibitors as antidepressants and antipsychotics: Clinical evidence." *Curr Opin Investig Drugs* 11 no. 1 (January 2010): 31–42.

Mutter, J., et al. "Comments on the article 'The toxicology of mercury and its chemical compounds' by Clarkson, et al." *Critical Reviews in Toxicology* 37 (2007): 537–49.

Navas-Acien, A., "Arsenic exposure and prevalence of type 2 diabetes in US adults." *JAMA* 300 no. 7 (2008): 814–22.

Perricone, C., et al. "Glutathione: A key player in autoimmunity." *Autoimmun Rev* 8 no. 8 (July 2009): 697–701.

Prasad, A. S., et al. "Zinc supplementation decreases incidence of infections in the elderly: Effect of zinc on generation of cytokines and oxidative stress 1,2,3." *Am J Clin Nutr* 85 (March 2007): 837–44.

Sagiv, S. K., Thurston, S. W., Bellinger, D. C., et al. "Prenatal exposure to mercury and fish consumption during pregnancy and attention-deficit/hyperactivity disorder–related behavior in children." *Arch Pediatr Adolesc Med* (2012): 1–9.

Shanker, A. H., et al. "Zinc and immune function: The biological basis of altered resistance to infection." *Am J Clin Nutr* 68 (1998): 447s–63s.

U.S. Food and Drug Administration. "FDA looks for answers on arsenic in rice." www.fda.gov/downloads/ForConsumers/ConsumerUpdates/UCM320040.pdf

Usberti, M., et. al. "Effects of a vitamin E-bonded membrane and of glutathione on anemia and erythropoietin requirements in hemodialysis patients." *Journal of Nephrology* 15 no. 5 (September–October 2002): 558–64.

Nine: Lyme, Functional Medicine, and Nutritional Therapies

Castagliuolo, I., et al. "Saccharomyces boulardii protease inhibits the effects of Clostridium difficile toxins A and B in human colonic mucosa." *Infection and Immunity* (January 1999): 302–7.

Chen, T., et al. "A new flavone isolated from rhizoma Smilacis glabrae and the structure requirements of its derivatives for preventing immunological hepatocyte damage." *Planta Med* 65 no. 1 (1999): 56–59.

Cooney, C., Dave, A. A., and Wolff, G. L. "Maternal methyl supplements in mice affect epigenetic variation and DNA methylation of offspring." *J Nutr* 132 no. 8 (2002): 2393s–2400s.

Docherty, J., et al. "Resveratrol selectively inhibits Neisseria gonnorhoeae and Neisseria meningitidis," *Journal of Antimicrobial Chemotherapy* 47 (2001): 243–44.

Dollnoy, D. C., Weinhouse, C., Jones, T. R., et al. "Variable histone modifications at the A(vy) metastable epiallele." *Epigenetics* 5 (2010): 637.

Dutta, A., et al. "Filiariasis properties of a wild herb, Andrographis paniculata." *J Helminthol* 56 (1982): 81–84.

Ferrante, A., et al. "Tetrandrine, a plant alkaloid, inhibits production of tumor necrosis factor-alpha by human monocytes." *Clin Exp Immunol* 80 no. 2 (1990): 232–35.

Ferrer, P., et al. "Inhibitor of cancer growth by resveratrol. Pterostilbene and quercetin inhibits metastatic melanoma growth and increases host survival." *Neoplasia* 7 no. 1 (January 2005): 37–47.

Fitzpatrick, F. "Plant substances active against mycobacterium tuberculosis." *Antibiotics and Chemotherapy* 4 no. 5 (1954): 528–36.

Fuks, F. "DNA methylation and histone modifications: Teaming up to silence genes." *Current Opinion in Genetics and Development* 15, no. 5 (2005): 490–95.

Guarente, L., and Franklin, H. "Epstein lecture: Sirtuins, aging, and medicine." *N Engl J Med* 364 (2011): 2235–43.

Hegde, V., et al. "Two new bacterial DNA primase inhibitors from the plant Polygonum cuspidatum." *Bioorg Med Chem Lett* 14 no. 9 (2004): 2275–77.

Hsieh, H.-Y., et al. "Epigenetics in traditional chinese pharmacy: A bioinformatic study at pharmacopoeia scale." *Evidence-Based Complementary and Alternative Medicine* 2010, 2011, http://www.hindawi.com/journals/eca/2011/816714/cta/. Accessed April 6, 2013.

Ignatowicz, E., et al. "Resveratrol, a natural chemopreventative agent against degerative diseases." *Polish Journal of Pharmacology* 53 (2001): 557–69.

Jiang, J., et al. "Immunomodulatory activity of the aqueous extract rom rhizome of Smilax glabra in the later phase of adjuvant-induced arthritis in rats." *J Ethnophamacol* 85 no. 1 (2003): 53–59.

Karlsson, J., et al. "Trans-resveratrol protects embryonic mesencephalic cells from tert-butyl hydroperoxide: Electron paramagnetic resonance spin trapping evidence for a radical scavenging mechanism." *Journal of Neurochem* 75 (2000): 141–50.

Kosuke, J., et al. "Potent enhancement of the sensitivity of Plasmodium falciparum to chloroquine by the bisbenzylisoquinoline alkaloid cepharanthin." *Antimicrobial Agents and Chemotherapy* 44 no. 10 (2000): 2706–8.

Koul, I., et al. "Effect of diterpenes from Andrographis paniculata on antioxidant defense system and lipid peroxidation." *Indian Jounal of Pharmacology* 26 no. 4 (1994): 296–300.

Krakowiak, P., et al. "Maternal metabolic conditions and risk for autism and other neurodevelopmental disorders." *Pediatrics* 2011–2583.

Lall, S. B., Singh, B., Gulati, K., Seth, S.D. "Role of nutrition in toxic injury." *Indian Journal of Experimental Biology* 37 (February 1999): 109–16.

Misra, P., et al. "Antimalarial acitivity of Andrographis paniculaa against Plasmodium NK 65 in Mastomys natalensis." *Int J Pharmalcol* 30 (1992): 263–74.

Navarro, M., et al. "Antibacterial, antiprotozoal, and antioxidant activity of five plants used in Izabal for infectious diseases." *Phytother Res* 17 no. 4 (2003): 325–29.

Packer, L., Tritschler, H. J., and Wessel, K. "Neuroprotection by the metabolic antioxidant alpha-lipoic acid." *Free Radic Biol Med* 22 nos. 1–2 (1997): 359–78.

Patrick, L. "Comparative absorption of calcium sources and calcium citrate malate for the prevention of osteoporosis." *Alt. Med. Review* 4 no. 2 (1999).

———. "Mercury toxicity and antioxidants: Part 1: Role of glutathione and alpha-lipoic acid in the treatment of mercury toxicity." *Altern Med Rev* 6 (December 7, 2002): 456–71.

Patrick, L. "Toxic metals and antioxidants: Part II. The role of antioxidants in arsenic and cadmium toxicity." *Altern Med Rev* 8 no. 2 (May 2003): 106–28.

Pinto, M., et al. "Resveratrol is a potent inhibitor of the dioxygenase activity of lipoxygenase." *J Agric Food Chem* 47 no. 12 (1999): 4842–46.

Roony, P. J., et al. "A short review of the relationship between intestinal permeability and inflammatory joint disease." *Clin Exp Rheum* 8 (1990): 75–83.

Singh, Y., et al. "Mixed function oxidases in response to quality and quantity of dietary protein." *Biochem Int* 17 no. 1 (July 1988): 1–8.

Skinner, M., Manikkam, M., and Guerrero-Bosagna, C. "Epigenetic transgenerational actions of environmental factors in disease etiology." *Trends Endocrinol Metab* 21 (2010): 214–22.

Soleas, G. J., Diamandis, E. P., and Goldberg, D. M. "Resveratrol: A molecule whose time has come? And gone?" *Clin Biochem* 30 no. 2 (March 1997): 91–113.

Suzuki, T., et al. "Epigenetic control using natural products and synthetic molecules." *Current Medicinal Chem* 11 (2006): 935–58.

Tjellström, B., et al. "Oral immunoglobulin treatment in Crohn's disease." *Acta Paediatr* 86 no. 2 (February 1997) 221–23.

U.S. Department of Agriculture. National Agricultural Library and National Academy of Sciences, Institute of Medicine, Food and Nutrition Board. "Dietary reference intakes for energy, carbohydrate, fiber, fat, fatty acids, cholesterol, protein, and amino acids (macronutrients)." (2005): chapt. 7: http://www.nal.usda.gov/fnic/DRI//DRI_Energy/339-421.pdf.

Valenzano, D. R., et al. "Resveratrol prolongs lifespan and retards the onset of age related markers in a short lived vertebrate." *Curr Biol* 16 no. 3 (February 7, 2006): 296–300.

Wang, T., et al. "Andrographolide reduces inflammation-mediated dopaminergic neurodegeneration in mesencephalic neuron-glial cultures by inhibiting microglial activation." *J Pharmacol Exp Ther* 308 no. 3 (2004): 975–83.

Weinhouse, C., et al. "An expression microarray approach for the identification of metastable epialleles in the mouse genome." *Epigenetics* 6 no. 9 (2011): 1105–13.

Ten: Lyme and Mitochondrial Dysfunction

Ash, M., and Nicolson, G. "Mechanisms of membrane repair and the novel role of oral phospholipids (lipid replacement therapy) and antioxidants to improve membrane function." *Open Access* (October 2012): www.nleducation.co.uk.

Balaban, R. S., et al. "Mitochondria, oxidants, and aging." *Cell* 120 (2005): 483–95.

Cohen, B. H., et al. "Mitochondrial cytopathy in adults: What we know so far." *Cleve. Clin. J. Med.* 68 (2001): 625–26, 629–42.

Conley, K. E., et al. "Ageing, muscle properties and maximal O(2) uptake rate in humans, pt. 1." *J. Physiol* 526 (2000): 211–17.

Einat, H., et al. "Increased anxiety-like behaviors and mitochondrial dysfunction in mice with targeted mutation of the Bcl-2 gene: Further support for the involvement of mitochondrial function in anxiety disorders." *Behav. Brain. Res* 165 (2005): 172–80.

Fattal, O., et al. "Review of literature on major mental disorders in patients with mitochondrial diseases." *Psychosomatics* 47 (2006): 1–7.

Fosslien, E. "Mitochondrial medicine-molecular pathology of defective oxidative phosphorylation." *Ann. Clin. Lab. Sci* 31 (2001): 25–67.

Fukui, H., et al. "The mitochondrial impairment, oxidative stress and neurodegeneration connection: Reality or just an attractive hypothesis?" *Trends Neurosci* 31 (2008): 251–56.

Gu, M., et al. "Mitochondrial DNA transmission of the mitochondrial defect in Parkinson's disease." *Ann Neurol* 44 (1998): 177–86.

Howitz, K. T., et al. "Small molecule activators of sirtuins extend Saccharomyces cerevisiae lifespan." *Nature* 425 (2003): 191–96.

Koike, K. "Molecular basis of hepatitis C virus-associated Hepatocarcinogenesis: Lessons from animal model studies." *Clin. Gastroenterol. Hepatol* 3 (2005): S132–35.

Lamkanfi, M., and Dixit, V. M. "Modulation of inflammasome pathways by bacterial and viral pathogens." *J Immunol* 187 (2011): 597–602.

Lieber, C. S., et al. "Model of nonalcoholic steatohepatitis." *Am. J. Clin. Nutr* 79 (2004): 502–9.

Muoio, D. "Metabolism and vascular fatty acid transport." *NEJM* 363 (July 15, 2010): 3.

Neustat, J., et al. "Medication-induced mitochondrial damage and disease." *Mol. Nutr. Food Res* 52 (2008): 780–88.

Nicolson, G. "Lipid replacement as an adjunct to therapy for chronic fatigue, anti-aging and restoration of mitochondrial function." *JANA* 2003 6 (3) 22–28.

Nicolson, G. "Metabolic syndrome and mitochondrial function: Molecular replacement and antioxidant supplements to prevent membrane peroxidation and restore mitochondrial function." *Journal of Cellular Biochemistry* (2007): 1352–1369.

Nicolson, G., et al. "Lipid replacement therapy with a glycophospholipid formulation with NADH and CoQ10 significantly reduces fatigue in intractable chronic fatiguing illnesses and chronic Lyme disease patients." *International Journal of Clinical Medicine* 3 (2012): 163–70.

Peppa, M., et al. "Glucose, advanced glycation end products, and diabetes complications: What is new and what works. "*Clinical Diabetes* 21 no. 4 (October 2003): 186–87.

Puddu, R., et al. "Mitochondrial dysfunction as an initiating event in atherogenesis: A plausible hypothesis." *Cardiology* 103 (2005): 103–41.

Soleas, G. J., Diamandis, E. P., and Goldberg, D. M. "Resveratrol: A molecule whose time has come? And gone?" *Clin Biochem*. 30 no. 2 (March 1997): 91–113.

Stavrovskaya, I. G., et al. "The powerhouse takes control of the cell: Is the mitochondrial permeability transition a viable therapeutic target against neuronal dysfunction and death?" *Free Radic. Biol. Med* 38 (2005): 687–97.

Stork, C., et al. "Mitochondrial dysfunction in bipolar disorder: Evidence from magnetic resonance spectroscopy research." *Mol. Psychiatry* 10 (2005): 900–19.

Sullivan, P. G., et al. "Mitochondrial aging and dysfunction in Alzheimer's disease." *Prog Neuropsychopharmacol Biol Psychiatry* 29 (2009): 407–10.

Valenzano, D. R., Terzibasi, E., Genade, T., et al. "Resveratrol prolongs lifespan and retards the onset of age-related markers in a short-lived vertebrate." *Curr Biol* 16 vol. 3 (February 7, 2006): 296–300.

Wallace, D. C. "A mitochondrial paradigm of metabolic and degenerative diseases, aging and cancer: A dawn for evolutionary medicine." *Annu. Rev. Genet* 39 (2005): 359–407.

Yunus, M. R. B., et al. "Primary fibromyalgia syndrome and myofascial pain syndrome: Clinical features and muscle pathology." *Arch. Phys. Med. Rehabil* 69 (1988): 451–54.

Eleven: Lyme and Hormones

Anisman, H., et al. "Neuroimmune mechanisms in health and disease: 2." *Disease. Can Med Assoc* 1 no. 8 (October 15, 1996): 155.

Berczi, I., et al. "Hormones in self-tolerance and autoimmunity: A role in the pathogenesis of rheumatoid arthritis?" *Autoimmunity* 16 (1993): 45–46.

Berczi, I., et al. "The pituitary gland, psychoneuroimmunology and infectious disease." In Friedman, H., Klein, T. W., Friedman, A. L., eds., *Psychoneuroimmunology, Stress and Infection.* Boca Raton, FL: CRC Press, 1996. pp. 79–109.

Bourdeau, I., et al. "Loss of brain volume in endogenous Cushing's syndrome and its reversibility after correction of hypercortisolism." *J of Clin Endocrinology and Metabolism* 87 (2000): 1949.

Clauw, D. J., et al. "Chronic pain and fatigue syndromes: Overlapping clinical and neuroendocrine features and potential pathogenic mechanisms." *Neuroimmunomodulation* 4 (1997): 134–53.

Dandona, P., et al. "Hypogonadotrophic hypogonadism in type 2 diabetes, obesity and the metabolic syndrome." *Curr Mol Med* 8 no. 8 (December 2008): 816–18.

Gooren, I. "Androgen deficiency in the aging male: Benefits and risks of androgen supplementation." *J Steroid Biochem Mol Biol* 85 nos. 2–5 (June 2003): 349–55.

Haddad, R. M., et al. "Testosterone and cardiovascular risk in men: A systematic review and meta-analysis of randomized placebo-controlled trials." *Mayo Clin Proc* 82 no. 1 (January 2007): 29–39.

Hedner, L. P., et al. "Endogenous iridocyclitis relieved during treatment with bromocryptine." *Am J Ophthalmol* 100 (1985): 618–19.

Izquierdo, M., et al. "Effects of strength training on muscle power and serum hormones in middle-aged and older men." *J App Physiol* 90 no. 4 (2001): 1497–1507.

Jalali, G. R., et al. "Impact of oral zinc therapy on the level of sex hormones in male patients on hemodialysis." *Ren Fail* 32 no. 4 (May 2010): 417–19.

Khaw, K. T., et al. "Endogenous testosterone and mortality due to all causes, cardiovascular disease, and cancer in men: European prospective investigation into cancer in Norfolk European Prospective Investigation into Cancer (EPIC-Norfolk) Prospective Population Study." *Circulation.* 116 no. 23 (December 4, 2007): 2694–2701.

Laaksonen, D. E., et al. "Sex hormones, inflammation and the metabolic syndrome: A population-based study." *Eur J Endocrinol* 149 no. 6 (December 2003): 1–8.

Maggio, M., et al. "25(OH)D serum levels decline with age earlier in women than in men and less efficiently prevent compensatory hyperparathyroidism in older adults." *J Endocrinol Invest* Suppl Proceedings 28 no. 11 (2005): 116–19.

Makhsida, N., et al. "Hypogonadism and metabolic syndrome: Implications for testosterone therapy." *J Urol* 174 no. 3 (September 2005): 827–34.

Morley, J. E., Charlton, E., Patrick, P., Kaiser, F. E., Cadeau, P., McCready, D., and Perry, H. M., III. "Validation of a screening questionnaire for androgen deficiency in aging males." *Metabolism* 49 (2000): 1232–42.

Muller, M., et al. "Endogenous sex hormones and metabolic syndrome in aging men." *J Clin Endocrinol Metab* 90 no. 5 (May 2005): 2618–23.

Nagata, C., et al. "Inverse association of soy product intake with serum androgen and estrogen concentrations in Japanese men." *Nutr Cancer* 36 no. 1 (2000): 14–18.

Nicolson, G., et al. "Diagnosis and integrative treatment of intracellular bacterial infections in chronic fatigue, and fibromyalgia syndromes, Gulf War Illness, rheumatoid arthritis and other chronic illnesses." *Clin Prac of Alt Med* 1 no. 1 (2000): 92–102.

Ohlsson, C., et al. "Low serum levels of dehydroepiandrosterone sulfate predict all-cause and cardiovascular mortality in elderly Swedish men." *J Clin Endocrinol Metab* 95 no. 9 (September 2010): 4406–14; electronic publishing: July 7, 2012.

Pilz, S., Frisch, S., Koertke, H., et al. "Effect of vitamin D supplementation on testosterone levels in men." *Hormone and Metabolic Research*, December 10, 2010.

Russell, I. J. "Neurochemical pathogenesis of fibromyalgia syndrome." *J Musculoskel Pain.* 4 (1996): 61–92.

Sapolsky, R. "Why stress is bad for your brain." *Science* 273 (1996): 749–50.

Shores, M. M., et al. "Low serum testosterone and mortality in male veterans." *Arch Intern Med* 166 no. 15 (August 14, 2006): 1660–65.

Takihara, H., et al. "Zinc sulfate therapy for infertile males with or without varicocelectomy." *Urology* 29 no. 6 (June 1987): 638–41.

Tang, Y. J., et al. "Serum testosterone level and related metabolic factors in men over 70 years old." *J Endocrinol Invest* 30 no. 6 (June 2007): 451–58.

Traish, A. M., et al. "The dark side of testosterone deficiency: II. Type 2 diabetes and insulin resistance." *J Androl* 30 no. 1 (January–February 2009): 23–32.

Wick, G., et al. "Immunoendocrine communication via the hypothalamo-pituitary adrenal axis in autoimmune diseases." *Endocr Rev* 14 (1993): 539–63.

Wolfe, F., et al. "The prevalence and characteristics of fibromyalgia in the general population." *Arthritis Rheum.* 38 (1995): 19–28.

Twelve: Lyme and the Brain

Ackerman, R., et al. "Chronic neurologic manifestations of Erythema migrans borreliosis." *Ann NY Acad Sci* 539 (1988): 16–23.

Al-Chalabi, A., et al. "Recent advances in amyotrophic lateral sclerosis." *Current Opinion in Neurology* 13 no. 4 (August 2000): 397–405.

Avery, R. A., Frank, G., and Eppes, S. C. "Diagnostic utility of Borrelia burgdorferi cerebrospinal fluid polymerase chain reaction in children with Lyme meningitis." *Pediatr Infect Dis J.* 24 no. 8 (August 2005): 705–8.

Battistini, S., et al. "Severe familial ALS with a novel exon 4 mutation (L106F) in the SOD1 gene." *Journal of the Neurological Sciences* 293 no. 1 (June 2010): 112–15.

Breitschwerdt, E. B., et al. "Molecular evidence of perinatal transmission of *Bartonella vinsonii* subsp. *berkhoffii* and *B. henselae* to a child." *Journal of Clin Microbiol* (April 14, 2010).

Breitschwerdt, E. B., et al. "*Bartonella* sp. bacteremia in patients with neurological and neurocognitive dysfunction." *Journal of Clinical Microbiology* 46 no. 9: 2856–61.

Coyle, P. K., et al. "Detection of Borrelia burgdorferi-specific antigen in antibody-negative cerebrospinal fluid in neurologic Lyme disease." *Neurology* 45 (1995): 2012–15.

Coyle, P. K. "Neurologic Lyme disease." *Semin Neurol* 12 (1992): 200–8.

Dantzer, R. "Cytokine-induced sickness behavior: A neural immune response to activation of innate immunity." *Eur J Pharmacol.* 500 nos. 1–3 (October 1, 2004): 399–411.

Dantzer, R. "Innate immunity at the forefront of psychoneuroimmunology." *Brain Behav Immun* 18 no. 1 (January 2004): 1–6.

Dattwyler, R. J., et al. "Failure of tetracycline therapy in early Lyme disease." *Arthritis Rheum* 30 no. 4 (April 1987): 448–50.

Fallon, B. A., et al. "A randomized, placebo controlled trial of repeated IV antibiotic therapy for Lyme encephalopathy." *Neurology* 70 no. 13 (March 2008): 992–1003.

Fallon, B. A., et al. "Functional brain imaging and neuropsychological testing in Lyme disease." *Clinical Infectious Diseases* 25 supp. 1 (1997): 857–63.

Fallon, B. A., et al. "The neuropsychiatric manifestations of Lyme borreliosis." *Psychiatric Quarterly* 63 (1992): 95–115.

Fallon, B. A., et al. "The under diagnosis of neuropsychiatric Lyme disease in children and adults." *Psychiatr Clin North Am* 21 no. 3 (September 1998): viii, 693–703.

Fallon, B. A., et al. "Inflammation and central nervous system Lyme disease." *Neurobiology of Disease*, 37 (2010): 534–41.

Fattal, O., et al. "Review of literature on major mental disorders in patients with mitochondrial diseases." *Psychosomatics* 47 (2006): 1–7.

Gasior, M., et al. "Neuroprotective and disease-modifying effects of the ketogenic diet." *Behavorial Pharmacology* (2006 Sept.) 17 (5–6): 431–39.

Hajek, T., et al. "Higher prevalence of antibodies to Borrelia burgdorferi in psychiatric patients than in healthy subjects." *Am J Psychiatry* 159 (February 2002): 297–301.

Halpern, J. J., et al. "Nervous system abnormalities in Lyme disease." *Ann NY Acad Sci* 539 (1988): 24–34.

Koranyi, E. K. "Somatic illness in psychiatric patients." *Psychosomatics* 21 (1980): 887–91.

Krause, P. J., et al. "Concurrent Lyme disease and babesiosis, evidence for increased severity and duration of illness." *JAMA* 275 no. 21 (June 5, 1996).

Krupp, L. B., et al. "An overview of chronic fatigue syndrome." *J Clin Psychiatry* 52 (1991): 403–10.

Krupp, L. B., et al. "Cognitive functioning in late Lyme borreliosis." *Arch Neurol* 48 (1991): 1125–29.

Logigian, E. L., Kaplan, R. F., and Steere, A. C. "Chronic neurologic manifestations of Lyme disease." *N Engl J Med* 323 (1999): 1438–44.

Logigian, E. L., Kaplan, R. F., and Steere, A. C. "Successful treatment of Lyme encephalopathy with intravenous ceftriaxone." *J Infect Dis* 180 (1999): 377–83.

Millet, Gregory E., et al. "If it goes up, must it come down? Chronic stress and the hypothalamic pituitary adrenocortical axis in humans." *Psych Bulletin* 133 (2007): 25–45.

Myers, J. S. "Proinflammatory cytokines and sickness behavior." *Oncology Nursing Forum* (2008).

Nicolson, G. L., et al. "Evidence of Mycoplasma, spp., Chlamydia pneumonia, and human herpesvirus 6 co-infections in blood of patients with autistic spectrum disorders." *Journal of Neuroscience Research* (2007, April 85): 1143–48.

Nicolson, G. L., Nasralla, M., Haier, J., and Pomfret, J. "High frequency of systemic mycoplasmal infections in Gulf War veterans and civilians with Amyotrophic Lateral Sclerosis (ALS)." *J. Clin. Neurosci* 9 (2002): 525–29.

Nields, J. A., and Fallon, B. A. "Differential diagnosis and treatment of Lyme disease, with special reference to psychiatric practice." *Directions in Psychiatry* 1998; 18: 209–27.

Pachner, A. R. "Borrelia burgdorferi in the nervous system: The new 'great imitator.'" *In Lyme Disease and Related Disease and Related Disorders. Annals of the New York Academy of Sciences* 539 (1988): 56–64.

Pachner, A. R. "Early disseminated Lyme disease: Lyme meningitis. *Am J Med* 98 no. 4A (1995): 305–75.

Picha, D., Moravcova, L., Zdarsky, E., et al. "PCR in lyme neuroborreliosis: a prospective study." *Acta Neurol Scand* 112 no. 5 (November 2005) 287–92.

Ratnasamy, N., et al. "Central nervous system manifestations of human erhlichiosis." *Clin Infect Dis* 23 no. 2 (August 1996): 314–19.

Schaller, J. L,. et al. "Do *Bartonella* infections cause agitation, panic disorder, and treatment resistant depression?" *MedGenMed* 9 no. 3 (September 13, 2007): 54.

Schutzer, S. E., et al. "Distinct cerebrospinal fluid proteomes differentiate post-treatment Lyme disease from chronic fatigue syndrome." *PLoS ONE* 6 no. 2 (February 23, 2011): e17287.

Steere, A. C., Berardi, V. P., Weeks, K. E., et al. "Evaluation of the intrathecal antibody response to Borrelia burgdorferi as a diagnostic test for Lyme neuroborreliosis." *J Infect Dis* 161 no. 6 (June 1990): 1203–9.

Tselis, A., et al. "Behavioral consequences of infections of the central nervous system: With emphasis on viral infections." *J Am Acad Psychiatry Law* 31 (2003): 289–98.

Yang, L., et al. "Brain amyloid imaging—FDA approval of Florbetapir F18 injection." *N Engl J Med* 367 (September 6, 2012): 885–87.

Zhao, Z., et al. "A ketogenic diet as a potential novel therapeutic intervention in amyotrophic lateral sclerosis." *BMC Neuroscience* (2006 Apr. 3): 7:29.

Thirteen: Lyme and Sleep Disorders

Ayas, N. T., et al. "A prospective study of sleep duration and coronary heart disease in women." *Archives of Internal Medicine* 163 no. 2 (Jan. 27, 2003): 205–209.

Benzing, T., et al. "Interaction of 14-3-3 protein with regulator of G protein signaling 7 is dynamically regulated by tumor necrosis factor-α." *J Biol Chem* 277 (2002): 32954–62.

Carskadon, M. A., et al. "Guidelines for the multiple sleep latency test (MSLT): A standard measure of sleepiness." *Sleep* 9 (1986): 519–24.

Chiao, J. W. "Immune modulating activity mediated by Borrelia burgdorferi." Abstract. 7th Intl Conf on Lyme Borreliosis. 1994.

Clinton, J. M., et al. "Biochemical regulation of sleep and sleep biomarkers." *J Clin Sleep Med* 7 supp. 5 (October 15, 2011): 538–42.

Covelli, V., et al. "Interleukin-1 β and β-endorphin circadian rhythms are inversely related in normal and stress-altered sleep." *Int J Neurosci* 63 (1992): 299–305.

Entzian, P., et al. "Obstructive sleep apnea syndrome and circadian rhythms of hormones and cytokines." *Am J Respir Crit Care Med* 153 (1996): 1080–96.

Feldman, M., et al. "Role of cytokines in rheumatoid arthritis." *Annual Review of Immunology* 14 (1996): 397–440.

Fujino, Y., et al. "A prospective cohort study of shift work and the risk of ischemic heart disease in Japanese male workers." *American Journal of Epidemiology* 164 (July 15, 2006): 128–35.

Gliklich, R. E., et al. "Health status in patients with disturbed sleep and obstructive sleep apnea." *Otolaryngology—Head and Neck Surgery* 122 (2000): 542–46.

Haack, M., et al. "Chronic sleep restriction leads to elevations in IL-6 and pain symptoms in healthy volunteers." *J Pain* 5 no. 3 (April 2004): supp. 1.

Haack, M., et al. "Chronic sleep restriction leads to elevations in IL-6 and pain symptoms in healthy volunteers." *J Pain* 5 no. 3 (April 2004): supp. 1.

Hublin, C., et al. "Sleep and mortality: A population-based 22-year follow-up study." *Sleep* 30 (2007): 1245–53.

Kapsimlis, F., et al. "Cytokines and normal sleep." *Curr Opin Pulm Med* Nov; 11 no. 6: 481–84.

Krause, P. J., Telford, S., Spielman, A., et al. "Concurrent Lyme disease and babesiosis: Evidence for increased severity and duration of illness." *JAMA* 275 (2006): 1657–60.

Libby, P., et al. "Inflammation and atherosclerosis." *Circulation* 105 (2002): 1135–43.

Lorton, D., et al. "Bidirectional communication between the brain and the immune system: Implications for physiological sleep and disorders with disrupted sleep." *Neuroimmunomodulation* 13 nos. 5–6 (2006): 357–74; published online: August 6, 2007.

Mallon, L., et al. "Sleep complaints predict coronary artery disease mortality in males: A 12-year follow-up study of middle-aged Swedish population." *Journal of Internal Medicine* 251 (March 2002): 207–16.

Moldofsky, H. "Adv management of sleep disorders in fibromyalgia." *Rheum Dis Clin North Am.* 28 (2002): 53–65.

Moldofsky, H. "Sleep and the immune system." *Int J Immunopharmacol* 17 (1995): 649–54.

Moldofsky, H. "Sleep, neuroimmune and neuroendocrine functions in fibromyalgia and chronic fatigue syndrome." *Adv Neuroimmunol* 5 (1995): 39–56.

Motivala, S. J. "Sleep and inflammation: psychoneuroimmunology in the context of cardiovascular disease." *Ann Behav Med* 42 no. 2 (October 2011): 141–52.

Mullington, J. M., et al. "Mediators of inflammation and their interaction with sleep: Relevance for chronic fatigue syndrome and related conditions." *Ann NY Acad Sci* 933 (2001): 201–10.

Parish, J. "Sleep-related problems in common medical conditions." *Chest* 135 no. 2 (February 2009): 563–72.

Sharma, S. K., Agrawal, S., Damodaran, D., et al. "CPAP for the metabolic syndrome in patients with obstructive sleep apnea." *N Engl J Med* 365 (2011): 2277–86.

Spath-Schwalbe, E., et al. "Sleep disruption alters nocturnal ACTH and cortisol secretory patterns." *Biol Psychiatry* 29 (1991): 575–84.

Theadom, A., et al. "Exploring the role of sleep and coping in quality of life in fibromyalgia." *J Psychosom Res* 62 (Feb. 2007): 145–51.

Thorpy, M. J., et al. "The clinical use of the Multiple Sleep Latency Test." *Sleep* 15 (1992): 268–76.

Vgontzas, A. N., et al. "IL-6 and its circadian secretion in humans." *Neuroimmunomodulation* 12 (2005): 131–40.

Wallace, D. J. "Is there a role for cytokine based therapies in fibromyalgia." *Curr Pharm Des* 12 (2006): 17–22.

Walsh, J. K., et al. "Effects of triazolam on sleep, daytime sleepiness, and morning stiffness in patients with rheumatoid arthritis." *J Rheumatol* 23 (1996): 245–52.

Fourteen: Lyme and Autonomic Nervous System Dysfunction/POTS

Garcia-Monoco, J. C., et al. "Experimental immunization with Borrelia burgdorferi induces development of antibodies to gangliosides." *Infection and Immunity* 63, no. 10 (1995): 4130–37.

Jacob, G., et al. "Hypovolemia in syncope and orthostatic intolerance: Role of the renin-angiotensin system." *Am J Med* 103 (1997): 1008–14.

Jordan, J., et al. "Increased sympathetic activation in idiopathic orthostatic intolerance: Role of systemic adrenoreceptor sensitivity." *Hypertension* 39 (2002): 173–178.

Karas, B., et al. "The postural orthostatic tachycardia syndrome: A potentially treatable cause of chronic fatigue, exercise intolerance, and cognitive impairment in adolescents." *PACE* 23 (2000): 344–51.

MedWatch: The FDA Safety Information and Adverse Event Reporting Program. United States Food and Drug Administration. "Safety labeling changes: Epogen/Procrit (epoetin alfa) and Aranesp (darbepoetin alfa)." August 11, 2011. http://www.fda.gov/Safety/MedWatch/Safety-Information/ucm267698.htm.

Raj, S. "The postural tachycardia syndrome (POTS): Pathophysiology, diagnosis and management." *Indian Pacing Electrophysiol J.* 6 no. 2 (April–June 2006): 84–99.

Rupprecht, T. A., et al. "Autoimmune-mediated polyneuropathy triggered by borrelial infection?" *Muscle and Nerve* 37 no 6 (2008): 781–85.

Staud, R. "Autonomic dysfunction in fibromyalgia syndrome: Postural orthostatic tachycardia." *Curr Rheumatol Rep* 10 no. 6 (December 2008): 463–66.

Stewart, J. M. "Microvascular filtration is increased in postural tachycardia syndrome." *Circulation.* 107 (June 10, 2003): 2816–22; published online: May 19, 2003.

Streeten, D. H., et al. "Excessive gravitational blood pooling caused by impaired venous tone is the predominant non-cardiac mechanism of orthostatic intolerance." *Clin Sci (Lond)* 90 (1996): 277–85.

Tanaka, M., et al. "Noradrenaline systems in the hypothalamus, amygdala and locus coeruleus are involved in the provocation of anxiety: Basic studies." *European Journal of Pharmacology* 405 nos. 1–3 (2000): 397–406.

Tani, H., et al. "Splanchnic-mesenteric capacitance bed in the postural tachycardia syndrome (POTS)." *Auton Neurosci.* 86 (2000): 107–13.

Thieben, M., et al. "Postural orthostatic tachycardia syndrome: The Mayo Clinic experience." *Mayo Clin Proc* 82 no. 3 (March 2007): 308–13.

Vernino, S., et al. "Autoantibodies to ganglionic AchR's in autoimmune autonomic neuropathies." *N Engl J Med* 343 (2000): 847–55.

Younger, D. S., et al. "Lyme neuroborreliosis: Preliminary results from an urban referral center employing strict CDC criteria for case selection." *Neurology Research International* June 2010.

Fifteen: Lyme and Allergies

Andresen, A. F. R. "Ulcerative colitis—an allergic phenomenon." *Am J Dig Dis* 9 (1942): 91.

Atherton, D. J., et al. "A double-blind controlled crossover trial of an antigen-avoidance diet in atopic eczema." *Lancet* 1 (1978): 401–3; cited by *Textbook of Natural Medicine*, vol. 1, 3rd ed., Pizzorno, J. E., Jr., et al., Elsevier Ltd: Philadelphia, 2006.

Berg, S. "Tackling the peanut allergy." *Asthma* 9 no. 4 (2004): 13–15, as cited by *Textbook of Natural Medicine* vol. 1, 3rd ed., Pizzorno, J. E., Jr., et al., Elsevier Ltd., 2006.

Butkus, S. N., et al. "Food allergies: Immunological reactions to food." *J Am Diet Assoc* 86 (1986): 601–8.

Carter, C. M., et al. "Effects of a few food diet in attention deficit disorder." *Arch Dis Child* 69 (1993): 564–68.

Edwards, A. M. "Food allergic disease." *Clin Exp Allergy* 25 (1995): 16–19.

Egger, J., et al. "Is migraine food allergy? A double-blind controlled trial of oligoantigenic diet treatment." *Lancet* 2 (1983): 865–69.

Egger, J., et al. "Controlled trial of oligoantigenic treatment in the hyperkinetic syndrome." *Lancet* 1 (1985): 540–45.

El Rafei, A., et al. "Diagnostic value of IgG4 measurement in patients with food allergy." *Ann Allergy* 62 (1989): 94–99.

Fagan, D. L., et al. "Monoclonal antibodies to immunoglobulin G4 induce histamine release from human basophils in vitro." *J Allergy Clin Immunol* 70 (1982): 399–404.

Fleischer, D. M., et al. "Peanut allergy: Recurrence and its management." *J Allergy Clin Immunol* 114 no. 5 (2004): 1195–1201.

Jang, A. S., et al. "Obesity in aspirin-tolerant and aspirin-intolerant asthmatics." *Respirology* 13 no. 7 (November 2008): 1034–38.

Kivity, S., et al. "Adult-onset food allergy." *Israel Medical Association Journal: IMAJ* 14 no. 1 (January 2012): 70–72.

Klimberg, V. S., et al. "Oral glutamine accelerates healing of the small intestine and improves outcome after whole abdominal radiation." *Arch Surg* 125 (1990) 1040–45.

Munro, J., et al. "Food allergy in migraine. Study of dietary exclusion and RAST." *Lancet* 2 (1980): 1–4.

Pizzorno, J. E., Jr., et al. *Textbook of Natural Medicine*, vol. 1, 3rd ed., Elsevier Ltd.: Philadelphia, 2006.

Rowe, A. H., et al. "Bronchial asthma due to food allergy alone in 95 patients." *JAMA* 169 (1959): 1158.

Russell, G. W., et al. "Biological activities of IgA." In Ogra, P. L., Mestecky, J., Lamm, M. E., et al., eds. *Mucosal Immunity*. San Diego, CA: Academic Press, 2004. pp. 225–40.

Savage, J., et al. "The natural history of peanut allergy: Extending our knowledge beyond childhood." *Journal of Allergy and Clinical Immunology* 120 iss. 3 (September 2007): 717–19.

Terfel, T. "Skin manifestations in food allergy." *Allergy* 56 supp. 67 (2001): 98–101.

Sixteen: Lyme and Gastrointestinal Health

Albrecht, J. "Roles of neuroactive amino acids in ammonia neurotoxicity." *Jnl of Neurosci* 51 no. 2 (January 15, 1998): 133–38.

Brown, J. P. "Role of gut bacterial flora in nutrition and health: A review of recent advances in bacteriological techniques, metabolism, and factors affecting flora composition." *CRC Crit Rev Food Sci Nutr* 8 no. 3 (1977): 229–336.

Burton Goldberg Group. *Alternative Medicine: The Definitive Guide*. WA: Future Medicine Pub: WA, 1993, p. 589.

Chen, W., Li, D., Paulus, B., et al. "High prevalence of Mycoplasma pneumoniae in intestinal mucosal biopsies from patients with inflammatory bowel disease and controls." *Dig Dis Sci* 46 no. 11 (2001): 2529–35.

Gibson, G., and Macfarlane G., eds. "Microbial ecology of the human large intestine." *Human colonic bacteria: Role in Nutrition, Physiology, and Pathology*. Boca Raton, FL: CRC Press, 1995, p. 292.

Dienst, F. T., Jr. "Tularemia. A perusal of three hundred thirty nine cases." *J La State Med Soc* 115 (1963): 114–24.

Domingue, G. J., Sr., and Woody, H. B. "Bacterial persistence and expression of disease." *Clin Microbiol Rev* 10 no. 2 (1997): 320–44.

FDA Drug Safety Communication Associated with Long-Term Use of Proton Pump Inhibitor drugs (PPIs) http://www.fda.gov/Drugs/DrugSafety/ucm245011.htm.

Ferran, C., et al. "Anti-tumor necrosis factor modulates anti-CD3 triggered T cell cytokine gene expression in vivo." *J Clin Invest* 93 (1994): 2189–96.

Johnson, D. H., and Cunha, B. A. "Atypical pneumonias. Clinical and extrapulmonary features of Chlamydia, Mycoplasma, and Legionella infections." *Postgrad Med* 93 no. 7 (1993): 69–72, 75–76, 79–86.

Lawley, T., et al. "Targeted restoration of the intestinal microbiota with a simple, defined bacteriotherapy resolves relapsing Clostridium difficile disease in mice." *PLOS Pathogens* 8 iss. 10 (October 2012).

Louie, T. J., et al. "Fidaxomicin versus vancomycin for Clostridium difficile infection." *NEJM* 364 (February 5, 2011): 5.

Malhotra, S. L. "Faecal urobilinogen levels and pH of stools in population groups with different incidence of cancer of the colon, and their possible role in its aetiology." *J R Soc Med* 75 no. 2 (1982): 709–14.

McFarland, L. V. "Meta-analysis of probiotics for the prevention of antibiotic associated diarrhea and the treatment of Clostridium difficile disease." *Am J Gastroenterol* 100 no. 4 (April 2006): 812–22.

Musso, G., et al. "Interactions between gut microbiota and host metabolism predisposing to obesity and diabetes." *Annu Rev Med* 2011; 62 (2011): 361–80.

Na, X., et al. "Probiotics in Clostridium difficile infection." *J Clin Gastroenterol* 45 supp. (November 2011): S154–S58.

Oprins, J. C., et al. "TNF-alpha potentiates the ion secretion induced by muscarinic receptor activation in HT29cl. 19A cells." *Am J Physiol Cell Physiol* 278 (2000): C463–C72.

Pimentel, M., et al. "Eradication of small intestinal bacterial overgrowth reduces symptoms of irritable bowel syndrome." *Am J Gastro* 95 (2000): 3503–6.

Reisinger, E., et al. "Diarrhea caused by primarily non-gastrointestinal infections." *Nat Clin Pract Gastroenerol Hepatol.* 2 no. 5 (2005): 216–22.

Roediger, W. E. "Intestinal mycoplasma in Crohn's disease." *Novartis Found Symp.* 263 (2004): 85–98.

Roediger, W. E., and Macfarlane, G. T. "A role for intestinal mycoplasmas in the aetiology of Crohn's disease?" *J Appl Microbiol* 92 no. 3 (2002): 377–81.

Saavedra, J. M., et al. "Human studies with probiotics and prebiotics: Clinical indications." *British Journal of Nutrition* 87 supp. 2 (2002): S241–S46.

Saulnier, D. M. A., et al. "Mechanisms of probiosis and prebiosis: Considerations for enhanced functional foods." *Curr Opin Biotechnol* 20 no. 2 (April 2009): 135–41.

United States Department of Health and Human Services, National Institutes of Health. "Opportunities and challenges in digestive diseases research: Recommendations of the National Commission on Digestive Diseases." NIH Publication 08-6514. Bethesda, MD: National Institutes of Health, 2009.

United States Department of Health and Human Services. National Institute of Diabetes and Digestive and Kidney Diseases. NIH publication 09-6433. Everhart, J. E., ed., *The Burden of Digestive Diseases in the United States.* Bethesda, MD: National Institutes of Health, 2008.

Van de Wetering, M. D., et al. "Severity of enterocolitis is predicted by IL-8 in pediatric oncology patients." *Eur J Cancer* 40 (2004): 571–78.

Vojdani, A., and Perlmutter, D. "Differentiation between celiac disease, nonceliac gluten sensitivity, and their overlapping with Crohn's disease: A case series." *Case Reports in Immunology* 2013, Article ID 248482, 9 pp.

Vrieze, A., et al. "Metabolic effects of transplanting gut microbiota from lean donors to subjects with metabolic syndrome." *EASD* (2010): abstract 90.

Weiss, G., Christensen, H. R., Zeuthen, L. H., et al. "H. Lactobacilli and bifidobacteria induce differential interferon-β profiles in dendritic cells." *Cytokine* 56 no. 2 (November 2011): 520–30.

Zaidi, S. A., et al. "Gastrointestinal and hepatic manifestations of tick-borne diseases in the United States." *Clin Infect Dis* 34 (2002): 1206–12.

Zimmer, C. "Tending the body's microbial garden." *New York Times* (June 18, 2012).

Seventeen: Lyme and Liver Dysfunction

Hashizume, H., et al. "Primary liver cancers with nonalcoholic steatohepatitis." *Eur J Gastroenterol Hepatol* 19 (2007): 827–34.

Horowitz, H. W., et al. "Liver function in early Lyme disease." *Hepatology* 23 no. 6 (June 1996): 1912–17.

Mizejewski, G. "Levels of alpha-fetoprotein during pregnancy and early infancy in normal and disease states." *Obstet Gynecol Surv* 58 no. 12 (December 2003): 804–26.

Nadelman, R. B., et al. "The clinical spectrum of early Lyme borreliosis in patients with culture confirmed erythema migrans." *Am J Med* 100 no. 5 (May 1996): 502–8.

Papadakis, M., et al. *Current Medical Diagnosis and Treatment.* New York: McGraw Hill: 2013, p. 675.

Runyon, B. A., et al. "The spectrum of liver disease in systemic lupus erythematosis. Report of 33 histologically proven cases and review of the literature." *Am J Med* 69 (1980): 187–94.

Shedlofsky, S. I., et al. "Hepatic dysfunction due to cytokines." In Kimball, E. S., ed., *Cytokines and Inflammation.* Boca Raton: CRC Press, 1991, pp. 235–61.

Shimizu, Y. "Liver in systemic disease." *World J Gastroenterol* 14 no. 76 (2008): 4111–19.

Silverman, J. F., et al. "Liver pathology in morbidly obese patients with and without diabetes." *Am J Gastroenterol* 85 (1990): 1349–55.

Smith, J., et al. "Low-dose naltrexone therapy improves active Crohn's disease." *Amer Jnl Gastroenterology* 102 (April 2007): 1–9.

Smith, J., et al. "Therapy with the opioid antagonist naltrexone promotes mucosal healing in active Crohn's disease: A randomized placebo-controlled trial." *Dig Dis Sci* March 8, 2011.

Tojo, J., et al. "Autoimmune hepatitis, accompanied by systemic lupus erythematosis." *Intern Med* 43 (2004): 258–62.

Wyngaarden, J. B., and Smith, L. H., Jr., eds., *Cecil Textbook of Medicine*, 17th ed. W. B. Saunders Company: Philadelphia, 1985.

Eighteen: Lyme and Pain

Aberer, E., et al. "Molecular mimicry and Lyme borreliosis: A shared antigenic determinant between Borrelia burgdorferi and human tissue." *Ann Neurol* 26 no. 6 (December 1989): 732–37.

Beck, G., et al. "Isolation of interleukin-1 from joint fluids of patients with Lyme disease." *J Rheumatol* 16 (1989): 802–6.

Beerman, C., Wunderli-Allenspach, H, et al. "Lipoproteins from Borrelia burgdorferi applied in liposomes and presented by dendritic cells induce CD8(+) T-lymphocytes in vitro." *Cell Immunology* 201 no. 2 (May 2000): 124–31.

Block, M. L., Zecca, L., and Hong, J. S. "Microglia-mediated neurotoxicity: Uncovering the molecular mechanisms." *Nature Reviews Neuroscience* 8 no. 1 (January 2007): 57–69.

Casjens, S. "Borrelia genomes in the year 2000." *J. Mol. Microbiol. Biotechnol* 2 no. 4 (2000): 401–10.

Cerhan, J. R., et al. "Antioxidant micronutrients and risk of rheumatoid arthritis in a cohort of older women." *American Journal of Epidemiology* 157 no. 4 (2003): 345–54.

Cree, B. A., et al. "Pilot trial of low dose naltrexone and quality of life in MS." Online *Annals of Neurology* 2010 19, February. Accessed April 7, 2013.

Das, U. N. "Angiotensin-II behaves as an endogenous pro-inflammatory molecule." *J Assoc Physicians India* 53 (May 2005): 472–76.

Davis, M. P., "Recent advances in the treatment of pain." F1000 *Med Reports* 2 (2010): 63.

Defosse, D. L., et al. "In vitro and in vivo induction of tumor necrosis factor alpha by Borrelia burgdorferi." *Infect. Immun* 60 (1992): 657–61.

Ferrante, A., et al. "Tetrandrine, a plant alkaloid, inhibits production of tumor necrosis factor-alpha by human monocytes." *Clin Exp Immunol* 80 no. 2 (1990): 232–35.

Fraser, C., et al. "Genomic sequence of a Lyme disease spirochete, Borrelia burgdorferi." *Nature* 390 (1997): 580–586.

Garon, C. F., Dorward, D. W., and Corwin, M. D. "Structural features of Borrelia burgdorferi—the Lyme disease spirochete: Silver staining for nucleic acids." *Scanning Electron Microscopy* 3 (1989): 109–15.

Gironi M., et al. "A pilot trial of low-dose naltrexone in primary progressive multiple sclerosis." *Multiple Sclerosis* 14 no. 8 (September 2008): 1076–83.

Lahesmaa, R., et al. "Immunopathogenesis of human inflammatory arthritis: Lessons from Lyme and reactive arthritis." *J. Infect. Dis* 170 (1994): 978–85.

Lindeberg, S., Jönsson, T., Granfeldt, Y., et al. "A Palaeolithic diet improves glucose tolerance more than a Mediterranean-like diet in individuals with ischaemic heart disease." *Diabetologia* (2007).

Lomaestro, B. M., et al. "Glutathione in health and disease: Pharmacotherapeutic issues." *Annals of Pharmacotherapy* 29 (1995): 1263–73.

Marshall, R. P., et al. "Angiotensin II and the fibroproliferative response to acute lung injury." *Am J Physiol Lung Cell Mol Physiol* 286 no. 1 (2003): 156–64.

Maurin, M., et al. "Phagolysosomal alkalinization and the bactericidal effect of antibiotics: The coxiella burnetti paradigm." *J Inf Dis* 166 (1992): 1097–1102.

Radolf, J. D., et al. "Analysis of Borrelia burgdorferi membrane architecture by freeze-fracture electron microscopy." *Journal of Bacteriology* 176 no. 1 (January 1994): 21–31.

Sommer, C., et al. "Recent findings on how proinflammatory cytokines cause pain: Peripheral mechanisms and inflammatory and neuropathic hyperalgesia." *Neuroscience Letters* 361 (2004): 184–87.

Szczepanski, A., and Benach, J. L. "Lyme borreliosis: Host responses to Borrelia burgdorferi." *Microbiol Rev* 55 no. 1 (March 1991): 21–34.

Trollmo, C., et al. "Molecular mimicry in Lyme arthritis demonstrated at the single cell level: LFA-1 alpha L is a partial agonist for outer surface protein A-reactive T cells." *J Immunol.* 166 no. 8 (April 15, 2001): 5286–91.

Weis, J. J., et al. "Biological activities of native and recombinant Borrelia burgdorferi outer surface protein A: Dependence on lipid modification." *Infect. Immun* 62 no. 10 (1994): 4632.

Whitmire, W. M., and Garon, C. F. "Specific and nonspecific responses of murine B cells to membrane blebs of Borrelia burgdorferi." *Infection & Immunity* 1993 61(1993): 1460–67.

Younger, D., et al. "Fibromyalgia symptoms are reduced by low dose naltrexone: A pilot study." *Pain Med* 10 no. 4 (May–June 2009): 663–72.

Nineteen: Lyme and Exercise

Alentorn-Geli, et al. "Six weeks of whole-body vibration exercise improves pain and fatigue in women with fibromyalgia." *Journal of Alternative and Complementary Medicine* 14 no. 8 (2008): 975–81.

Andreasen, A. K., et al. "The effect of exercise therapy on fatigue in multiple sclerosis." *Multiple Sclerosis Journal* 17 no. 9 (September 2011): 1041–54.

Black, S. A. "Diabetes, diversity, and disparity: What do we do with the evidence?" *American Journal of Public Health* 92 (2002): 543–48.

Booth, F., et al. "Exercise and gene expression: Physiological regulation of the human genome through physical activity." *Journal of Physiology* 3 no. 2 (2002): 399–411.

Broman, G., Quintana, M., Engardt, M., et al. "Older women's cardiovascular responses to deepwater running." *Journal of Aging and Phys Activ* 14 (2006) 29–40.

Brown, M., et al. "The role of changes in activity as a function of perceived available and expended energy and nonpharmacological treatment outcomes for ME/CFS." *Journal of Clinical Psychology* 67 no. 3 (2011): 253–60.

Burrascano, J. "Rehabilitation therapy as a support to treatment." LDF Conference Abstract. 1993 Atlantic City, N.J.

Center for Disease Control and Prevention. Morbidity and Mortality Weekly Report 60 (2011): 1641–45.

Cider, A., Svealv, B. G., Tang, M. S., et al. "Immersion in warm water induces improvement in cardiac function in patients with chronic heart failure." *Eur J Heart Fail* 8 no. 3 (2006): 308–13.

Crane, J. R., et al. "Massage therapy attenuates inflammatory signaling after exercise-induced muscle damage." *Sci. Transl. Med* (February 11, 2012).

Eaton, S. B., et al. "Evolutionary health promotion." *Preventive Medicine* 34 (February 2002): 109–18.

Edmonds, M., et al. "Exercise therapy for chronic fatigue syndrome." *Cochrane Database of Systemic Reviews* http://cfiols.best.vwh.net/cfs.inform/Exercise/edmonds.eta104.pdf (2004).

Folsom, A. R., Yatsuya, H., Nettleton, J. A., et al. ARIC Study Investigators. "Community prevalence of ideal cardiovascular health, by the American Heart Association definition, and relationship with cardiovascular disease incidence." *J Am Coll Cardiol.* 57 (2011): 1690–96.

Hu, F. B., et al. "Diet, lifestyle, and the risk of type-2 diabetes in women." *New England Journal of Medicine* 345 (Sept. 13, 2011): 790–97.

Hu, F. B., et al. "Physical activity and the risk of stroke in women." *JAMA* 283 (June 14, 2000): 2961–67.

Hu, F. B., et al. "Walking compared with vigorous physical activity and the risk of type 2 diabetes in women: A prospective study." *JAMA* 282(15), (1999): 1433–39.

Jason, L. A., et al. "The energy envelope theory and myalgic encephalomyelitis/chronic fatigue syndrome." *AAOHN Journal* 56 (2008): 189–95.

Jancin, B., and Kearney-Strouse, J. ed. "Heart healthy lifestyles also cut cancer risks." *Internal Medicine News.* February 15, 2012.

Kelm, M. "Flow-mediated dilatation in human circulation: Diagnostic and therapeutic aspects." *American Journal of Physiology* 282, (2002): H1–5.

Kremer, J. M., et al. "Fish oil fatty acid supplementation in active rheumatoid arthritis. A double blinded, controlled, crossover study." *Annals of Internal Medicine* 106 no. 4 (1987): 497–503.

Lane, A. M., et al. "The effects of exercise on mood changes: The moderating effect of depressed mood." *Journal of Sports Medicine and Physical Fitness* 41 no. 4 (2003): 539–45.

Lotshaw, A. M., Thompson, M., Sadowsky, S., et al. "Quality of life and physical performance in land- and water-based pulmonary rehabilitation." *Journal of Cardiopulmonary Rehab and Prev* 27 (2007) 247–51.

Martinez, M. E., et al. "Leisure time physical activity, body size, and colon cancer in women." Nurses' Health Study Research Group. *Journal of the National Cancer Institute* 89(13) (1997): 948–55.

Mock, V., et al. "Exercise manages fatigue during breast cancer treatment: A randomized controlled trial." *Psycho-Oncology* 14 (2005): 464–77.

Morrison, P. R., et al. "Cytochrome c protein-synthesis rates and mRNA contents during atrophy and recovery in skeletal muscle." *Biochemical Journal* 241 (1987): 257–63.

Moser, M. M. C. "Treatment for a 14-year-old girl with Lyme disease using therapeutic exercise and gait training." *Phys Ther* 91 (2011): 1412–23.

Naziroglu, M., et al. "Vitamins C and E treatment combined with exercise modulates oxidative stress markers in blood of patients with fibromyalgia: A controlled clinical pilot study." *Stress* 13 no. 6 (November 2010): 498–505.

Neill, J., et al. "Effectiveness of non-pharmacological interventions for fatigue and adults with multiple sclerosis, rheumatoid arthritis, or systemic lupus erythematosus: A systemic review." *Journal of Advanced Nursing* 56(6) (2006): 617–635.

Oken, B. S., et al. "Randomized controlled trial of yoga and exercise in multiple sclerosis." *Neurology* 62 (2004) 2058–64.

Tomassini, V., et al. "Comparison of the effects of acetyl L-carnitine and amantadine for the treatment of fatigue in multiple sclerosis: Results of a pilot, randomized, double-blind, crossover trial." *Journal of the Neurological Sciences* 218 no. 1–2 (2004): 103–8.

Zheng, D., et al. "Regulation of muscle GLUT-4 transcription by AMP-activated protein kinase." *Journal of Applied Physiology* 91 2001 (3) 1073–83.

Twenty: Meditation, Mind Training, and Medicine

Alexander, C. N., Robinson, P., Orme-Johnson, D. W., et al. "The effects of transcendental meditation compared to other methods of relaxation and meditation in reducing risk factors, morbidity, and mortality." *Homeostasis* 35 (1994), 243–263.

Carlson, L. E., Speca, M., Patel K. D., and Goodey, E. "One year pre-post intervention follow-up of psychological, immune, endocrine and blood pressure outcomes of mindfulness-based stress reduction (MBSR) in breast and prostate cancer outpatients." *Brain, Behavior, and Immunity* 21 (2007): 1038–49.

Carlson, L. E., Speca, M., Patel, K. D., and Goodey, E. (2003). "Mindfulness-based stress reduction in relation to quality of life, mood, symptoms of stress, and immune parameters in breast and prostate cancer out-patients." *Psychosomatic Medicine* 65 (4) (2003): 571–81.

Carrington, P., Collins, G. H., Benson, H., et al. "The use of meditation-relaxation techniques for the management of stress in a working population." *Journal of Occupational Medicine* 22 (1980): 221–31.

Coe, C. L. "All roads lead to psychoneuroimmunology." In Suls, J. M., Davidson, K. W., and Kaplan, R. M., eds., *Handbook of Health Psychology and Behavioral Medicine*. NY: Guilford Press, 2010. pp. 182–99.

Davidson, R. J., and McEwen, B. S. "Social influences on neuroplasticity: Stress and interventions to promote well-being." *Nature Neuroscience* 15 no. 5 (2012): 689–95.

Davidson, R. J., Kabat-Zinn, J., Schuacher, J., et al. "Alterations in brain and immune function produced by mindfulness meditation." *Psychosomatic Medicine* 65 (2003): 564–70.

Foley, E., Baillie, A., Huxter, M., et al. "Mindfulness-based cognitive therapy for individuals whose lives have been affected by cancer: A randomized controlled trial." *Journal of Consulting and Clinical Psychology* 78 (2010): 72–79.

Fredrickson, B., et al. "Open hearts build lives: Positive emotions, induced through loving-kindness meditation, build consequential personal resources." *Journal of Personality and Social Psychology* 95 no. 5 (2008): 1045–62.

Grossman P., et al. "Mindfulness-based stress reduction and health benefits. A meta-analysis." *Journal of Psychosomatic Research* 57 (2004): 35–43.

Karl, A., et al. "A meta-analysis of structural brain abnormalities in PTSD." *Neuroscience and Biobehavioral Reviews* 30 (2006) 1004–31.

Kiecolt-Glaser, J. K., et al. "Psychoneuroimmunology and psychosomatic medicine: Back to the future." *Psychosomatic Medicine* 64 (2002): 15–18.

Miller, G. E., and Chen, Z. "If it goes up, must it come down?" Chronic stress and the hypothalamic-pituitary-adrenocortical axis in humans." *Psychological Bulletin* 133 (2007): 25–45.

Robles, T. F., and Kiecolt-Glaser J. K. "Out of balance: A new look at chronic stress, depression, and immunity." *Current Directions in Psychological Science* 14 (2005): 111–15.

Rosenkranz, M. A., et al. "A comparison of mindfulness-based stress reduction and an active control in modulation of neurogenic inflammation." *Brain, Behavior, and Immunity*. Vol 27, January 2013, 174–184.

Segerstrom, S. C., and Miller, G. E. "Psychological stress and the human immune system: A meta-analysis study of 30 years of inquiry." *Psychological Bulletin* 130 (2004) 601–30.

Wallace, R. K., and Benson, H. "The physiology of meditation." *Scientific American* 226 (1972): 84–90.

Appendix A: Treatment Protocols for Lyme Disease–MSIDS for Health-Care Providers

Breitschwerdt, E. B., et al. "Molecular evidence of perinatal transmission of *Bartonella vinsonii* subsp. *berkhoffii* and *B. henselae* to a child." *Journal of Clinical Microbiology* (April 14, 2010).

Herbert, W. N., Seeds, J. W., Koontz, W. K., Cefalo, R. C., et al. "Rocky Mountain spotted fever in pregnancy: Differential diagnosis and treatment." *Southern Medical Journal* (1982).

Horowitz, R., et al. "Lyme disease and pregnancy." Abstract, Sixteenth International Scientific Conference on Lyme Disease (May 2003).

Lamas, G., et al. "Effect of disodium EDTA chelation regimen on cardiovascular events in patients with previous myocardial infarction." The TACT Randomized Trial, *Journal of the American Medical Association* 30 g(12) (2013): 1241–50.

MacDonald, A. "Human fetal borreliosis, toxemia of pregnancy, and fetal death." *Zentralbl Bakteriol Mikrobiol Hyg A.* (1986): 189–200.

Schmidt, B. L., et al. "Detection of Borrelia burgdorferi DNA by polymerase chain reaction in the urine and breast milk of patients with Lyme borreliosis." *Diagnostic Microbiology and Infectious Diseases* 21 (1995): 121–28.

Silver, H. "Lyme disease during pregnancy." *Infectious Disease Clinics of North America* vol. 11, no. 1 (March 1997).

Index